A·N·N·U·A·L E·D·I·T·I·O·N·S

P9-CBT-631

Nutrition

Sixteenth Edition

04/05

EDITOR

Dorothy Klimis-Zacas
University of Maine-Orono

Dorothy Klimis-Zacas is a Professor of Clinical Nutrition at the University of Maine and cooperating professor of nutrition and dietetics at Harokopio University, Athens, Greece. She teaches undergraduate and graduate classes in nutrition and its relation to health and disease for students of dietetics, nurses, and physicians.

Her current research interests relate to basic investigations in the area of trace mineral nutrition and its role in the development of atherosclerosis and to applied investigations that utilize nutritional interventions to reduce cardiovascular disease risk in adolescents both in the United States and in the Mediterranean region.

A Ph.D. and Fullbright Fellow, Dr. Klimis-Zacas is the author of numerous research articles and the editor of two books, *Manganese in Health and Disease* and the recently published second edition of *Nutritional Concerns for Women*. She is a member of Sigma Delta Epsilon, The American Society of Nutritional Sciences, The International Atherosclerosis Society, the American Dietetic Association, The Society for Nutrition Education, and The American Heart Association.

McGraw-Hill/Dushkin
2460 Kerper Blvd., Dubuque, Iowa 52003

Visit us on the Internet
http://www.dushkin.com

Credits

1. **Nutrition Trends**
   Unit photo—© 2004 by Sweet By & By/Cindy Brown.
2. **Nutrients**
   Unit photo—© 2004 by PhotoDisc, Inc.
3. **Diet and Disease: Through the Life Span**
   Unit photo—© 2004 by Cleo Freelance Photography.
4. **Obesity and Weight Control**
   Unit photo—© 2004 by PhotoDisc, Inc.
5. **Health Claims**
   Unit photo—© 2004 by Sweet By & By/Cindy Brown.
6. **Food Safety**
   Unit photo—© 2004 by Sweet By & By/Cindy Brown.
7. **World Hunger and Malnutrition**
   Unit photo—United Nations photo.

Copyright

Cataloging in Publication Data
Main entry under title: Annual Editions: Nutrition. 2004/2005.
1. Nutrition—Periodicals. I. Klimis-Zacas, Dorothy, *comp.* II. Title: Nutrition.
ISBN 0–07–286133–9   658'.05   ISSN 1055–6990

Sixteenth Edition

Cover image © 2004 Kevin Sanchez/Cole Group/Getty Images
Printed in the United States of America   1234567890QPDQPD0987654   Printed on Recycled Paper

Editors/Advisory Board

Members of the Advisory Board are instrumental in the final selection of articles for each edition of ANNUAL EDITIONS. Their review of articles for content, level, currentness, and appropriateness provides critical direction to the editor and staff. We think that you will find their careful consideration well reflected in this volume.

EDITOR

Dorothy Klimis-Zacas
University of Maine - Orono

Staff

To the Reader

In publishing ANNUAL EDITIONS we recognize the enormous role played by the magazines, newspapers, and journals of the public press in providing current, first-rate educational information in a broad spectrum of interest areas. Many of these articles are appropriate for students, researchers, and professionals seeking accurate, current material to help bridge the gap between principles and theories and the real world. These articles, however, become more useful for study when those of lasting value are carefully collected, organized, indexed, and reproduced in a low-cost format, which provides easy and permanent access when the material is needed. That is the role played by ANNUAL EDITIONS.

Since nutrition is an evolving science, it necessitates updating *Annual Editions: Nutrition* annually to keep up with the plethora of topics and controversies raised in the field. The main goal of this anthology is to provide the reader with up-to-date information by presenting current topics based on scientific evidence. *Annual Editions: Nutrition* also presents controversial topics in a balanced and unbiased manner. Where appropriate, international perspectives are presented. We hope that the reader will develop critical thinking and be empowered to ask questions and seek answers.

Consumers are thoroughly confused with the food choices that they have to make when they walk into a supermarket or visit a restaurant. Scientific information is misinterpreted by the news media intentionally or unintentionally which confuses and frustrates the public. We are presently experiencing obesity and diabetes epidemics, as result of large portion sizes and thus increased amounts of energy. Consumers are unaware, and do not necessarily relate large portions with higher calories, a problem which becomes critical for the youth. Additionally, there is conflicting information on several nutrition topics that appear on the news, in popular magazines and scientific journals, and over the Internet.

"Nutrition experts" and "health advisers" seem to sprout everywhere. We are at the parapet not only of a revolution in information technology but also of nutritional research. Information is distributed at a very fast pace, across continents, and without consideration of country borders. Thus, informing the consumer regularly with reliable and current nutrition information is the duty of the professional.

Annual Editions: Nutrition 04/05 is to be used as a companion to a standard nutrition text so that it may update, expand, or emphasize certain topics that are covered in the text or present a totally new subject not covered in a standard text.

To accomplish this, *Annual Editions: Nutrition 04/05* is composed of seven units that review current knowledge and controversies in the area of nutrition. The first unit describes current trends in the field of nutrition in the United States and the rest of the world, including the new dietary guidelines for the United States and the "New Food Guide Pyramid" an alternative to the U.S.D.A.'s traditional Food Guide Pyramid. Units two, three, and four include topics that focus on nutrients and recent research findings on the role nutrients play in degenerative disease and the obesity epidemic worldwide. Units five and six cover topics on health claims and focus on food safety, including subjects about which consumers are misinformed and are thus vulnerable to quackery. Finally, unit seven focuses on world hunger and malnutrition, including environmental sustainability and biotechnology. A *topic guide* will assist the reader in finding other articles on a given subject and *World Wide Web* sites will help in further exploring a particular topic.

Your input is most valuable to improving this anthology, which we update yearly. We would appreciate your comments and suggestions as you review the current edition.

Dorothy Klimis-Zacas
Editor

Contents

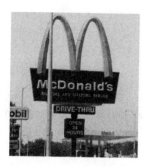

UNIT 1
Nutrition Trends

Seven articles examine the eating patterns of people today. Some of the topics considered include nutrients in our diet, eating trends, and how the food industry is making Americans overweight.

Unit Overview   xvi

The concepts in bold italics are developed in the article. For further expansion, please refer to the Topic Guide and the Index.

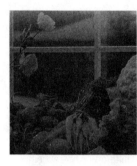

UNIT 2
Nutrients

Six articles discuss the importance of nutrients. Topics include the role of proteins, fats, carbohydrates, and vitamin and mineral supplements in our diet.

Unit Overview
28

The concepts in bold italics are developed in the article. For further expansion, please refer to the Topic Guide and the Index.

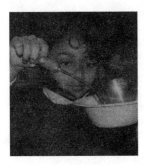

UNIT 3
Diet and Disease Through the Life Span

Five articles examine our health as it is affected by diet throughout our lives. Some topics include the links between diet and degenerative diseases, the human genome project, and nutrition for the elderly and athletes.

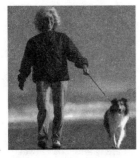

UNIT 4
Obesity and Weight Control

Seven articles examine weight management. Topics include the relationship between dieting and exercise, the effects of various diet plans, and the dangers of eating disorders.

The concepts in bold italics are developed in the article. For further expansion, please refer to the Topic Guide and the Index.

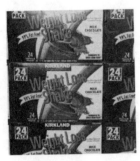

UNIT 5
Health Claims

Six unit articles examine some of the health claims made by today's "specialists." Topics
include data on supplements, misconceptions about energy bar claims, and nutrition myths
and misinformation.

Unit Overview　　120

The concepts in bold italics are developed in the article. For further expansion, please refer to the Topic Guide and the Index.

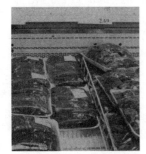

UNIT 6
Food Safety

Six articles in this section discuss the safety of food. Topics include food-borne illness, food additives, and genetically modified foods.

The concepts in bold italics are developed in the article. For further expansion, please refer to the Topic Guide and the Index.

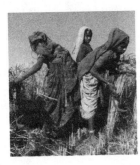

UNIT 7
World Hunger and Malnutrition

Ten articles discuss the world's food supply. Topics include global malnutrition, nutrition and infection, agricultural biotechnology, bioterrorism, and a sustainable world food supply.

The concepts in bold italics are developed in the article. For further expansion, please refer to the Topic Guide and the Index.

The concepts in bold italics are developed in the article. For further expansion, please refer to the Topic Guide and the Index.

Topic Guide

This topic guide suggests how the selections in this book relate to the subjects covered in your course. You may want to use the topics listed on these pages to search the Web more easily.

On the following pages a number of Web sites have been gathered specifically for this book. They are arranged to reflect the units of this *Annual Edition*. You can link to these sites by going to the DUSHKIN ONLINE support site at *http://www.dushkin.com/online/*.

ALL THE ARTICLES THAT RELATE TO EACH TOPIC ARE LISTED BELOW THE BOLD-FACED TERM.

World Wide Web Sites

The following World Wide Web sites have been carefully researched and selected to support the articles found in this reader. The easiest way to access these selected sites is to go to our DUSHKIN ONLINE support site at *http://www.dushkin.com/online/*.

AE: Nutrition 04/05

The following sites were available at the time of publication. Visit our Web site—we update DUSHKIN ONLINE regularly to reflect any changes.

General Sources

American Dietetic Association
http://www.eatright.org

This consumer link to nutrition and health includes resources, news, marketplace, search for a dietician, government information, and a gateway to related sites. The site includes a tip of the day and special features.

The Blonz Guide to Nutrition
http://www.blonz.com

The categories in this valuable site report news in the fields of nutrition, food science, foods, fitness, and health. There is also a selection of search engines and links.

CSPI: Center for Science in the Public Interest
http://www.cspinet.org

CSPI is a nonprofit education and advocacy organization that is committed to improving the safety and nutritional quality of our food supply. CSPI publishes the *Nutrition Action Healthletter*, which has monthly information about food.

Institute of Food Technologists
http://www.ift.org

This site of the Society for Food Science and Technology is full of important information and news about every aspect of the food products that come to market.

International Food Information Council Foundation (IFIC)
http://ific.org

IFIC's purpose is to be the link between science and communications by offering the latest scientific information on food safety, nutrition, and health in a form that is understandable and useful for opinion leaders and consumers to access.

U.S. National Institutes of Health (NIH)
http://www.nih.gov

Consult this site for links to extensive health information and scientific resources. Comprised of 24 separate institutes, centers, and divisions, the NIH is one of eight health agencies of the Public Health Service, which, in turn, is part of the U.S. Department of Health and Human Services.

UNIT 1: Nutrition Trends

Food Science and Human Nutrition Extension
http://www.fshn.uiuc.edu/

This extensive Iowa State University site links to latest news and reports, consumer publications, food safety information, and many other useful nutrition-related sites.

Food Surveys Research Group
http://www.barc.usda.gov/bhnrc/foodsurvey/home.htm

Visit this site of the Beltsville Human Nutrition Research Center Food Surveys research group first, and then click on USDA to keep up with nutritional news and information.

UNIT 2: Nutrients

Dole 5 A Day: Nutrition, Fruits & Vegetables
http://www.dole5aday.com

The Dole Food Company, a founding member of the "National 5 A Day for Better Health Program," offers this site to entice children into taking an interest in proper nutrition.

Food and Nutrition Information Center
http://www.nal.usda.gov/fnic/

Use this site to find dietary and nutrition information provided by various USDA agencies and to find links to food and nutrition resources on the Internet.

Nutrient Data Laboratory
http://www.nal.usda.gov/fnic/foodcomp/

Information about the USDA Nutrient Database can be found on this site. Search here for answers to FAQs, a glossary of terms, facts about food composition, and useful links.

NutritionalSupplements.com
http://www.nutritionalsupplements.com

This source provides unbiased information about nutritional supplements and prescription drugs, submitted by consumers with no vested interest in the products.

U.S. National Library of Medicine
http://www.nlm.nih.gov

This site permits you to search databases and electronic information sources such as MEDLINE, learn about research projects, and keep up on nutrition-related news.

UNIT 3: Diet and Disease Through the Life Span

American Cancer Society
http://www.cancer.org

Open this site and its various links to learn the concerns and lifestyle advice of the American Cancer Society. It provides information on alternative therapies, tobacco, other Web resources, and more.

American Heart Association (AHA)
http://www.americanheart.org

The AHA offers this site to provide the most comprehensive information on heart disease and stroke as well as late-breaking news. The site presents facts on warning signs, a reference guide, and explanations of diseases and treatments.

The Food Allergy and Anaphylaxis Network
http://www.foodallergy.org

The Food Allergy Network site, which welcomes consumers, health professionals, and reporters, includes product alerts and updates, information about food allergies, daily tips, and links to other sites.

Heinz Infant & Toddler Nutrition
http://www.heinzbaby.com

An educational section full of nutritional information and meal-planning guides for parents and caregivers as well as articles and reviews by leading pediatricians and nutritionists can be found on this page.

LaLeche League International
http://www.lalecheleague.org
> Important information to mothers who are contemplating breast feeding can be accessed at this Web site. Links to other sites are also possible.

Vegetarian Pages
http://www.veg.org
> The Vegetarian Pages Web site offers information on everything of interest to vegans, vegetarians, and others.

UNIT 4: Obesity and Weight Control

American Anorexia Bulimia Association/National Eating Disorders Association (AABA)
http://www.nationaleatingdisorders.org/
> The AABA is a nonprofit organization of concerned people dedicated to the prevention and treatment of eating disorders. It offers many services, including help lines, referral networks, school outreach, support groups, and prevention programs.

American Society of Exercise Physiologists (ASEP)
http://www.asep.org/
> The goal of the ASEP is to promote health and physical fitness. This extensive site provides links to publications related to exercise and career opportunities in exercise physiology.

Calorie Control Council
http://www.caloriecontrol.org
> The Calorie Control Council's Web site offers information on cutting calories, achieving and maintaining healthy weight, and low-calorie, reduced-fat foods and beverages.

Eating Disorders: Body Image Betrayal
http://www.bibri.com/home/index.htm
> This extensive collection of links leads to information on compulsive eating, bulimia, anorexia, and other disorders.

Shape Up America!
http://www.shapeup.org
> At the Shape Up America! Web site you will find the latest information about safe weight management, healthy eating, and physical fitness. Links include Support Center, Cyberkitchen, Media Center, Fitness Center, and BMI Center.

UNIT 5: Health Claims

Federal Trade Commission (FTC): Diet, Health & Fitness
http://www.ftc.gov/bcp/menu-health.htm
> This site of the FTC on the Web offers consumer education rules and acts that include a wide range of subjects, from buying exercise equipment to virtual health "treatments."

Food and Drug Administration (FDA)
http://www.fda.gov/default.htm
> The FDA presents this site that addresses products they regulate, current news and hot topics, safety alerts, product approvals, reference data, and general information and directions.

National Council Against Health Fraud (NCAHF)
http://www.ncahf.org
> The NCAHF does business as the National Council for Reliable Health Information. At its Web page it offers links to other related sites, including Dr. Terry Polevoy's "Healthwatcher Net."

QuackWatch
http://www.quackwatch.com
> Quackwatch Inc., a nonprofit corporation, provides this guide to examine health fraud. Data for intelligent decision making on health topics are also presented.

UNIT 6: Food Safety

American Council on Science and Health (ACSH)
http://www.acsh.org/food/
> The ACSH addresses issues that are related to food safety here. In addition, issues on nutrition and fitness, alcohol, diseases, environmental health, medical care, lifestyle, and tobacco may be accessed on this site.

Centers for Disease Control and Prevention (CDC)
http://www.cdc.gov
> The CDC offers this home page, from which you can obtain information about travelers' health, data related to disease control and prevention, and general nutritional and health information, publications, and more.

FDA Center for Food Safety and Applied Nutrition
http://vm.cfsan.fda.gov
> It is possible to access everything from this Web site that you might want to know about food safety and what government agencies are doing to ensure it.

Food Safety Project (FSP)
http://www.extension.iastate.edu/foodsafety/
> FSP's site contains food safety lessons, 10 steps to a safe kitchen, consumer control points, and food law.

National Food Safety Programs
http://vm.cfsan.fda.gov/~dms/fs-toc.html
> Data from the Food and Drug Administration, U.S. Department of Agriculture, Environmental Protection Agency, and Centers for Disease Control and Prevention expanding on the government policies and initiatives regarding food safety are presented on this site.

USDA Food Safety and Inspection Service (FSIS)
http://www.fsis.usda.gov
> The FSIS, part of the U.S. Department of Agriculture, is the government agency "responsible for ensuring that the nation's commercial supply of meat, poultry, and egg products is safe, wholesome, and correctly labeled and packaged."

UNIT 7: World Hunger and Malnutrition

Population Reference Bureau
http://www.prb.org
> A key source for global population information, this is a good place to pursue data on nutrition problems worldwide.

World Health Organization (WHO)
http://www.who.int/en/
> This home page of the World Health Organization will provide you with links to a wealth of statistical and analytical information about health and nutrition around the world.

WWW Virtual Library: Demography & Population Studies
http://demography.anu.edu.au/VirtualLibrary/
> A multitude of important links to information about global poverty and hunger can be found here.

UNIT 1
Nutrition Trends

Unit Selections

Key Points to Consider

- What sort of similarities are there among the diets in communities around the world?

- What foods make up a diet that prevents illness?

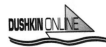 **Links: www.dushkin.com/online/**
These sites are annotated in the World Wide Web pages.

Food Science and Human Nutrition Extension
   http://www.fshn.uiuc.edu/
Food Surveys Research Group
   http://www.barc.usda.gov/bhnrc/foodsurvey/home.html

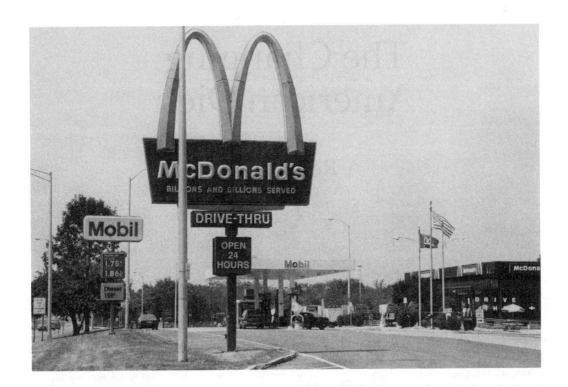

Consumers worldwide are bombarded daily with messages about nutrients and health. They are presented with large servings in restaurants and in supermarkets and it is up to them to be aware that they are eating more calories and to resist eating larger portions. The first unit describes current trends and developments in the field of nutrition and explores the roles of the food industry, agribusiness and other special interest groups and institutions, in contributing to the U.S. obesity epidemic. It also presents the nature of the "new" dietary guidelines and dietary allowances, describes a "new" type of pyramid, alternate to the USDA's Food Guide Pyramid. The first article describes how Americans are doing with their eating. Since the 70s, Americans are now eating more cheeses, breads, chicken and vegetables but have also increased their soda consumption dramatically. The good news is that they have decreased beef and whole milk consumption. Finally it addresses the challenges of nutritionists to educating consumers toward healthful sustainable diets that will not only improve quality of life but will also benefit the environment and support local agriculture.

Americans can refer to the 2000 U.S. Dietary Guidelines for guidance to construct a healthy diet. Focusing on building a healthy base, choosing sensibly and for the first time advising the population to aim for fitness are the basic premises of the New Dietary Guidelines. Keeping foods safe is also added for the first time to the 2000 Dietary Guidelines.

The Traditional USDS Food Guide Pyramid focuses on meat and dairy, does not give advice on cholesterol and saturated fat and does not distinguish among types of carbohydrates. Drs. Willet and Stampfer offer an alternative with the "New Food Guide Pyramid" which encourages the consumption of healthy

fats, and whole grain foods, exercise, and distinguishes among carbohydrates.

The next three articles describe the role the food industry plays in American life styles, the role of agribusiness and government in School Lunch Programs and their contribution to the increase of the obesity epidemic especially among youth, and offer ways we may reverse those trends.

Large portions of food are the norm in many eateries. The incidence of obesity in the United States is on the rise. It seems that the message of professionals to reduce fat calories has been misinterpreted by Americans. Most Americans think that eating certain types of food while avoiding other is more critical to weight management than reducing their portion sizes and thus, caloric intake. Americans depend increasingly on the food industry to offer them ready-prepared ready to eat foods and are falling prey to "Meal Deals" that deceptively make them think they are getting a bargain. This leads to obesity, heart disease and diabetes. Another complex relationship that contributes to the above degenerative diseases is the relationship among farmers, the government, schools and the directors of the School Lunch Programs. Agricultural producers "get rid" of high-saturated fat foods such as meat and dairy to School Lunch Programs. This contributes to the obesity crisis seen in kids.

The importance and immediacy of nutritionists educating consumers toward a healthful diet that will benefit the environment, support local economy and agriculture and prevent disease is discussed in the last article of this unit, and presents Joan Gassow a professor of Nutrition at Columbia and a homesteader, as an example to follow.

1

The Changing American Diet:

A Report Card

BY BONNIE LIEBMAN

What are Americans eating? Are we turning towards vegetarian diets or indulging in more steak? Are we getting fat on fat-free ice cream, cake, and cookies or rewarding ourselves with fat-laden cheesecake, ice cream, and pastries? Are we eating more fruits and vegetables or more french fries?

Since the early 1900s, the U.S. Department of Agriculture has been tracking the amount of food available for Americans to eat. (The numbers over-estimate what we actually swallow, since some food never gets sold, some spoils, and some gets left on our plate. But they're valid for year-to-year comparisons.)

Every few years, we use that data to size up the American diet. The "grades" look not just at what we're eating, but whether we're moving in the right direction. Here's our latest report card.

Beverages: D

In 1977, soda became the most popular American beverage, and it never looked back. We now drink roughly 50 gallons of soda per person per year. And that doesn't include the eight gallons of uncarbonated soda that masquerades as "fruit" drinks. Of the healthier beverages—milk, fruit *juice*, and bottled water—only water is clearly climbing. The bottom line: The soft-drink industry keeps filling our ever-larger cups with its high-calorie sugar water, and we keep drinking as though there were no (bathroom scale to get on) tomorrow.

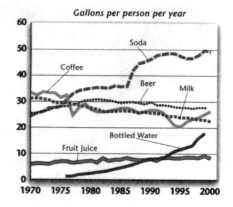

Gallons per person per year

Dairy Products: D

We're eating only slightly less ice cream than we did in 1970. And most of it is as fatty as it was 30 years ago (except for Ben & Jerry's and Häagen-Dazs, which are even fattier).

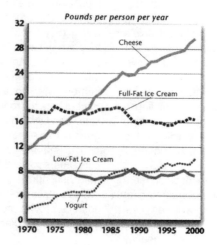

Pounds per person per year

As for cheese: The sky's the limit. We eat more than twice as much as we did in 1970. Cheese has now passed beef as our number-one source of saturated fat. Pizza and cheeseburgers started the trend back in the 1960s. But now cheese is everywhere: in your tacos and nachos, your soups and salads, your rice and potatoes, your chicken and fish... and your arteries.

Flour & Cereal: B

We're eating more flour than we did in the 1970s (in the U.S., flour means wheat). Some goes into breads, bagels, pasta, and pancakes; some ends up in cakes, cookies, Cinnabons, doughnuts, and other sweets.

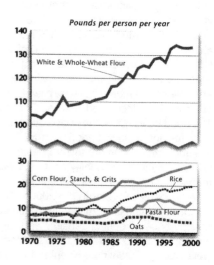

Pounds per person per year

Are all those carbs making us fat? You bet they are ... along with all the fat, protein, and alcohol we scarf down. And only a tiny fraction of the wheat flour is whole-grain, the kind that may help lower the risk of heart disease and diabetes.

Added Fats & Oils: B

The big trends in fats and oils are clear: Since 1970, we've been eating slightly less butter and margarine, more shortening, and (much) more oil.

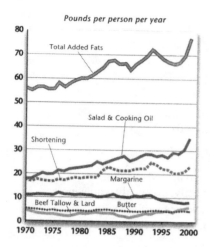

Pounds per person per year

Shortening, butter, and some margarines have saturated or trans fat, which clogs arteries. Oils don't. But all fats have calories…and that's one thing we don't need more of. Some people blame America's obesity epidemic on a low-fat diet (see "Big Fat Lies," November 2002). Can you find the low-fat diet on this graph?

Sweeteners: F

We now produce 152 pounds of added sugars each year for every man, woman, and child in America. That's 25 percent more than in 1970. Soft drinks account for a third of our intake. So-called "fruit" drinks supply another ten percent, while cookies, cakes, and other sweet baked goods contribute 14 percent (thank you, Mrs. Fields and Cinnabon). Candy, breakfast cereals, and ice cream each chip in about five percent. Does the tiny dip in 2000 signal the end of our runaway sweet tooth? Stay tuned.

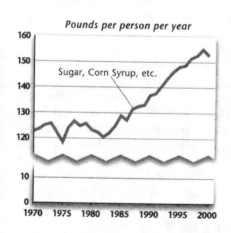

Pounds per person per year

Meat, Poultry, & Seafood: B

Beef and pork were neck-and-neck for the first half of the 20th century. But in the 1950s, beef started a steep climb that finally peaked in the mid-1970s. Chicken's growth keeps clucking along. But we still eat far more red meat (111 pounds per person) than poultry and seafood (83 pounds) each year.

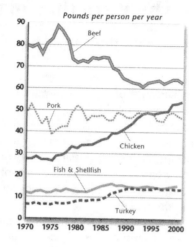

Pounds per person per year

Fruits & Vegetables: A

We're eating more fruits and vegetables than we did 30 years ago. On the upswing are bell peppers, broccoli, carrots, cucumbers, mushrooms, onions, spinach, squash, and tomatoes (but not brussels sprouts, cabbage, celery, or sweet potatoes). Also rising are bananas, grapes, mangos, melons, papayas, pears, pineapples and strawberries (but not apples, apricots, cherries, grapefruit, oranges, peaches, or plums). We still don't eat enough fruits and vegetables, but at least we're moving in the right direction.

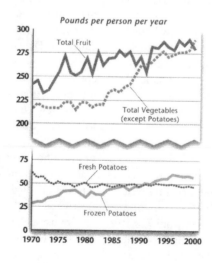

Pounds per person per year

Milk: C

Whole milk is down (that's good). So is reduced-fat (2 percent) milk (also good). But low-fat (1 percent) and skim (fat-free) aren't replacing the fattier milks. And we still drink more than twice as much of the two fattier milks than their two low-fat cousins.

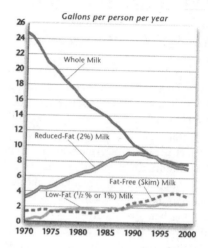

Gallons per person per year

Heather Jones DeMino helped compile the information for this article. Source: Economic Research Service, U.S. Department of Agriculture. (To access the U.S.D.A.'s per capita food consumption database on-line, go to www.ers.usda.gov/data/foodconsumption.)

The 2000 Dietary Guidelines for Americans:
What are the changes and why were they made?

RACHEL K. JOHNSON, PhD, MPH, RD; EILEEN KENNEDY, DSc, RD

The Dietary Guidelines for Americans form the foundation of US federal nutrition policy. Each federal nutrition program in the United States uses the Dietary Guidelines as one part of the nutrition standard. Therefore, every day the guidelines directly impact 21.4 million Americans receiving food stamps, 26 million children who participate in the school lunch program, 7 million children participating in the school breakfast program, and approximately 7.4 million women, infants, and children receiving benefits under the Special Supplemental Program for Women, Infants, and Children (WIC). The Food Guide Pyramid (1), the most widely distributed and best-recognized nutrition education device ever produced in the United States, is based in part on the US Dietary Guidelines.

The National Nutrition Monitoring and Related Research Act of 1990 (2) mandates that the guidelines be reviewed by the US Department of Agriculture (USDA) and the US Department of Health and Human Services (HHS) every 5 years. Hence, in 1998 the secretaries of USDA and HHS appointed an 11-member committee (Figure 1) to review the 1995 Dietary Guidelines for Americans and recommend what changes, if any, should be made in the 2000 guidelines. The Dietary Guidelines Advisory Committee was charged by the secretaries with answering the following question: "What should Americans eat to stay healthy?" The committee rigorously reviewed the peer-reviewed scientific literature, found that substantial new knowledge was available, and agreed that revision of the 1995 guidelines was needed. The aim of this paper is to discuss the changes in the 2000 guidelines and present the scientific rationale for these changes. The final Dietary Guidelines for Americans were released by the President on May 27, 2000.

GENERAL

Major revisions were made in the presentation of the guidelines using 3 basic messages: Aim for fitness, Build a healthy base, and Choose sensibly for good health (ABC). The committee recommended increasing the number of guidelines from 7 to 10 and believed the ABCs for good health would help organize the guidelines in a memorable, meaningful way. The guidelines are intended for healthy children (aged 2 years and older) and adults of any age.

1. Aim for fitness
- Aim for a healthy weight.

- Be physically active each day.

2. Build a healthy base
- Let the Pyramid guide your food choices.
- Eat a variety of grains daily, especially whole grains.
- Eat a variety of fruits and vegetables daily.
- Keep foods safe to eat.

3. Choose sensibly
- Choose a diet that is low in saturated fat and cholesterol and moderate in total fat.
- Choose beverages and foods to moderate your intake of sugars.
- Choose and prepare foods with less salt.
- If you drink alcoholic beverages, do so in moderation.

SPECIFIC RECOMMENDED GUIDELINES

Aim for fitness

Aim for a healthy weight The change in this guideline was aimed at improving the clarity of the wording. The word "balance" in the 1995 guideline (Figure 2) was interpreted by some focus group participants to mean that it was acceptable to be overweight as long as physical activity and energy intake were balanced. The word "improve" was construed by some to mean to increase weight and by others to decrease weight (3). The committee believed the new guideline combined the message into one actionable phrase.

The new guideline contains easy-to-use information on how to evaluate body weight. This includes a nomogram to simply calculate body mass index (BMI) (Figure 3) and gives instructions on how to measure waist circumference. Using the 1998 National Institutes of Health National Heart, Lung, and Blood guidelines for the identification, evaluation, and treatment of overweight and obesity, consumers are guided through a process of using their BMI, waist circumference, and other risk factors to determine if they are at a healthy weight (4).

Although the evidence that overweight and obesity lead to adverse health outcomes is indisputable (5), there is less agreement about the management of obesity. This is especially true with regard to whether the emphasis should be on weight maintenance or weight loss. The committee recommended that if people are overweight, they should aim for a loss of about 10%

of their weight over 6 months. This is based on evidence that weight reductions of 5% to 15% reduce risk factors for obesity-associated conditions (6), and that people's initial goal should be to lose 10% of their weight over a period of about 6 months (4). Emphasis is placed on consumption of foods that are low in energy density as a means to control energy intake. This recommendation is based on a group of studies that demonstrated the energy density of foods plays a role in daily energy consumption (7–9). Hence, consumers are urged to make grains (especially whole grains), fruits, and vegetables the mainstays of their diet. People are urged to choose sensible portion sizes and cautioned that if a food is labeled low-fat, it does not necessarily mean the food is low in energy.

The number of children in the United States who are overweight has more than doubled over the past decade (10), and parents are advised to see a health care professional for evaluation and intervention if they are concerned about their child's weight. Parents are also urged to limit the time children spend in sedentary activities like watching television or playing video and computer games. One-fourth of all children in the United States watch 4 or more hours of television each day, and hours of television watched is positively associated with increased BMI and skinfold thickness (11).

Be physically active each day A new guideline on physical activity was added because the benefits of physical activity go well beyond energy balance and weight management (12). Over the past 5 years, 9 national position papers or reports have been published documenting the importance of moderate physical activity for good health (4,12–19). These reports indicate that being physically active for 30 to 45 minutes per day reduces the risk of developing heart disease, hypertension, colon cancer, and type 2 diabetes mellitus. These conditions are major contributors to morbidity and mortality in the United States. Furthermore, physical activity is related to improvements in flexibility, bone mass density, risk of hip fractures in women, depression and anxiety, and health-related quality of life. In children, physical activity improves aerobic endurance and muscular strength as well as BMI, blood lipids, blood pressure, and bone health (13,20).

The committee also recommended the addition of this guideline because physical activity levels in both US children and adults have declined and are much lower, on average, than what is recommended for good health and weight management (4,13,18,19). Hence, improvements in physical activity levels are needed in every age group. The committee followed standards supported by the Centers for Disease Control and Prevention and the American College of Sports Medicine (12) and recommended that adults be physically active at least 30 minutes most days-preferably all days of the week. Children are urged to be physically activity at least 60 minutes per day (13,21).

Build a healthy base

Let the Pyramid guide your food choices The wording of the 1995 guideline "Eat a variety of foods" was changed to the new wording based on 3 lines of evidence. First, a critical concept to be conveyed by this guideline is nutritional adequacy. Choosing foods from all the Pyramid food groups improves nutrient adequacy (22,23). Thus, the committee felt that the recommendation to use the Food Guide Pyramid was better justified than simply a broad recommendation to eat a variety of foods. The second issue confronting the committee was that guidance to consume a variety of foods might promote overconsumption of energy. A limited number of controlled feeding studies demonstrated that more food is eaten at a meal if a variety of foods are available than if the selection is more limited (24). In addition, a 1999 analysis of nationwide food consumption data suggested that a wide variety of sweets, snacks, condiments, entrees, and carbohydrates, coupled with a small variety of vegetables, was positively associated with increased energy intakes and body fatness (25).

The last consideration by the committee was that the 1995 guideline was unclear to consumers. Focus group participants responded that variety in the 1995 guideline was too vague to guide consumers to take specific actions. There was no definition of variety, or of a desirable level of variety (3). On the other hand, many focus group respondents stated that the Food Guide Pyramid was the most useful part of the US Dietary Guidelines (26). The overall literature on effects of variety in the diet was viewed by the committee as mixed. Revised wording stressing the Food Guide Pyramid better reflected the goal of this guideline.

Choose a variety of grains daily, especially whole grains The 1995 guideline "Choose a diet with plenty of grain products, vegetables, and fruits" was split into 2 separate guidelines. These separate guidelines were recommended for several reasons: increasing attention to grains as distinct from vegetables and fruits, simplification of the messages, and clarification that there are distinct advantages to the 2 broad categories of plant foods. The committee added the important phrase "especially whole grains" for 2 major reasons: a) some research has shown that consumption of whole grains lowers risk for cardiovascular disease and some forms of cancer (27), and b) intake of whole grains is very low in the United States, with intakes averaging only half a serving per person per day (28). The committee considered whether increasing the intake of whole grains at the expense of enriched, folate-fortified refined grains would decrease the intake of some micronutrients (iron, folate, and zinc) to undesirably low levels. An analysis of dietary intakes using data from the 1994–1996 USDA Continuing Survey of Food Intakes of Individuals data demonstrated that substituting 3 servings of whole grains for enriched, folate-fortified refined grains did not adversely affect nutrient intake levels.

Choose a variety of fruits and vegetables Very few Americans meet intake recommendations for these 2 food groups (29). Fruits are purposely listed before vegetables because fewer people meet the recommended intake of fruits. The revised wording of this guideline focuses on the importance of variety within the fruit and vegetables groups and avoids the use of the word "diet" which many consumers considered to be suggestive of restrictions (26). Numerous ecological studies, prospective studies, and case-controlled studies showed an association between fruit and vegetable intake and decreased risk of cardiovascular disease. In addition, several case-control studies indicate that intakes of selected fruits or vegetables are associated with lower incidence of some cancers. Increased intake of fruits and vegetables has also been associated with decreased blood pressure (30).

Keep food safe to eat The committee added this guideline because it promotes actionable measures that can be taken by consumers and public officials to keep Americans healthy. The 1995 guidelines did not mention food safety (Figure 2). The proposed new guideline covers the following topics: a) healthful eating requires that food be safe, b) foodborne illness is a major preventable public-health problem in the United States, and c) consumers can apply simple food-handling practices to minimize their risk of foodborne illness. The proposed new guideline emphasizes 7 simple messages that consumers can apply whenever they are preparing, serving, and storing food:

- Clean.
- Wash hands and food surfaces often.
- Separate. Separate raw, cooked, and ready-to-eat foods while storing and preparing.
- Cook. Cook foods to a safe temperature.
- Chill. Refrigerate perishable foods promptly.
- Follow the label.
- Serve safely.

1995: Dietary Guidelines

- Eat a variety of foods
- Balance the food you eat with physical activity— maintain or improve your weight
- Choose a diet with plenty of grain products, vegetables, and fruits
- Choose a diet low in fat, saturated fat, and cholesterol
- Choose a diet moderate in sugars
- Choose a diet moderate in salt and sodium
- If you drink alcoholic beverages, do so in moderation

2000: Dietary Guidelines

Aim for Fitness
- Aim for a healthy weight
- Be physically active each day

Build a healthy base
- Let the pyramid guide your food choices.
- Eat a variety of grains daily, especially whole grains.
- Eat a variety of fruits and vegetables daily.
- Keep foods safe to eat.

Choose sensibly
- Choose a diet that is low in saturated fat and cholesterol and moderate in total fat.
- Choose beverages and foods to moderate your intake of sugars.
- Choose and prepare foods with less salt.
- If you drink alcoholic beverages, do so in moderation.

FIG 2: The 1995 and the recommended 2000 Dietary Guidelines for Americans.

- If in doubt, throw it out.

Each of these messages is consistent with well-founded principles of microbiology and sanitation (31,32). The first 4 messages (clean, separate, cook, chill) are, in essence, identical to the Fight BAC! messages of the Partnership for Food Safety Education (33). The last 3 bullets in the guideline provide additional advice to consumers to ensure that food will be safe and wholesome.

Choose sensibly

Choose a diet low in saturated fat and cholesterol and moderate in total fat The wording of this guideline was changed from the 1995 guideline to emphasize the importance of reducing intake of saturated fat and cholesterol. There is robust evidence that diets high in saturated fat and cholesterol contribute to the development of coronary heart disease. It is now well accepted that lowering serum low-density lipoprotein (LDL) cholesterol levels will reduce the risk for coronary heart disease (34). The guideline text also emphasizes the importance of reducing *trans*-fatty acid intakes. *Trans*-fatty acids are included because of an impressive body of evidence indicating

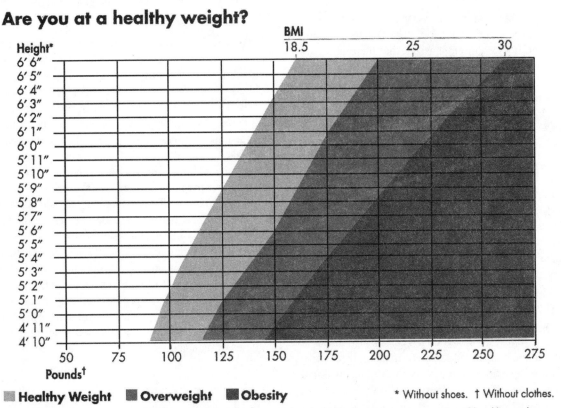

Are you at a healthy weight?

Healthy Weight **Overweight** **Obesity**   * Without shoes. † Without clothes.

The BMI (weight-for-height) shown above for adults are not intended to indicate exact categories of healthy and unhealthy weights. Instead, they are intended to show that health risk increases at higher levels of overweight and obesity. Even within the healthy BMI range, weight gains can carry health risks for adults.

Directions: Find your weight on the bottom of the graph. Go straight up from that point until you come to the line that matches your height. Then look to find your weight group.

➢ BMI of 25 defines the upper boundary of healthy weight
➢ BMI of higher than 25 to 30 defines overweight
➢ BMI of higher than 30 defines obesity

that they raise serum LDL cholesterol levels as well as lower serum high-density lipoprotein (HDL) cholesterol.

An important change in this guideline is the placement of total fat after saturated fat and cholesterol. In addition, the wording recommends a diet termed "moderate" in total fat.

Although the guideline continues to recommend a diet with 30% or less of energy from total fat, the committee believed the phrase, "moderate in total fat" best reflects this concept.

Research in laboratory animals, short-term studies in humans, and some epidemiological evidence suggest that high-fat diets contribute to obesity. More recently, however, data from both experimental and population studies question the strength of the relationship between dietary fat and body weight. Indeed, the committee was concerned that emphasizing low-fat diets for weight control had left the erroneous impression that low-fat diets, without energy reductions, would lead to weight loss. This belief may have led to overconsumption of total energy. In

fact, although the percentage of fat in the US diet has fallen, total fat intake is not lower than in the recent past because of apparent increased intakes of energy (37).

The committee emphasized that all the guidelines, including the fat guideline, apply to children beginning at age 2 years. Current recommendations for adults do not need to be modified for children who are 2 years of age or older. Studies support the safety for children of diets that are low in saturated fat and cholesterol and moderate in total fat, as long as energy needs are met (38–40).

Choose beverages and foods to moderate your intake of sugars The Dietary Guideline for sugars emphasizes moderating the intake of sugars for 2 reasons. First, the focus group research indicated that consumers understand the word "moderate" to mean some but not too much (26). This, in fact, is the intent of the guideline. Second, the concept of a moderate intake is consistent with the theme of moderation in the fat and alcohol guidelines.

The principle diet and health association for the sugars guideline continues to be dental caries. The Dietary Guidelines Advisory Committee report emphasized that there is no compelling evidence that sugars affect children's behavior. In addition, there is little evidence linking sugars with the etiology of noninsulin dependent diabetes. Finally, there is little evidence that diets high in sugars are associated with obesity. However, this lack of association may be confounded by the pervasive problem of underreporting of food intake (41), which is more prevalent and severe among overweight and obese people (42–44). To further complicate the issue, the intakes of food high in added sugar are known to be underreported to a greater extent than other foods (45). Thus, it is difficult to draw conclusions about associations between self-reported sugar intake and BMI. Because the data on total sugars, added sugars and nutrient density, and sugar intake and obesity provided ambiguous patterns, the advisory committee strongly advised the government to pursue more research in these areas.

For the first time, however, the word "beverages" was added to the wording of the guidelines to emphasize that they are a major source of sugars in the US diet. There is also discussion in the text distinguishing added sugars from naturally occurring sugars. This was done because focus group participants found it confusing when the 1995 guideline promoted the consumption of fruits and low-fat dairy products—which are high in the naturally occurring sugars fructose and lactose—while at the same time promoting a diet moderate in sugar. Added sugars are defined as all sugars used as ingredients in processed and prepared foods such as bread, cake, soft drinks, jam, and ice cream, as well as sugars eaten separately. Sugars occurring naturally in foods such as fruit and milk are excluded (46). The most important source of added sugars in the American diet is nondiet soft drinks, which account for one third of all intake of added sugars (47). Nondiet soft drinks, sugars and sweets (such as candies), sweetened grains (cakes, cookies, pies), fruit aides and fruit drinks, flavored milk and other sweetened milk products (ice cream) provide more than three fourths of the total intake of added sugars (47). Soft drink consumption is associated with lower intakes of several "shortfall" nutrients (folate, vitamin A, and calcium) (48) and may be inversely associated with intakes of calcium-rich beverages, such as milk (49–51). Hence, the guideline text cautions consumers not to let soft drinks or other sweets crowd out other foods needed to maintain health, such as low-fat milk or other good sources of calcium.

Choose and prepare foods with less salt The intent of this guideline is unchanged from the 1995 guideline. However, the new wording is framed in terms of choosing foods rather than a diet. This is meant to convey a clearer meaning and to avoid the erroneous interpretation that the guideline refers to either prescribed "special diets" or to weight-reduction diets. Reference to food preparation ("choose and prepare foods") was proposed to highlight the particular importance of food preparation practices in determining the sodium content of foods. "Less" is substituted for "moderate" because of its greater clarity for consumers who find the term "moderate" difficult to interpret. "Sodium" was dropped from the guideline for simplicity; salt is the more familiar term.

If you drink alcoholic beverages, do so in moderation The committee recommended retaining the 1995 wording of this guideline. The text now places more emphasis on the adverse effects of excess alcohol intake and adds information on the increased risk of breast cancer associated with alcohol intake. Moderate drinking is clearly defined as one drink per day for women and 2 drinks per day for men, and the text is reworded to make it clear that the different limits are based on both metabolism and body size. The guideline strengthens the language concerning pregnant women by saying "women who may become pregnant or who are pregnant" should not drink.

The principal benefit of moderate alcohol intake is the lowered risk of cardiovascular disease. However, the text now clarifies that this benefit occurs mainly in men older than age 45 and women older than age 55. Moderate consumption provides little, if any, benefit to younger people. This age specificity is based on the age- and sex-specific rates of coronary heart disease (52) and on the age-specific relative risks related to moderate alcohol consumption obtained from prospective cohort studies of men and women in the United States(53–55).

CONCLUSION

The impact of the Dietary Guidelines for Americans is wide ranging. Not only are the Dietary Guidelines used as the basis of nutrition standards for the federal government's food and nutrition programs, but the guidelines also form the basis for nutrition education messages for the general public. Each edition of the Dietary Guidelines continues to reflect the overwhelming consensus of science to answer the question posed at the beginning of this commentary: "What should Americans eat to stay healthy?"

A systematic campaign to promote the Dietary Guidelines will also be launched by USDA and HHS. Consumption patterns based on the Dietary Guidelines for Americans will lead to major improvements in public health and nutrition for the United States. Dietetics professionals have a key role to play in promoting the Dietary Guidelines as one component of healthful lifestyles.

References

1. Welsh S, Davis C, Shaw A. Development of the Food Guide Pyramid. *Nutr Today.* 1992;27:12–23.
2. Federation of American Societies for Experimental Biology, Life Sciences Research Office. Third Report of Nutrition Monitoring in the United States, vol 1. Washington, DC: US Government Printing Office; 1995.
3. *Dietary Guidelines for Americans Focus Group Study: Final Report.* Washington, DC: ILSI Human Nutrition Institute; 1998.

4. National Institutes of Health, National Heart, Lung, and Blood Institute. *Clinical Guidelines on the Identification, Evaluation, and Treatment of Overweight and Obesity in Adults.* Washington, DC: US Dept of Health and Human Services, Public Health Service; 1998.

5. National Institute of Diabetes and Digestive and Kidney Diseases. National Task Force on Prevention and Treatment of Obesity. Obesity and Health Risk. *Arch Intern Med.* In press.

6. Goldstein DJ. Beneficial health effects of modest weight loss. *Int J Obes Relat Metab Disord.* 1992;16:397–415.

7. Bell EA, Castellanos VH, Pelkman CL, Thorwart ML, Rolls BJ. Energy density affects energy intake in normal-weight women. *Am J Clin Nutr.* 1998;67:412–420.

8. Rolls BJ, Hill JO. Carbohydrates and weight management. ILSI North America. Washington, DC: ILSI Press; 1998.

9. Stubbs RJ, Ritz P, Coward WA, Prentice AM. Covert manipulation of the ratio of dietary fat to carbohydrate and energy density: effect on food intake and energy balance in free-living men eating ad libitum. *Am J Clin Nutr.* 1995;62:330–337.

10. Troiano RP, Flegel KM. Overweight children and adolescents; description, epidemiology, and demographics. *Pediatrics.* 1998;101:497–504.

11. Andersen RE, Crespo CJ, Bartlett SJ, Cheskin LJ, Pratt M. Relationship of physical activity and television watching with body weight and level of fatness among children: results from the Third National Health and Nutrition Examination Survey. *JAMA.* 1998;279:938–942.

12. Pate RR, Pratt M, Blair SN, Haskell WL, Macera CA, Bouchard C, Buchner D, Ettinger W, Heath GW, King AC, Kriska A, Leon AS, Marcus BH, Morris J, Paffenbarger RS, Patrick K, Pollack ML, Rippe JM, Sallis J, Wilmore JH. Physical activity and public health—a recommendation from the Centers for Disease Control and Prevention and the American College of Sports Medicine. *JAMA.* 1995; 273:402–407.

13. Centers for Disease Control and Prevention. Guidelines for school and community health programs to promote lifelong physical activity among young people. *MMWR.* 1997:46:1–34.

14. Mazzeo RS, Cavanagh P, Evans WJ, Fiatrone M, Hagberg J, McAuley E, Startzell J. Exercise and physical activity for older adults. *Med Sci Sports Exerc.* 1998;30:992–1008.

15. National Institutes of Health Consensus Development Panel on Physical Activity and Cardiovascular Health. Physical activity and cardiovascular health. *JAMA.* 1996;276:241–246.

16. Pollock ML, Evans WJ. Resistance training for health and disease: introduction. *Med Sci Sports Exerc.* 1999;31:10–11.

17. Pollock ML, Gaesser GA, Butcher JD, Despres J-P, Dishman RK, Franklin BA, Garber CE. The recommended quantity and quality of exercise for developing and maintaining cardiorespiratory and muscular fitness, and flexibility in healthy adults. *Med Sci Sports Exerc.* 1998:30:975–991.

18. *Physical Activity and Health: A Report of the Surgeon General.* Atlanta, Ga: US Department of Health and Human Services, Centers for Disease Control and Prevention, National Center for Chronic Disease Prevention and Health Promotion; 1996.

19. *Healthy People 2010 Objectives: Draft for Public Comment.* Washington, DC: US Department of Health and Human Services, Office of Public Health and Science; 1998.

20. Ulrich CM, Georgiou CC, Snow-Harter CM, Gillis DE. Bone mineral density in mother-daughter pairs: relations to lifetime exercise, lifetime milk consumption, and calcium supplements. *Am J Clin Nutr.* 1996;63:72–79.

21. Health Education Authority. Young and active? Young people and health-enhancing physical activity—evidence and implications. In: Biddle S, Sallis J, Cavill N, eds. *Health Education Authority.* London, England: Trevelyan House; 1998.

22. Kant AK, Schatzkin A, Block G, Ziegler RG, Nestle M. Food group intake patterns and associated nutrient profiles of the US population. *J Am Diet Assoc.* 1991;91:1532–1537.

23. Krebs-Smith SM, Smicklas-Wright H, Guthrie HA, Krebs-Smith J. The effects of variety in food choices on dietary quality. *J Am Diet Assoc.* 1987;87:897–903

24. Rolls BJ. Experimental analyses of the effects of variety in a meal on human feeding. *Am J Clin Nutr.* 1985:42:932–939.

25. McCrory MA, Fuss PJ, McCallum JE, Yao M, Vinken AG, Hays NP, Roberts SB. Dietary variety within food groups: association with energy intake and body fatness in men and women. *Am J Clin Nutr.* 1999;69:440–447.

26. Report of the Initial Focus Groups on Nutrition and Your Health: Dietary Guidelines for Americans. 4th ed. US Dept of Agriculture, Center for Nutrition Policy and Promotion; 1999.

27. Jacobs DR, Meyer KA, Kushi LH, Folsom AR. Whole grain intake may reduce the risk of ischemic heart disease death in postmenopausal women: the Iowa Women's Health Study. *Am J Clin Nutr.* 1998;68:248–257.

28. Albertson A, Tobelmann R. Consumption of grain and whole-grain foods by an American population during the years 1990–1992. J Am Diet Assoc. 1995:95:703–704.

29. Krebs-Smith SM, Cook A, Subar AF, Cleveland L, Friday J. US adults' fruit and vegetable intakes, 1989 to 1991: a revised baseline for the Healthy People 2000 objective. *Am J Public Health.* 1995;85:1623–1629.

30. Appel LJ, Moore TJ, Obarzanek E, Vollmer WM, Svetkey LP, Sacks FM, Bay GA, Vogt TM, Cutler JA, Windhauser MM, Lin PH, Karanja N. A clinical trial of the effects of dietary patterns on blood pressure. DASH Collaborative Research Group. *N Engl J Med.* 1997;336:1117–1124.

31. Council for Agricultural Science and Technology. Foodborne pathogens: Risks and consequences. Task Force Report No 122. 1994; 18.

32. Institute of Medicine. *Emerging Infections: Microbial Threats to Health in the United States.* Washington, DC: National Academy Press; 1992.

33. Partnership for Food Safety Education. Fight Bad Keep Food Safe from Bacteria. Available at: http://www.fight-bac.org. Accessed May 3, 2000.

34. Gould AL, Rossouw JE, Santanello NC, Heyse FJ, Furberg CD. Cholesterol reduction yields clinical benefit: impact of statin trials. *Circulation*. 1998; 97:946–952.

35. Grundy SM. Overview: 2nd International Conference on Fats and Oil Consumption in Health and Disease: How we can optimize dietary composition to combat metabolic complications and decrease obesity. *Am J Clin Nutr*. 1998;67(suppl):497S–499S.

36. Krause RM. Triglycerides and atherogenic lipoproteins: rationale for lipid management, *Am J Med*. 1998;105(suppl):58S–62S.

37. Anand RS, Basiotis PP. Is total fat consumption really decreasing? *Nutr Insights*. USDA Center for Nutrition Policy and Promotion: April 1998.

38. Lauer RM, Obarzanek E, Kwiterovich PO, Kimm SYS, Hunsburger SA, Barton BA, van Horn L, Stevens VJ, Lasser NL, Robson AM, Franklin FA, Simons-Morton DG. Efficacy and safety of lowering dietary intake of fat and cholesterol in children with elevated low density lipoprotein cholesterol: the dietary intervention study in children. *JAMA*. 1996;273:1429–1435.

39. Niinikoski H, Viikari J, Ronnemaa T, Helenius H, Eero J, Lapinleimu H. Regulation of growth in 7–36 month old children by energy and fat intake in the prospective, randomized STRIP trial. *Pediatrics*. 1997:100:810–816.

40. Obarzanek, E, Hunsberger SA, van Horn L, Hartmuller VV, Barton BA, Stevens FJ. Safety of a fat reduced diet: the Dietary Intervention Study in Children. *Pediatrics*. 1997;100:51–59.

41. Black AE, Prentice, AM, Goldberg GR, Jebb SA, Bingham SA, Livingstone BE, Coward AW. Measurements of total energy expenditure provide insights into the validity of dietary measurements of energy intake. *J Am Diet Assoc*. 1993:93:572–579.

42. Bandini LG, Schoeller DA, Cyr HN, Dietz WH. Validity of reported energy intake in obese and nonobese adolescents. *Am J Clin Nutr*. 1990:52:421–425.

43. Lichtman SW, Pisareka K, Berman ER, Pestones M, Dowling H, Offenbacher E, Weisel H, Heshka S, Matthews DE, Heymefield DB. Discrepancy between self-reported and actual caloric intake and exercise in obese subjects. *N Eng J Med*. 1992;327:1893–1898.

44. Prentice A, Black A, Coward W, Davies H, Goldberg G, Murgatroyd P, Ashford J, Sawyer M, Whitehead R. High levels of energy expenditure in obese women. *BMJ*. 1986;292:983–987.

45. Poppitt SD, Swann D, Black AE, Prentice AM. Assessment of selective underreporting of food intake by both obese and non-obese women in a metabolic facility, *Int J Obesity*. 1998:22:303–311.

46. Cleveland LE, Cook DA, Krebs-Smith S, Friday J. Method for assessing food intakes in terms of servings based on food guidance. *Am J Clin Nutr*. 1997:65 (suppl): 1254S–1263S.

47. Guthrie JF, Morton JF. Food sources of added sweeteners in the diets of Americans. *J Am Diet Assoc*. 2000;100:43–48.

48. Harnack L, Stang J, Story M. Soft drink consumption among US children and adolescents: nutritional consequences, *J Am Diet Assoc*. 1999:99:438–441.

49. Guenther PM. Beverages in the diets of American teenagers. *J Am Diet Assoc*. 1986;86:493–495.

50. Skinner JD, Carruth BR, Moran J. Houck K. Coletta F. Fruit juice intake is not related to children's growth. *Pediatrics*. 1999;103:58–64.

51. Guthrie JF. Dietary patterns and personal characteristics of women consuming recommended amounts of calcium. *Fam Econ Nutr Rev*. 1996:9:33–49.

52. *Health, United States, 1999 with Health and Aging Chartbook*. National Center for Health Statistics: Hyattville, Md; 1999.

53. Fuchs CS, Stampfer MJ, Colditz GA, Giovannucci EL, Manson JE, Kawachi I, Hunter DJ, Hankinson SE, Hennekens CH, Rosner B, Speizer FE, Willett WC. Alcohol consumption and mortality among women. *N Engl J Med*. 1995;332:1245–1250.

54. Rimm EB, Giovannucci EL, Willett WC, Colditz GA, Ascherio A, Rosner B, Stampfer MJ. Prospective study of alcohol consumption and risk of coronary disease in men. *Lancet*. 1991;338:464–468.

55. Thun MJ, Peto R, Lopez AD, Monaco JH, Henley J, Health C, Doll R. Alcohol consumption and mortality among middle-aged and elderly US Adults. *N Engl J Med*. 1997;337:1705–1714.

Every member of the Year 2000 Dietary Guidelines Advisory Committee (Figure 1) contributed countless hours to the report upon which this manuscript is based. We are indebted to them. We thank the dedicated staff members from HHS (Linda Meyers, PhD; Kathryn McMurry, MS; and Joan Lyon, MS) and USDA (Shanthy Bowman, PhD; Carol Davis, MS, RD; and Alyson Escobar, MS, RD) who assisted with the preparation of the report. We are grateful to Carol Suitor, PhD RD, for her expert editorial assistance throughout the process of preparing the report.

R. K. Johnson is associate dean of research at the College of Agriculture and Life Sciences and professor of nutrition at the University of Vermont, Burlington. Eileen Kennedy is the Deputy Under Secretary for Research, Education, and Economics at the US Department of Agriculture.
Address correspondence to Rachel K. Johnson, 108 Morrill Hall, Burlington, VT 05405.

REBUILDING

the

Food Pyramid

The dietary guide introduced a decade ago has led people astray. Some fats are healthy for the heart, and many carbohydrates clearly are not.

By Walter C. Willett and Meir J. Stampfer

In 1992 the U.S. Department of Agriculture officially released the Food Guide Pyramid, which was intended to help the American public make dietary choices that would maintain good health and reduce the risk of chronic disease. The recommendations embodied in the pyramid soon became well known: people should minimize their consumption of fats and oils but should eat six to 11 servings a day of foods rich in complex carbohydrates—bread, cereal, rice, pasta and so on. The food pyramid also recommended generous amounts of vegetables (including potatoes, another plentiful source of complex carbohydrates), fruit and dairy products, and at least two servings a day from the meat and beans group, which lumped together red meat with poultry, fish, nuts, legumes and eggs.

Even when the pyramid was being developed, though, nutritionists had long known that some types of fat are essential to health and can reduce the risk of cardiovascular disease. Furthermore, scientists had found little evidence that a high intake of carbohydrates is beneficial.

Since 1992 more and more research has shown that the USDA pyramid is grossly flawed. By promoting the consumption of all complex carbohydrates and eschewing all fats and oils, the pyramid provides misleading guidance. In short, not all fats are bad for you, and by no means are all complex carbohydrates good for you. The USDA's Center for Nutrition Policy and Promotion is now reassessing the pyramid, but this effort is not expected to be completed until 2004. In the meantime, we have drawn up a new pyramid that better reflects the current understanding of the relation between diet and health. Studies indicate that adherence to the recommendations in the revised pyramid can significantly reduce the risk of cardiovascular disease for both men and women.

How did the original USDA pyramid go so wrong? In part, nutritionists fell victim to a desire to simplify their dietary recommendations. Researchers had known for decades that saturated fat—found in abundance in red meat and dairy products—raises cholesterol levels in the blood. High cholesterol levels, in

turn, are associated with a high risk of coronary heart disease (heart attacks and other ailments caused by the blockage of the arteries to the heart). In the 1960s controlled feeding studies, in which the participants eat carefully prescribed diets for several weeks, substantiated that saturated fat increases cholesterol levels. But the studies also showed that polyunsaturated fat—found in vegetable oils and fish—reduces cholesterol. Thus, dietary advice during the 1960s and 1970s emphasized the replacement of saturated fat with polyunsaturated fat, not total fat reduction. (The subsequent doubling of polyunsaturated fat consumption among Americans probably contributed greatly to the halving of coronary heart disease rates in the U.S. during the 1970s and 1980s.)

The notion that fat in general is to be avoided stems mainly from observations that affluent Western countries have both high intakes of fat and high rates of coronary heart disease. This correlation, however, is limited to saturated fat. Societies in which people eat relatively large portions of monounsaturated and polyunsaturated

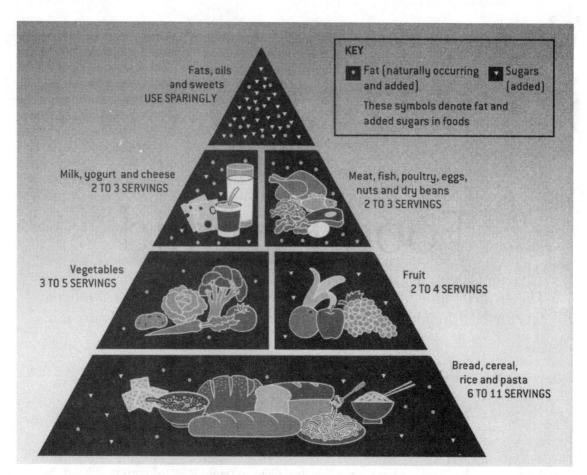

Old Food Pyramid conceived by the U.S. Department of Agriculture was intended to convey the message "Fat is bad" and its corollary "Carbs are good." These sweeping statements are now being questioned.

For information on the amount of food that counts as one serving, visit www.nal.usda.gov: 8001/py/pmap.htm

fat tend to have lower rates of heart disease [*see illustration on next page*]. On the Greek island of Crete, for example, the traditional diet contained much olive oil (a rich source of monounsaturated fat) and fish (a source of polyunsaturated fat). Although fat constituted 40 percent of the calories in this diet, the rate of heart disease for those who followed it was lower than the rate for those who followed the traditional diets of Japan, in which fat made up only 8 to 10 percent of the calories. Furthermore, international comparisons can be misleading: many negative influences on health, such as smoking, physical inactivity and high amounts of body fat, are also correlated with Western affluence.

Unfortunately, many nutritionists decided it would be too difficult to educate the public about these subtleties. Instead they put out a clear, simple message: "Fat is bad." Because saturated fat represents about

40 percent of all fat consumed in the U.S., the rationale of the USDA was that advocating a low-fat diet would naturally reduce the intake of saturated fat. This recommendation was soon reinforced by the food industry, which began selling cookies, chips and other products that were low in fat but often high in sweeteners such as high-fructose corn syrup.

When the food pyramid was being developed, the typical American got about 40 percent of his or her calories from fat, about 15 percent from protein and about 45 percent from carbohydrates. Nutritionists did not want to suggest eating more protein, because many sources of protein (red meat, for example) are also heavy in saturated fat. So the "Fat is bad" mantra led to the corollary "Carbs are good." Dietary guidelines from the American Heart Association and other groups recommended that people get at least half their calories from carbohydrates and

no more than 30 percent from fat. This 30 percent limit has become so entrenched among nutritionists that even the sophisticated observer could be forgiven for thinking that many studies must show that individuals with that level of fat intake enjoyed better health than those with higher levels. But no study has demonstrated long-term health benefits that can be directly attributed to a low-fat diet. The 30 percent limit on fat was essentially drawn from thin air.

The wisdom of this direction became even more questionable after researchers found that the two main cholesterol-carrying chemicals—low-density lipoprotein (LDL), popularly known as "bad cholesterol," and high-density lipoprotein (HDL), known as "good cholesterol"—have very different effects on the risk of coronary heart disease. Increasing the ratio of LDL to HDL in the blood raises the risk, whereas decreasing

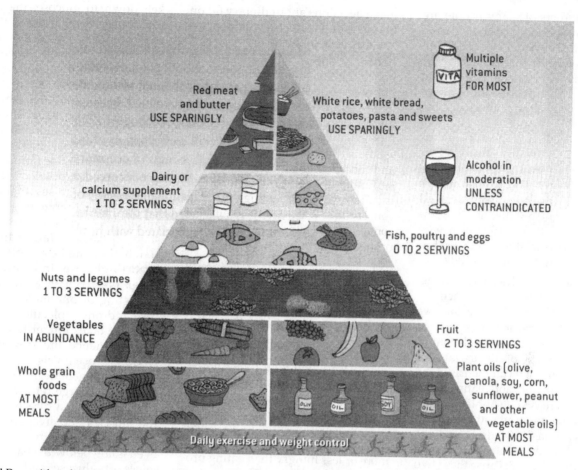

New Food Pyramid outlined by the authors distinguishes between healthy and unhealthy types of fat and carbohydrates. Fruits and vegetables are still recommended, but the consumption of dairy products should be limited.

the ratio lowers it. By the early 1990s controlled feeding studies had shown that when a person replaces calories from saturated fat with an equal amount of calories from carbohydrates the levels of LDL and total cholesterol fall, but the level of HDL also falls. Because the ratio of LDL to HDL does not change, there is only a small reduction in the person's risk of heart disease. Moreover, the switch to carbohydrates boosts the blood levels of triglycerides, the component molecules of fat, probably because of effects on the body's endocrine system. High triglyceride levels are also associated with a high risk of heart disease.

The effects are more grievous when a person switches from either monounsaturated or polyunsaturated fat to carbohydrates. LDL levels rise and HDL levels drop, making the cholesterol ratio worse. In contrast, replacing saturated fat with ei-ther monounsaturated or polyunsaturated fat improves this ratio and would be expected to reduce heart disease. The only fats that are significantly more deleterious than carbohydrates are the trans-unsaturated fatty acids; these are produced by the partial hydrogenation of liquid vegetable oil, which causes it to solidify. Found in many margarines, baked goods and fried foods, trans fats are uniquely bad for you because they raise LDL and triglycerides while reducing HDL.

THE BIG PICTURE

TO EVALUATE FULLY the health effects of diet, though, one must look beyond cholesterol ratios and triglyceride levels. The foods we eat can cause heart disease through many other pathways, including raising blood pressure or boosting the tendency of blood to clot. And other foods can prevent heart disease in surprising ways; for instance, omega-3 fatty acids (found in fish and some plant oils) can reduce the likelihood of ventricular fibrillation, a heart rhythm disturbance that causes sudden death.

The ideal method for assessing all these adverse and beneficial effects would be to conduct large-scale trials in which individuals are randomly assigned to one diet or another and followed for many years. Because of practical constraints and cost, few such studies have been conducted, and most of these have focused on patients who already suffer from heart disease. Though limited, these studies have supported the benefits of replacing saturated fat with polyunsaturated fat, but not with carbohydrates.

The best alternative is to conduct large epidemiological studies in which the diets of many people are periodically assessed and the participants are monitored for the development of heart disease and other conditions. One of the best-known examples of this research is the Nurses' Health Study, which was begun in 1976 to evaluate the effects of oral contraceptives but was soon extended to nutrition as well. Our group at Harvard University has followed nearly 90,000 women in this study who first completed detailed questionnaires on diet in 1980, as well as more than 50,000 men who were enrolled in the Health Professionals Follow-Up Study in 1986.

After adjusting the analysis to account for smoking, physical activity and other recognized risk factors, we found that a participant's risk of heart disease was strongly influenced by the type of dietary fat consumed. Eating trans fat increased the risk substantially, and eating saturated fat increased it slightly. In contrast, eating monounsaturated and polyunsaturated fats decreased the risk—just as the controlled feeding studies predicted. Because these two effects counterbalanced each other, higher overall consumption of fat did not lead to higher rates of coronary heart disease. This finding reinforced a 1989 report by the National Academy of Sciences that concluded that total fat intake alone was not associated with heart disease risk.

But what about illnesses besides coronary heart disease? High rates of breast, colon and prostate cancers in affluent Western countries have led to the belief that the consumption of fat, particularly animal fat, may be a risk factor. But large epidemiological studies have shown little evidence that total fat consumption or intakes of specific types of fat during midlife affect the risks of breast or colon cancer. Some studies have indicated that prostate cancer and the consumption of animal fat may be associated, but reassuringly there is no suggestion that vegetable oils increase any cancer risk. Indeed, some studies have suggested that vegetable oils may slightly reduce such risks. Thus, it is reasonable to

make decisions about dietary fat on the basis of its effects on cardiovascular disease, not cancer.

Finally, one must consider the impact of fat consumption on obesity, the most serious nutritional problem in the U.S. Obesity is a major risk factor for several diseases, including type 2 diabetes (also called adult-onset diabetes), coronary heart disease, and cancers of the breast, colon, kidney and esophagus. Many nutritionists believe that eating fat can contribute to weight gain because fat contains more calories per gram than protein or carbohydrates. Also, the process of storing dietary fat in the body may be more efficient than the conversion of carbohydrates to body fat. But recent controlled feeding studies have shown that these considerations are not practically important. The best way to avoid obesity is to limit your total calories, not just the fat calories. So the critical issue is whether the fat composition of a diet can influence one's ability to control caloric intake. In other words, does eating fat leave you more or less hungry than eating protein or carbohydrates? There are various theories about why one diet should be better than another, but few long-term studies have been done. In randomized trials, individuals assigned to low-fat diets tend to lose a few pounds during the first months but then regain the weight. In studies lasting a year or longer, low-fat diets have consistently not led to greater weight loss.

CARBO-LOADING

NOW LET'S LOOK at the health effects of carbohydrates. Complex carbohydrates consist of long chains of sugar units such as glucose and fructose; sugars contain only one or two units. Because of concerns that sugars offer nothing but "empty calories"—that is, no vitamins, minerals or other nutrients—complex carbohydrates form the base of the USDA food pyramid. But refined carbohydrates, such as white bread and white rice, can be very quickly bro-

ken down to glucose, the primary fuel for the body. The refining process produces an easily absorbed form of starch—which is defined as glucose molecules bound together—and also removes many vitamins and minerals and fiber. Thus, these carbohydrates increase glucose levels in the blood more than whole grains do. (Whole grains have not been milled into fine flour.)

Or consider potatoes. Eating a boiled potato raises blood sugar levels higher than eating the same amount of calories from table sugar. Because potatoes are mostly starch, they can be rapidly metabolized to glucose. In contrast, table sugar (sucrose) is a disaccharide consisting of one molecule of glucose and one molecule of fructose. Fructose takes longer to convert to glucose, hence the slower rise in blood glucose levels.

A rapid increase in blood sugar stimulates a large release of insulin, the hormone that directs glucose to the muscles and liver. As a result, blood sugar plummets, sometimes even going below the baseline. High levels of glucose and insulin can have negative effects on cardiovascular health, raising triglycerides and lowering HDL (the good cholesterol). The precipitous decline in glucose can also lead to more hunger after a carbohydrate-rich meal and thus contribute to overeating and obesity.

In our epidemiological studies, we have found that a high intake of starch from refined grains and potatoes is associated with a high risk of type 2 diabetes and coronary heart disease. Conversely, a greater intake of fiber is related to a lower risk of these illnesses. Interestingly, though, the consumption of fiber did not lower the risk of colon cancer, as had been hypothesized earlier.

The best way to avoid obesity is to LIMIT YOUR TOTAL CALORIES, not just the fat calories.

Overweight, inactive people can become resistant to insulin's effects and therefore require more of the hormone to regulate their blood sugar. Recent evidence indicates that the adverse metabolic response to carbohydrates is substantially worse among people who already have insulin resistance. This finding may account for the ability of peasant farmers in Asia and elsewhere, who are extremely lean and active, to consume large amounts of refined carbohydrates without experiencing diabetes or heart disease, whereas the same diet in a more sedentary population can have devastating effects.

EAT YOUR VEGGIES

HIGH INTAKE OF FRUITS and vegetables is perhaps the least controversial aspect of the food pyramid. A reduction in cancer risk has been a widely promoted benefit. But most of the evidence for this benefit has come from case-control studies, in which patients with cancer and selected control subjects are asked about their earlier diets. These retrospective studies are susceptible to numerous biases, and recent findings from large prospective studies (including our own) have tended to show little relation between overall fruit and vegetable consumption and cancer incidence. (Specific nutrients in fruits and vegetables may offer benefits, though; for instance, the folic acid in green leafy vegetables may reduce the risk of colon cancer, and the lycopene found in tomatoes may lower the risk of prostate cancer.)

The real value of eating fruits and vegetables may be in reducing the risk of cardiovascular disease. Folic acid and potassium appear to contribute to this effect, which has been seen in several epidemiological studies. Inadequate consumption of folic acid is responsible for higher risks of serious birth defects as well, and low intake of lutein, a pigment in green leafy vegetables, has been associated with greater risks of

cataracts and degeneration of the retina. Fruits and vegetables are also the primary source of many vitamins needed for good health. Thus, there are good reasons to consume the recommended five servings a day, even if doing so has little impact on cancer risk. The inclusion of potatoes as a vegetable in the USDA pyramid has little justification, however; being mainly starch, potatoes do not confer the benefits seen for other vegetables.

Another flaw in the USDA pyramid is its failure to recognize the important health differences between red meat (beef, pork and lamb) and the other foods in the meat and beans group (poultry, fish, legumes, nuts and eggs). High consumption of red meat has been associated with an increased risk of coronary heart disease, probably because of its high content of saturated fat and cholesterol. Red meat also raises the risk of type 2 diabetes and colon cancer. The elevated risk of colon cancer may be related in part to the carcinogens produced during cooking and the chemicals found in processed meats such as salami and bologna.

Poultry and fish, in contrast, contain less saturated fat and more unsaturated fat than red meat does. Fish is a rich source of the essential omega-3 fatty acids as well. Not surprisingly, studies have shown that people who replace red meat with chicken and fish have a lower risk of coronary heart disease and colon cancer. Eggs are high in cholesterol, but consumption of up to one a day does not appear to have adverse effects on heart disease risk (except among diabetics), probably because the effects of a slightly higher cholesterol level are counterbalanced by other nutritional benefits. Many people have avoided nuts because of their high fat content, but the fat in nuts, including peanuts, is mainly unsaturated, and walnuts in particular are a good source of omega-3 fatty acids. Controlled feeding studies show that nuts improve blood cholesterol ratios, and epidemiological studies indicate that they lower the risk of heart disease and diabetes. Also, people who eat nuts are actually

less likely to be obese; perhaps because nuts are more satisfying to the appetite, eating them seems to have the effect of significantly reducing the intake of other foods.

Yet another concern regarding the USDA pyramid is that it promotes over-consumption of dairy products, recommending the equivalent of two or three glasses of milk a day. This advice is usually justified by dairy's calcium content, which is believed to prevent osteoporosis and bone fractures. But the highest rates of fractures are found in countries with high dairy consumption, and large prospective studies have not shown a lower risk of fractures among those who eat plenty of dairy products. Calcium is an essential nutrient, but the requirements for bone health have probably been overstated. What is more, we cannot assume that high dairy consumption is safe: in several studies, men who consumed large amounts of dairy products experienced an increased risk of prostate cancer, and in some studies, women with high intakes had elevated rates of ovarian cancer. Although fat was initially assumed to be the responsible factor, this has not been supported in more detailed analyses. High calcium intake itself seemed most clearly related to the risk of prostate cancer.

More research is needed to determine the health effects of dairy products, but at the moment it seems imprudent to recommend high consumption. Most adults who are following a good overall diet can get the necessary amount of calcium by consuming the equivalent of one glass of milk a day. Under certain circumstances, such as after menopause, people may need more calcium than usual, but it can be obtained at lower cost and without saturated fat or calories by taking a supplement.

A HEALTHIER PYRAMID

ALTHOUGH THE USDA'S food pyramid has become an icon of nutrition over the past decade, until recently no studies had evaluated the health of individuals who followed its guidelines. It very likely has some benefits, especially from a high intake of fruits and vegetables. And a decrease in total fat intake would tend to reduce the consumption of harmful saturated and trans fats. But the pyramid could also lead people to eat fewer of the healthy unsaturated fats and more refined starches, so the benefits might be negated by the harm.

To evaluate the overall impact, we used the Healthy Eating Index (HEI), a score developed by the USDA to measure adherence to the pyramid and its accompanying dietary guidelines in federal nutrition programs. From the data collected in our large epidemiological studies, we calculated each participant's HEI score and then examined the relation of these scores to subsequent risk of major chronic disease (defined as heart attack, stroke, cancer or nontraumatic death from any cause). When we compared people in the same age groups, women and men with the highest HEI scores did have a lower risk of major chronic disease. But these individuals also smoked less, exercised more and had generally healthier lifestyles than the other participants. After adjusting for these variables, we found that participants with the highest HEI scores did not experience significantly better overall health outcomes. As predicted, the pyramid's harms counterbalanced its benefits.

Because the goal of the pyramid was a worthy one—to encourage healthy dietary choices—we have tried to develop an alternative derived from the best available knowledge. Our revised pyramid emphasizes weight control through

exercising daily and avoiding an excessive total intake of calories. This pyramid recommends that the bulk of one's diet should consist of healthy fats (liquid vegetable oils such as olive, canola, soy, corn, sunflower and peanut) and healthy carbohydrates (whole grain foods such as whole wheat bread, oatmeal and brown rice). If both the fats and carbohydrates in your diet are healthy, you probably do not have to worry too much about the percentages of total calories coming from each. Vegetables and fruits should also be eaten in abundance. Moderate amounts of healthy sources of protein (nuts, legumes, fish, poultry and eggs) are encouraged, but dairy consumption should be limited to one to two servings a day. The revised pyramid recommends minimizing the con sumption of red meat, butter, refined grains (including white bread, white rice and white pasta), potatoes and sugar.

Trans fat does not appear at all in the pyramid, because it has no place in a healthy diet. A multiple vitamin is suggested for most people, and moderate alcohol consumption can be a worthwhile option (if not contraindicated by specific health conditions or medications). This last recommendation comes with a caveat: drinking no alcohol is clearly better than drinking too much. But more and more studies are showing the benefits of moderate alcohol consumption (in any form: wine, beer or spirits) to the cardiovascular system.

Men and women eating in accordance with THE NEW PYRAMID had a lower risk of major chonic disease.

Can we show that our pyramid is healthier than the USDA's? We created a new Healthy Eating Index that measured how closely a person's diet followed our recommendations. Applying this revised index to our epidemiological studies, we found that men and women who were eating in accordance with the new pyramid had a lower risk of major chronic disease [*see illustration on opposite page*]. This benefit resulted almost entirely from significant reductions in the risk of cardiovascular disease—up to 30 percent for women and 40 percent for men. Following the new pyramid's guidelines did not, however, lower the risk of cancer. Weight control and physical activity, rather than specific food choices, are associated with a reduced risk of many cancers.

Of course, uncertainties still cloud our understanding of the relation between diet and health. More research is needed to examine the role of dairy products, the health effects of specific fruits and vegetables, the risks and benefits of vitamin supplements, and the long-term effects of diet during childhood and early adult life. The interaction of dietary factors with genetic predisposition should also be investigated, although its importance remains to be determined.

Another challenge will be to ensure that the information about nutrition given to the public is based strictly on scientific evidence. The USDA may not be the best government agency to develop objective nutritional guidelines, because it may be too closely linked to the agricultural industry. The food pyramid should be rebuilt in a setting that is well insulated from political and economic interests.

WALTER C. WILLETT and *MEIR J. STAMPFER* are professors of epidemiology and nutrition at the Harvard School of Public Health. Willett chairs the school's department of nutrition, and Stampfer heads the department of epidemiology. Willett and Stampfer are also professors of medicine at Harvard Medical School. Both of them practice what they preach by eating well and exercising regularly.

Our Ready-prepared Ready-to-eat-Nation

Ready-to-eat/ready-prepared foods loom larger in most Americans' eating repertoires than they realize. One of our nutrition-business experts takes a look at how we got there and what is likely next.

James E. Tillotson, PhD, MBA

Given Americans' often self-confessed obsessive interest with their food, recent changes in their daily diet lead to questions of where their true interests lie. We see this demonstrated in a paradox of the public's acknowledgment of their changing lifestyles. Last August was the 20th anniversary of IBM's development of the personal computer. With this milestone, there was also much celebration over reaching the 50% level in American homes owning and using at least one computer—certainly a milestone in our changing lifestyles.

Yet at approximately this same point in history, we now spend 50% of our total food dollars for ready-prepared ready-to-eat foods of all kinds, a marked change in our relationship to our daily diet. This 50% milestone has been reached with surprisingly little public notice. We live in a time when ever busier, more time-pressed, affluent young and older Americans, often in dual-career homes, increasingly avoid the drudgery of grocery shopping and food preparation and opt to become the steady breakfast, lunch, dinner, and snacking "guests" of the food industry in its multiple new business formats.

Scanning the US Consumer Food Sales for 1998, which totaled some $690 billion nationally, according to the US Department of Agriculture (USDA), we see in Figure 1 that retail ready-prepared foods, supplied by all restaurants and food service outlets, accounted for $352 billion of the total $690 billion annual consumer sales, or 51% of all retail food dollars Americans spent in 1998. Concurrently, total store food sales were $338 billion, or 49% of total retail food sales, some $14 billion less than total food service and restaurant sales. The diagram's overlapping area between food stores and food service sales is the result of traditional food stores—mainly supermarkets—attempting to compete for sales by also offering their own ready-prepared take-out foods in addition to traditional grocery items.

These numbers are part of a continuing trend that started in the early 1990s: retail fresh ready-prepared food purchases have risen above the 50% level, now outselling traditional grocery food sales. In spite of a multitude of ever-more-convenient retail food products by the food processing industry, the consumer trend has been away from food requiring further preparation and toward fresh food fully prepared. Such food appeals because it combines services, including ingredient procurement, full preparation, and often even delivery with no clean-up required! For consumers, this is the ultimate in convenience in satisfying hunger: just pay and eat!

Half of American food dollars go to ready-prepared ready-to-eat foods.

Increasingly, Americans with more money than time have stopped preparing their own meals and become willing customers for commercial organizations that take over this daily chore. Today, even when Americans cook, we are obsessed with time- and labor-saving products. According to a 2000 survey of 2000 US households conducted by the NPD Group's Kitchen Audit, 44% of weekday home meals are prepared in 30 minutes or less. Even in traditional families (2-parent households with a stay-at-home mom), average food preparation time is between 31 and 45 minutes per weekday evening meal. Speed and food have become synonymous in modern lifestyles.

"Ingredients" are increasingly semiprepared foods. Although we still choose our foods, the fabrication and contents are increasingly delegated to others. From a food-policy perspective, one wonders about how effective tools such as the Food Guide Pyramid, which stresses basic ingredients, will be in the future.

Modern attraction to fresh fully-prepared ready-to-eat foods is part of a natural progression in commercial foods during the past 150 years, as we moved from retail commodity to packaged and now ready-to-eat foods. Historically, this began in the Industrial Revolution in the mid-19th century, when many people left agriculture to work in industrial jobs, requiring food they could get in the city in exchange for their industrial wages. Thus our vast food-processing, distribution, and marketing system developed. There have been 3 eras in this system: retail commodity food products (mid-19th century through the 1930s), the growth of packaged and branded convenience foods (1930s-1980s), and the present growth of ready-prepared ready-to-eat foods.

All 3 eras are marked by ever-increasing consumer service combined with decreasing effort in final food preparation. Over time, food preparation has increasingly been delegated out of the home. It is unlikely that this trend can now be reversed. We are reaching the ultimate stage of this product progression, with increasing shift from various levels of self-prepared food to ready-to-eat food eaten at home or out.

This new eating pattern may be unavoidable in an industrial nation, but hopefully it may also be integrated successfully with progressive new health policies. This will be a difficult task, as we recall McDonald's™ failed attempt with the nutritionally correct "91% fat-free" McLean Deluxe™ hamburgers; the chain is believed to have lost as much as $100 million for this noble effort.

Actual 1999-2000 sales data confirm the trend. According to The Food Institute, in the calendar year 1999, real food sales (deflated) in grocery stores rose 2.95% nationally, whereas food sales in eating and drinking outlets rose twice as fast, growing 6.98%. Again, in the year 2000, national eating and drinking establishment sales outdistanced national grocery store food sales growth: 4.52% vs. 1.93%. These markedly different growth rates have been the recent norm. Given the social, economic, and technologic motivating factors, this trend is likely to continue.

In addition, it has and will continue to influence the composition of our diet. We are at the 50% purchase level, but total caloric intake from ready-prepared foods probably somewhat trails this, taking into account its inherently greater labor costs. Current estimates place total average caloric intake for all fresh ready-prepared foods in the range between the mid-30 to low 40 percent level for the (mythical) average consumer. Obviously as purchase level increases, caloric intake from ready-prepared foods is also projected to rise.

Social commentaries, such as Eric Schlosser's Fast Food Nation, Noreena Hertz's The Silent Takeover, Naomi Kleins' No Logo: Taking Aim at the Brand Bullies, and others, can castigate the food industry and its highly effective branding and promotional efforts but fall silent on alternatives acceptable to the consumer, given the economic and social dynamics presently driving this trend. As a one-time director of an industrial food product development group, I quickly learned that in spite of government nutrition policies and guidelines, nutritionists' advice, and activists' laments, the American public buys what meets its fancy, taste, and economic needs, despite all good advice and good intentions. The market—always the consumer—leads the industry, not the reverse. The food industry survives only by satisfying the market, and the market today is increasingly receptive to ready-prepared ready-to-eat foods.

Work habits are a strong motivation for public "wants." According to the International Labor Organization, today's Americans work the most hours—1979 hours per year, on average—of all industrial nations. Why? The root causes are complex. Some reasons include mothers with young children who tend to start working sooner and for longer hours than mothers in the past, many low-wage workers are forced by economic need to work 2 and 3 jobs, and the growing salaried professionals who work 60 plus hours each week.

In addition, Americans' take the shortest annual vacation time in all industrialized nations, resulting in an average working year of about 49½ weeks! These American work patterns favor ready-prepared foods as a necessary time-management tool. Those who lament, "Who has time to cook?" reflect what is true for many.

Ready-prepared foods are also being tailor-made for current American lifestyles. Last July, the Institute of Food Technologists' biannual list of the Top Ten Trends in consumer food demands, listed at the top, Do-It-For-Me, commenting that "premade meals and take-out rule the roost."

Coupled with this is the rising trend in eating out. Eating out is one of our favorite forms of entertainment and fits the modern lifestyle, work schedule, and increasing affluence. Favored by remarkably low basic food costs in America, the average American spends less than 10% of his or her total disposable income for all food, according to recent government figures. "Eating out" is now an everyday event for many Americans.

---

3 eras:
- *19th century to 1930s—retail commodity foods*
- *1930s to 1980s—packaged branded convenience foods*
- *Today—ready-prepared ready-to-eat*

The National Restaurant Association, a trade group representing 844,000 US restaurants, recently reported that in 2000 the average number of restaurant meals purchased per person was 141. This is up from 113 times per person in 1984, a 25% increase. The 2000 figures are projected to fall to 137 per person in 2001, due to the current economic softening and the September 11 tragedy, but the restaurant industry still expects to set a new total sales record. Total national restaurant dollar sales are up from $119.6 billion in 1980 to $239.3 billion in 1990 and projected to reach $399 billion in 2001. This is a 234% increase in 22 years.

The rapid growth of chain restaurants, particularly the quick-service types, have been at the forefront of America's "eating out" pattern. Before the first McDonald's™ fast-food outlets in the 1940s, restaurants were primarily single-establishment businesses. Chains introduced new mass-feeding technologies and used modern marketing techniques, mass advertising, and promotion, developed by packaged-goods companies, to gain remarkable growth. By 1998, the top 20 restaurant chains (eg, KCF™, Denny's™, Pizza Hut™, Burger King™, Wendy's™, Subway™, McDonald's™, etc), had 79,922 outlets with combined retail sales of $56 billion, some 23% of all restaurant sales in that year.

There are many reasons these chains appeal: they offer popular American foods with dependable quality, quick courteous service, clean convenient outlets and long business hours, moderate pricing, and overwhelming portion sizes. Their foods are a perfect fit for Americans' busy lifestyles and growing desire and need for food service. Commonly offering "around-the-clock" service, these chains meet our "all-hours" eating patterns, rather than the 3-meals-a-day pattern of the past. The fast-food industry estimates presently the availability of one fast-food outlet for approximately every 1400-1500 Americans. McDonald's™ claims that more than 40 million people eat at all of its domestic outlets every day.

Increasingly, restaurants and food-service outlets, not supermarkets, are projected to become the major destination of consumer dollars in the future. In the 1950s restaurant sales represented 25% of all domestic retail food sales, this increased to 44% in 1999, and industry projections suggest that by 2010 53% of all US retail sales will be made at restaurants alone.

This strong market move to restaurant and other fresh ready-prepared food opens new questions for food policy. The Nutrition Labeling and Education Act (NLEA) of 1990 established mandatory nutrition labeling for all packaged foods. At that time, restaurants and nonpackaged ready-prepared foods were for the most part exempted due to a combination of difficulty in implementation, practicality, and adroit industry lobbying. As restaurant and food service ready-prepared food becomes increasingly a major portion of the American diet, do we move back to a pre-1990 NLEA era in consumer knowledge about what they are eating? One is left to wonder whether policies, much heralded as "the answer" at their inception only a decade ago, and implementation costs in the billions can quickly become "worn out" because of the lightning-fast changes in social and economic conditions of our food system.

Let us return to our opening paradox, the comparison between PCs and ready-prepared foods. Interestingly, while current IT industry projections for significant increases in home PC penetration are guarded, food industry projections see no barriers to an ever-increasing percentage of our total diet being sold in ready-prepared ready-to-eat forms. In spite of all the buzz about our new information technology age, in the years ahead it is likely that the percent of ready-prepared food intake will well outdistance the home penetration of PCs with many Americans! One could wonder, whimsically, if, as in the past one used the home to "prepare" food while getting information (newspapers, magazines, books, radio, and television) delivered, in the future one will use the home to "prepare" one's information, using the PC, while having fresh ready-prepared ready-to-eat food delivered!

The 50% PC home penetration figure has had apparently little influence on our long-term well-being (barring the influence of reduced physical activity plus the random chance through PC overuse of things such as repetitive carpal tunnel syndrome). Yet one wonders if the present 50% purchase level of ready-prepared ready-to-eat foods in our daily eating habits, with further increases sure, will prove to be as benign.

James E. Tillotson, PhD, MBA, is currently professor of food policy and international business at Tufts University. Before returning to the academic world, he worked in industry, holding various research and development positions in the food and chemical sectors.

Unhappy Meals

School lunches are loaded with fat—

and the beef and dairy industries are making sure it stays that way.

Barry Yeoman

Every weekday at lunch, courtesy of the federal government, more than 27 million schoolchildren sit down to the nation's largest mass feeding. If we took a giant snapshot of their trays on a typical day—say, Tuesday, September 24—here's what the continent-wide photo would look like:

In Lynnwood, Washington, we would see kids eating sausage with Belgian waffle sticks and syrup. In Clovis, California, bacon cheeseburgers. In La Quinta, California, Canadian bacon and cheese rolls. In Rexburg, Idaho, cheese nachos and waffles. In Fort Collins, Colorado, "homemade" pigs in a blanket. In Bryan, Texas, cheeseburgers, chicken-fried steak, and pizza. In Hot Springs, Arkansas, country steak with creamed potatoes. In Cedar Falls, Iowa, mini-corndogs. In Lafayette, Indiana, beef ravioli with cheesy broccoli. In Columbus, Ohio, egg rolls with tater tots. In Kingstree, South Carolina, sloppy joes with onion rings. In Richmond, Virginia, chili cheese nachos. In Gatesville, North Carolina, three-meat subs with Fritos. In Orwigsburg, Pennsylvania, cheese steak on rolls with buttered pasta. And in Fitchburg, Massachusetts, pretzels with cheese sauce.

Here and there, we'd also see baked chicken and salads. But by and large, school cafeterias coast to coast offer an artery-clogging menu of beef, pork, cheese, and grease. "Whenever I see children clinically, I ask them if they buy lunch at school or bring it from home," says Patricia Froberg, a nutritionist at Connecticut Children's Medical Center in Hartford. "If they say, 'I get it at school,' I cringe."

At a time when weight-related illnesses in children are escalating, schools are serving kids the very foods that lead to obesity, diabetes, and heart disease. That's because the National School Lunch Program, which gives schools more than $6 billion each year to offer low-cost meals to students, has conflicting missions. Enacted in 1946, the program is supposed to provide healthy meals to children, regardless of income. At the same time, however, it's designed to subsidize agribusiness, shoring up demand for beef and milk even as the public's taste for these foods declines.

Under the program, the federal government buys up more than $800 million worth of farm products each year and turns them over to schools to serve their students. The U.S. Department of Agriculture, which administers the system, calls this a win-win situation: Schools get free ingredients while farmers are guaranteed a steady income. The trouble is, most of the commodities provided to schools are meat and dairy products, often laden with saturated fat. In 2001, the USDA spent a total of $350 million on surplus beef and cheese for schools—more than double the $161 million spent on all fruits and vegetables, most of which were canned or frozen. On top of its regular purchases, the USDA makes special purchases in direct response to industry lobbying. In November 2001, for example, the beef industry wrote to Agriculture Secretary Ann Veneman, complaining that a decline in travel after September 11, along with a lowered demand for beef in Japan, was suppressing sales of their product. The department responded two months later with a $30 million "bonus buy" of frozen beef roasts and ground beef for schools.

"Basically, it's a welfare program for suppliers of commodities," says Jennifer Raymond, a retired nutritionist in Northern California who has worked with schools to develop healthier menus. "It's a price support program for agricultural producers, and the schools are simply a way to get rid of the items that have been purchased."

All in all, schools obtain almost 20 percent of their food from the commodities program—and they depend on the handouts to meet tight budgets. "School districts are under intense budgetary pressure, and oftentimes nutrition is at the bottom of the priority list," says David Ludwig, director of the obesity program at Children's Hospital in Boston. School nutrition directors face increasing mandates from their higher-ups to break even, or even make a profit, and therefore have no choice but to accept surplus commodities. "They help shape our menus significantly, especially if you're going to run a program successfully financially," says Christy Koury, director of child nutrition for schools in Freeport, Texas, where menus run heavy on hamburgers, cheese-stuffed pizza sticks, and pepperoni calzones.

School nutrition officials like Koury consider the free food so vital to their budgets that they have sometimes overlooked good nutrition to side with the beef and dairy industries, forming a powerful alliance that has blocked efforts to serve healthier meals to students. The National School Lunch Program is up for reauthorization this year for the first time since 1998, but given the interests backing the current system, few expect Congress to approve any meaningful reforms. Kit's understood that commodity programs exist," says Graydon Forrer, former director of consumer affairs for the USDA, "and that commodity programs will continue to exist."

THE KINDERGARTNERS arrive first at the Chapman Elementary School cafeteria in Huntsville, Alabama, holding Popsicle sticks painted with their names and payment codes. They grab green plastic trays and pick out half-pint cartons of chocolate and plain milk. Then cafeteria workers pile the lunch entree directly onto the trays: tortilla chips heaped with ground beef and smothered with melted yellow cheese. The kids grab apple halves and cornbread, and a few take the side order of watery chili beans. "I like the meat," declares second-grader Matthew Miller. "I like the cheese and I like the apples," adds classmate Tanner Teets. Another boy tears open a packet of salty taco sauce and sucks it straight from the foil.

The lunches at Huntsville's public schools tend to run heavy on beef and cheese—items the federal government regularly delivers to their doorstep. Like all 99,000 schools and childcare centers that participate in the National School Lunch Program, Huntsville's schools depend on the agricultural commodities they receive throughout the year. Today's nachos are made from surplus ground beef. So were the spaghetti sauce and the taco salad on this month's menu. Surplus ham contributed to a barbecue lunch, and surplus cheese was used on sandwiches. A roast-beef lunch was fashioned from surplus meat, even though child-nutrition director Carol Wheelock says the kids don't particularly like roast beef.

Wheelock knows that a beef-filled menu isn't the healthiest thing children can eat. If she could afford to refuse the commodities, she says, she would buy leaner meats like turkey and chicken. But like others who oversee school lunches, she tries not to complain about the commodities program. "I treat it as a challenge," she says. "We have to put our thinking cap on and come up with ways to use the commodities that we're given."

In 2001, the USDA spent $350 million on surplus beef and cheese for schools—and officials say such high-fat meals are contributing to the growing health crisis among kids.

Wheelock's dilemma is repeated in districts across the country. School boards, coping with tight budgets, aren't willing to spend more for better nutrition. Huntsville, for example, left 50 teaching slots empty this year to trim its $187 million budget. "The school food service is held hostage, because they can't go into the open market and buy healthy foods and stay profitable," says Raymond, the retired nutritionist.

Schools rely on the commodities program for another reason: It fits neatly into the decades-old method they have traditionally used to prepare school meals. Known as "food-based menu planning," the system mandates specific servings of meat, dairy, vegetable, and grain on each child's plate—without bothering to determine the meal's total nutritional value. "It's been done that way for so long," says Suzanne Havala Hobbs, a former spokeswoman for the American Dietetic Association who teaches nutrition at the University of North Carolina. "There's just resistance to change."

The USDA insists that school lunches are getting healthier. "There have been tremendous moves to reduce the fat content in school meals," says department spokeswoman Jean Daniel. In recent years, the government has lowered the acceptable fat levels for ground beef and pork, introduced light cheeses and ground turkey, and eliminated tropical oils from its peanut butter.

For the most part, though, fat levels remain dangerously high. Based on USDA recommendations, an adolescent girl who eats a 730-calorie lunch should receive no more than 24 grams of fat, and no more than 8 grams of saturated fat. Yet one portion of USDA surplus chuck roast, plus a glass of whole milk, delivers 31 grams of fat, including 14 grams of saturated fat. Buttered rolls and a side dish of cheesy broccoli bump those figures even higher. And if a school wants to cut animal fat by eliminating whole milk, it can't: Federal law requires that schools continue offering it as long as 1 percent of the students purchase it.

As a result, school lunches routinely fail the government's own nutritional standards. By law, schools are supposed to restrict fat content in lunches to 30 percent of the calories served each week. But according to the USDA, 81 percent of schools exceed that limit. Worse, 85 percent fail the standard for saturated tat, a leading contributor to coronary disease. Half of all schools serve whole milk, which further drives up the saturated-fat content. On any given day, less than 45 percent of schools serve cooked vegetables other than potatoes—which are often prepared in the form of french fries—and less than 10 percent serve legumes, a healthy, low-fat form of protein.

School food directors say they have to serve fatty meals to satisfy the tastes of children raised on McDonald's and Domino's. "They'd love to have pizza and french fries every day," says Wheelock, the Huntsville official. "You can't eliminate french fries." Adding fat is sometimes the only way to get kids to eat green vegetables. "A little bit of cheese on broccoli they love," she says. "The benefit from eating the broccoli will far outweigh a little additional fat."

But all that cheese adds up. Public schools serve more than 4 billion meals every year—a number that would make many fast-food chains envious—and officials say all those lunches are contributing to the growing health crisis among kids. According to the Centers for Disease Control and Prevention, obesity rates have doubled in children and tripled in adolescents since 1980, spurring an epidemic of type II diabetes, once considered an adult-onset condition. Obesity has also been associated with heart disease, arthritis, and certain cancers, and researchers have found fatty streaks in the blood vessels of children as young as 10.

"USDA needs to relate the current crisis in kids' health to the meals that are being served, especially to poor kids, because that's the population that's most vulnerable," says Antonia Demas, director of the Food Studies Institute, a child-nutrition group based in upstate New York. Because low-income children often eat both breakfast and lunch at school, "they get at least two-thirds of their calories from school each day, and they're the population really showing an increase in the diet-related diseases."

USDA INSIDERS acknowledge privately that the commodities program works against kids' health. "This was never talked about publicly," says Forrer, the department's consumer affairs director under President Clinton. "It was talked about after work, over beer: If you were designing a system for health and nutrition, you wouldn't cordon off part of it and say, 'This will serve the commodities community.' But you've got to dance very lightly around the commodities people. They've got the power."

Agribusiness has wielded that power to make sure schools continue serving fatty foods. The National Cattlemen's Beef Association, the political arm of the red-meat industry, spends $400,000 a year on lobbying and has given nearly $3 million in federal campaign contributions since 1990, according to the nonpartisan Center for Responsive Politics. Its former lobbyist, Dale Moore, now serves in the Bush administration as chief of staff to Agriculture Secretary Veneman, while another former lobbyist, Elizabeth Johnson, serves as Veneman's senior adviser on nutrition issues. Though most of the association's financial support has gone to Republicans, its aims have been embraced by both parties. "I think it's clear USDA and cattlemen have a shared agenda," then-Agriculture Secretary Dan Glickman, a Democrat, told the organization at its 1999 convention. "We've got to sell, sell, sell."

Given the industry's clout, USDA officials are careful to include agribusiness representatives in almost every discussion about the school lunch program. In the mid-1990s, a group of health advocates met with the USDA to ask that schools be allowed to serve soy products like veg-

gie burgers. According to one participant, a department official asked them, "Have you spoken with the Cattlemen about this? Until the Cattlemen go for this, we aren't going to be able to move on it." Soy alternatives were eventually allowed, but only after the beef industry group was consulted.

Such access put beef and dairy lobbyists in a good position to help defeat the most significant effort to reform the program. Shortly after President Clinton took office, he appointed a consumer activist named Ellen Haas to oversee the Agriculture Department's nutrition programs. Haas was no government insider. She had headed the nonprofit Public Voice for Food and Health Policy, which frequently criticized the government for compromising the quality of school lunches. Clinton hoped that Haas would use her energy to reform the system from the inside.

Haas, an intense, dark-haired woman who talks quickly and always seems in a hurry, plunged into her charge immediately. She went on a nationwide tour to build support for reform among physicians, parents, and food-service workers, and she cultivated allies in Congress. Rather than attack the commodities program directly, however, she proposed a rule requiring schools to meet USDA limits on fat. To achieve that goal, schools would have to scrap their old, "food-based" method of planning menus and adopt a healthier way of preparing lunches. Known as "nutrient-based menu planning," the new system would require schools to calculate the nutritional content of meals and ensure that they meet federal standards.

The proposed reform would have come at some cost to the beef and dairy industries. The reductions in cheese would have cost farmers up to $200 million annually, and school beef offerings might have dropped by more than 125 million pounds. "Obviously, any trade association is going to worry about things like that," says Elizabeth Johnson, the former Cattlemen's lobbyist. The group quietly began lobbying against the reform; one beef lobbyist later told Havala Hobbs, the University of North Carolina dietitian, that fighting the proposal "was my primary focus for six months to a year."

Given the industry's clout, USDA includes agribusiness in almost every discussion about the school lunch program.

Beef producers were worried about more than the loss in revenues, though, fearing that a redesigned lunch program would change children's lifelong eating habits. "If they were taught, even subliminally, that beef wasn't a part of a healthy school meal, they would internalize that and eat less beef—or not eat beef as they grow up," one insider said, expressing industry's concerns.

THE PROPOSED REFORM also angered those responsible for planning school lunches. The American School Food Service Association, an $8-million-a-year organization whose 55,000 members oversee student meals, joined with the beef and dairy industries in opposing Haas' efforts. The group feared the proposed changes would require costly computers and training to analyze school menus without providing adequate funding. "The policy goal was absolutely right on target," says Marshall Matz, the association's lobbyist. "But it's a big, diverse country, and a system that will work in Los Angeles or New York, which have a lot of resources, will not necessarily work in rural South Dakota." Matz feared that some districts, frustrated by the new rules, would leave the National School Lunch Program altogether, leaving the poorest children without free or low-cost meals.

Haas and her staff dismissed the food-service association as nothing more than "the lunchroom ladies," but she underestimated her opponents. Nearly 200,000 workers serve school lunches to kids nationwide, and the group has an effective political machine that organizes letter-writing campaigns and dispatches members to lobby Washington. "It's a very potent and universal constituency," says Neal Flieger, former deputy administrator of USDA's Food and Nutrition Service. "Teachers, food-service workers, postal workers, and cops are the only constituencies that appear in every congressional district in America" The association also has close ties to the food industry. Its foundation is funded by companies like Heinz, Land O'Lakes, Tyson Foods, and Pizza Hut. Matz, its lobbyist, is a well-connected former congressional aide whose firm also lobbies for the National Meat Association, General Mills, Kraft Foods, McDonald's, and the National Frozen Pizza Institute.

Matz promoted alternative legislation allowing schools to use "any reasonable approach" to menu planning—a move that would effectively preserve the status quo, While school nutrition directors descended on Capitol Hill, Matz aggressively worked his own network to defeat the reform. "He set up endless meetings with staff to convince them that what Ellen was doing was too extreme," recalls Ed Barron, a senior Democratic congressional staffer. Haas soon found herself frozen out by legislators and abandoned by the Clinton administration. Says a key USDA staffer, "We were told by the White House, 'You have to live with this.'"

Although Congress did set fat limits for school lunches, it created no effective mechanism for reaching those standards—and no penalty for failing. "It was a baby step forward, but our problems are so drastic that far greater

changes are needed before we see a substantial improvement in kids' health," says dietitian Havala Hobbs. Even Matz, the food-service lobbyist, regrets the battle. "Good God, we spent two years arguing about process," he says. "Those years were a lost opportunity."

This year, Congress will take up the National School Lunch Program for the first time in five years. But industry representatives and health experts agree there will be no serious effort to prevent schools from serving children so many cheeseburgers, pizzas, and french fries. Instead, most of the debate is expected to center on who serves up those items. The food-service association estimates that 30 percent of all public high schools currently sell Burger King, Domino's Pizza, and other brand-name fast food in their cafeterias alongside federally subsidized meals, and many more dispense chips and sodas in vending machines down the hall. Nutrition experts want the USDA to regulate corporate vendors in schools, but such "competitive" foods appeal to cash-strapped districts, many of which are eager to accept money from fast-food companies to open franchises right on campus.

The debate over fast food is sure to grab headlines, but nutrition advocates warn that it will do nothing to improve the unhealthy meals currently served to the nation's children every weekday. "If Johnny can't read by first grade, parents are going to be up in arms," says Connie Holt, a dietitian who teaches at Widener University in Pennsylvania. "But if he gains five pounds in first grade and doesn't eat well, nobody's going to say anything. All of the health problems we're seeing in the adult world, we have an opportunity to make a difference—but only if we approach school lunch differently."

The Hidden Health Costs of Meal Deals

Much food for only a little more money—that's the "deal" that American eateries and food retailers are offering us. But overweight, obesity and chronic disease are the real price we pay for these food bargains.

Just before lunch, Katie Weigle went into a fast food restaurant in Washington, D.C., and ordered a cheeseburger. "For just $1.40 more you can get a meal package—cheeseburger, fries and a Coke," the server said. "Sounds too good to be true," Katie replied. The server responded, "As a matter of fact, for just 58 cents more, you can super size that meal… "

So Katie walked out the door with a bag containing a 4-ounce hamburger, a large order of French fried potatoes and a large Coke. It was a bargain. The trouble was her lunch now contained 1,380 calories, or about 700 more calories than a woman her size requires at lunch.

That's how "value marketing" works. Restaurants and food retailers offer you a lot more food for just a little more money. Since food, as opposed to labor, rent or utilities, is their smallest cost, they make money on such deals. Customers are happy, too. They pay a little less per unit and get an enormous portion of food.

Everything would be hunky dory, if they didn't eat all those extra calories. Seventy percent of respondents to a recent AICR survey, however, said they eat everything they are served in a restaurant all or most of the time. So a decade or two of "value marketing" may help explain why 64 percent of Americans are now overweight or obese.

Survey Counts the Health Cost

Of course, Katie didn't eat that 1,380-calorie lunch. She brought it back to AICR along with her sales slip. Her purchase was part of a study conducted by health organizations nationwide. They were attempting to quantify just how much damage "value marketing" does. Here are some of their results:

- At Cinnabon, when one Minibon (300 calories) was ordered, the clerk said, "it's only 48 cents more for a classic Cinnabon (670 calories)." So our researchers paid 24 percent more for 123 percent more calories.

- At 7-Eleven, researchers asked for a "Gulp" of Coke (150 calories) and left the store with a "Double Gulp" (600 calories) for only 37 cents more. That's a 42 percent increase in price for 400 percent more calories.
- At movie theaters, researchers asked for a medium popcorn without butter (900 calories) and were told you can get a large (1,160 calories) for only 60 cents more. That's 23 percent more money for 260 more calories.
- Researchers found a whopping big "deal" at McDonald's. There they paid 8 cents less to buy the large value meal (Quarter Pounder with cheese, large fries and large Coke at 1,380 calories) than to buy the Quarter Pounder, small fries and small Coke (890 calories). That is, they spent 8 cents less to purchase 490 calories more.

The list goes on, but the pattern is the same: customers are manipulated into paying a little bit more for many more calories than they can afford to eat.

How to Fight Back

Say "small," say "half" and share. When ordering, always insist on the smallest size. At times that is difficult. "Small" has grown so large in our eateries that it often has names like "tall" or "supreme." Just say, "Which is the smallest size? That's the one I want."

At table service restaurants, order the half size, if it's available. If not, cut the meal in two and tell the server to put half in a doggie bag. If you can set half aside before it is served, you'll be spared any temptation.

When all other strategies fail, order one meal and share it. Even if the restaurant makes you pay for the extra set up, you'll save money and leave feeling comfortably full. In an age when candy bars are 3.7 ounces instead of 2, bagels are 4.5 ounces instead 1.5 and sodas are 62 ounces instead of 8, the best way to ensure your health may be to share every food item you buy with a friend or loved one.

Moving Toward Healthful Sustainable Diets

Nutritionists have increasingly been focusing on the challenge of moving consumers toward healthful diets and simultaneously helping them to make the connection between healthy food and a healthy environment. Simply stated, to foster food sustainability, consumers will need to choose minimally processed and minimally packaged foods. In addition, when possible, they should buy locally produced foods to support regional agriculture and local economies, preserve farmland, and use less energy and other natural resources.

BARBARA STORPER, MS, RD

Nutritionists have increasingly been focusing on the challenge of moving consumers toward healthful diets and simultaneously helping them to understand that what's good for their health may well be good for the health of the planet. Promoting food sustainability and ecologic harmony as an essential function of the nutrition professional was first proposed more than 20 years ago by Dr Joan Gussow, Mary Swartz Rose Professor Emeritus of Nutrition Education at Teachers College, Columbia University, and Dr Kate Clancy, Director of The Agriculture Policy Project at the Henry A. Wallace Institute for Sustainable Agriculture. Today, their message falls on receptive ears, as nutritionists better understand the connection between agriculture, the environment, hunger, health, and, ultimately, food security.

Drs Gussow and Clancy first introduced the term "food sustainability" to the nutrition profession in an article published in 1986 by the *Journal of Nutrition Education* entitled, "Dietary Guidelines for Sustainability."[1] They explained how the US Dietary Guidelines, the government's model for promoting health, can also be used as the framework by which nutritionists can promote sustainable diets. The article still serves today as a seminal treatise, calling the profession to promote a diet that is healthy for the individual, the rest of the world, and the planet.

Dr Gussow is still on the forefront of this mission today, promoting the sustainability advantages of "whole foods"—foods that are minimally processed and packaged. Nutritionally, whole foods fit more easily into a healthful diet than their processed and packaged counterparts because they are naturally higher in fiber and lower in fat, sodium, sugar, and additives. Globally, whole foods also bypass the high energy costs of food processing. In general, more profit stays with the farmer, helping farmers to make a livable income, thus staving off the alarming decline of the small and family farm in this country. Last, but far from least, Gussow claims that whole foods taste better, give people more opportunity to prepare them the way they like, and allow people to feel more connected to the food's origin.

> *To foster sustainability, consumers should choose minimally processed and minimally packaged foods and, when possible, buy locally produced foods to support regional agriculture that preserves farmland and is less energy intensive*

What's even better, she proclaims in her newest book, *This Organic Life: Confessions of a Suburban Homesteader*[2] is for people to eat locally produced food, and whenever possible, grow their own. The important current issue, says Gussow, is learning how to produce food for everyone in a way that's sustainable, and we are not doing that. What we are doing, she continues, is overproducing food globally while destroying the environment and our capacity for future food production. Supermarkets "trick" the consumer by selling foods from around the world all year long so that consumers on the East Coast expect summer produce in the winter, such as strawberries in January. The economic and environmental costs associated with these practices, however, are invisible to most consumers.

For Gussow, localization of the food supply remains the optimal approach to foster sustainability. The need to relocalize our food supply is urgent now, according to Gussow, because of the increasing harm caused by agribusiness practices—their emphasis on monocultures (ie, growing single crops over large areas) and their continued dependence on pesticides. She claims that our present agricultural system downplays the health and environmental hazards of pesticides, which are being used today at a far greater rate than when Rachel Carson's[3] *Silent Spring* first exposed their alarming consequences.

SUSTAINABILITY AND MODERN FARMING PRACTICES

Gussow uses the example of a potato to explain why current farming practices are not sustainable. There are 5,000 known varieties of the potato plant. Peruvian Indians in the Andes knew and used 3,000 of them. Yet, today, only 6 are grown commercially in the United States. Why? According to Gussow, it is to meet the demands of a processing industry that requires uniformity. The fast-food industry, in particular, prefers a single variety, the Russet, for its shape. The Russet potato is long enough so that when made into French Fries, the fries can extend beyond the edges of the cardboard container, creating the visual appearance consumers expect. Yet, she claims that limiting a nation's reliance on a few varieties of a crop is precisely what devastated Ireland's economy in the 1840s, when blight struck the two varieties of potatoes on which the entire nation depended for its food supply.

She also argues that monoculture also depletes the soil, creating an increased dependence on fertilizers and pesticides, manufactured from nonrenewable fossil fuels. This overdependence on pesticides, in turn, increases the health problems for growers and consumers of pesticide-ridden produce here and abroad.

Returning to a more locally produced food supply will not only help the environment but also, according to Gussow, make the public more aware of the link between their food and the health and environmental consequences of modern farming methods. Buying locally not only supports small farms and helps to maintain local economies but also helps neighbors stay in business and ultimately promotes sustainable communities.

It is surprising, according to Gussow, that the United States ranks as one of the leading food importers in the world! She believes that emphasizing local agriculture here may also help poor people in other countries who are steadily being pushed off their own lands when large agribusiness firms establish production sites for luxury and out-of-season foods for US tables. Ironically, she notes, the fruits and vegetables we eat out of season are often produced in countries with poor sanitation and questionable hygienic practices. Why eat a fruit from a country where one would not drink the water? Eating locally may offer a safe and healthy alternative to the consequences of a global marketplace.

MOVING TOWARD SUSTAINABLE DIETS

Here are some ways nutritionists can help to promote sustainability:

- Recommend that a certain portion of the weekly grocery money be used exclusively for foods that are produced locally and sold in farmers markets or through farms that establish memberships with local residents.

- Learn about and promote seasonal foods that can be grown locally in the consumer's own region and teach people how to cook these foods—or how to cook at all!

- Have your own backyard garden and encourage public organizations, schools, hospitals, etc, to build community gardens and use the foods grown for feeding programs.

Here are some creative resources nutrition educators can use to promote food sustainability with school-age children:

- LIFE Program (Linking Food and the Environment) a project of Teacher's College, Columbia University promotes the "Food Triangle"—a take-off on the Food Pyramid. Using a triangle, the project staff divide foods into three groups— "plant foods," "animal foods," and "man-made foods"—to help children learn about how their food choices affect their environment and their health. They also use hands-on activities such as gardening, cooking, shopping, composting, and recycling.

- "Earth Friends" is a minidiscovery museum housed at Teacher's College where classes from New York City schools visit and learn about food from farm to table in a series of games, exhibits, and cooking activities. Contact David Russo, Project Coordinator, 212-678-3955.

- "Cookshop" is a classroom curriculum designed by the New York Community Food Resource Center to help students and teachers cook a variety of locally grown wholesome foods that will then be introduced in the school cafeteria. Evaluations show dramatic increases in consumption of these previously unfamiliar foods when students learn about them first in class. Contact Toni Liquori at 212-894-8074 or tliquori@cfrcnyc.org.

- "Close Encounters with Agriculture," a Cooperative Extension Service of the University of Maryland Program links elementary school children with class activities and field trips to agricultural areas to learn about animals, horticulture, and farming.

- "Field to Table," a Cornell University Extension Project helps students to identify and increase their consumption of locally grown fruits and vegetables based on the Northeast Regional Food Guide.

- "From Land to Landfill" is a program developed by nutritionists at Purdue University using a systems approach to integrate health and nutrition into core subject areas.

- "FOODPLAY" is this author's traveling nutrition theater show that tours schools nationally and uses juggling, theater, music, magic, and audience participation to encourage children to make food choices that are good for their health and the health of the planet. Contact Barbara Storper at 800-FOODPLAY or http://www.foodplay.com.

Barbara Storper, MS, RD, is the Director of FOODPLAY Productions, an Emmy Award-winning nutrition media organization that produces national touring school theater shows, video kits, media campaigns, and resources to improve children's health. Ms Storper holds degrees in both journalism and nutrition and has received the first Outstanding Young Nutrition Educator in the Country Award and Media Partnership from the Society for Nutrition Education.

Corresponding author: Barbara Storper, MS, RD, FOODPLAY Productions, 221 Pine St, Florence, MA 01062 (e-mail: barbara@foodplay.com).

REFERENCES

1. Gussow JD, Clancy K. Dietary guidelines for sustainability. *J Nutr Edu.* 1986; 18:1–15.
2. Gussow JD. *This Organic Life: Confessions of a Suburban Homesteader.* White River Junction, Vt: Chelsea Green Publishing Company; 2001.
3. Carson R. *The Silent Spring.* Boston: Houghton Mifflin; 1994..

From *Nutrition Today*, March/April 2003, pp.57-59. © 2003 by Lippincott Williams and Wilkins. Reprinted by permission.

UNIT 2
Nutrients

Unit Selections

Key Points to Consider

- Check out several labels from foods containing fats and oils that you eat frequently. Can you tell how much trans-fat each contains?

- Determine the percentage of your average daily calories that is contributed by total fat and saturated fat. What do your calculations tell you about potential health risks?

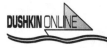 **Links: www.dushkin.com/online/**
These sites are annotated in the World Wide Web pages.

Dole 5 A Day: Nutrition, Fruits & Vegetables
http://www.dole5aday.com

Food and Nutrition Information Center
http://www.nal.usda.gov/fnic/

Nutrient Data Laboratory
http://www.nal.usda.gov/fnic/foodcomp/

NutritionalSupplements.com
http://www.nutritionalsupplements.com

U.S. National Library of Medicine
http://www.nlm.nih.gov

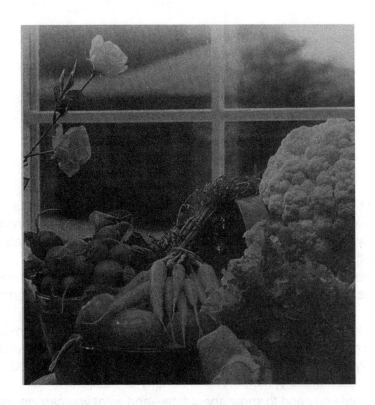

This unit focuses on the most recent advances that have been reported on nutrients and their role in health and disease. With the onset and development of new technologies in the area of nutrition, the plethora of information on the role of certain nutrients, and the speed with which information is printed and disseminated, even the professional has a hard time keeping up with the data. The media report any sensational, even erroneous data, which confuses the public and creates many misunderstandings. Preliminary reports have to undergo rigorous testing in animal models and clinical trials before they are accepted and implemented by scientific community.

Additionally, how individuals will respond to dietary changes will depend on their genetic make-up along with other environmental factors. Thus, the National Academy of Sciences has a difficult task in trying to establish exact amounts of nutrients that will cover the requirements but not create toxicity in the long run for the majority of the population.

The articles in this unit have been selected to present current knowledge about nutrients resulting from state-of-the-art research, as well as controversies brewing at the present time. Articles related to nutrient function and their effects on chronic disease such as cardiovascular disease, obesity, and osteoporosis are included.

An area of perennial controversy concerns fats and the types of fat. Americans have focused on single ingredients, attempting to exclude them from food. This has resulted in the proliferation of low-fat products that are not necessarily low in calories. Two articles present current scientific finding about types of fats. Trans-fatty acids that arise from food processing, which convert liquid oils to solid margarines, are as harmful to heart health as saturated fat. Current scientific findings on trans-fat are discussed and practical advice is offered in adding fish oil to our diet. Trans-fatty labeling becomes mandatory by the FDA beginning in 2006.

Consumers have misinterpreted the advice to choose a diet low in fat to mean eliminating all fat from their diet. As research evolves, a diet moderate in total fat is being advised, especially incorporating omega-3 fatty acids found in fish such as tuna and salmon. Omega-3 fatty acids promote heart health and eye health and have beneficial effects on the immune system.

Osteoporosis is a debilitating disease whose incidence is steadily increasing worldwide as the population is getting older and pollution gets worse in major cities around the world. Carol Coughlin updates us on the role of nutrients in osteoporosis prevention. Not only do we need optimal levels of calcium in our diet but also a lot of other nutrients (such as vitamins D, K, and B12) and minerals such as phosphorus, magnesium, boron, and fluoride to maintain adequate bone mass throughout life. Dr. Hollick emphasizes the role of vitamin D not only for prevention of osteoporosis, but also blood pressure, cancer and diabetes.

The importance of vitamins is of great interest to consumers since vitamins have been touted to cure and/or prevent disease. As the baby boomers are aging, diseases that affect their eyes such as macular degeneration and cataracts are on the rise. Several antioxidant vitamins and phytochemicals may have a protective effect in these age-related eye disorders. Finally, new evidence is presented on folic acid and its relation to cancer and cardiovascular disease.

Face the **FATS**

"I still don't know what kind of oil to buy," says Michelle LaFountain of Glens Falls, New York. "Some people recommend monos like olive or canola oil. Others say polys like soybean or corn oil are better. With advice about fats changing so frequently, I'm very confused."

Ms. LaFountain isn't the only one to get that glazed look whenever she's in the oil aisle. Who wouldn't be confused by the steady stream of mixed messages?

Diet books range from virtually fat-free (Ornish) to high-fat (Atkins). The media publish conflicting reports on saturated, monounsaturated, polyunsaturated, trans, omega-3, and other fats. Ads plug fish oil, DHA, and flaxseed oil supplements to boost immunity, memory, and healthy circulation.

Here's what you need to know about fats—and what you can ignore. For one thing, Ms. LaFountain, the oil aisle isn't your biggest problem.

By Bonnie Liebman

Heart disease, stroke, breast cancer, prostate cancer, colon cancer, obesity. Is there *any* illness that hasn't been blamed on too much fat?

It's now clear that fat is not a monolithic enemy. The only exception: When it comes to obesity, *all* fats are suspect because all are equally high in calories. And when it comes to cancer, *no* fats appear to be at fault, though some fatty *foods*, like red meats, may be.

"Red meat is associated with colon and prostate cancer, but probably not because of its fat," says epidemiologist Edward Giovannucci of the Harvard School of Public Health.

That leaves heart disease and stroke, where it's not *how much* fat that matters. It's how much of *which* fat.

"It's become clearer which kinds of fat are desirable and which aren't," says William Connor of the Oregon Health & Science University in Portland.

Here's the latest on fats and cardiovascular health. The story may be more complicated than it was ten years ago, but it's also more encouraging.

BAD FATS: SATURATED & *TRANS*

"There's a new fat to fear," warned "The New Bad Fat," an article in the March 2002 issue of *Marie Claire* magazine. "Read on to find out when cheesecake can actually be your healthiest choice!"

A slice of cheesecake (which can have a day's worth of saturated fat) is better than frosted yellow cake, the article claimed, because it has less *trans* fat. That's the wrong message, say researchers.

"It would be a great tragedy to worry so much about *trans* that people forget about saturated fat," says Connor. Most *trans* fat is created when manufacturers turn liquid oils into more solid fats like shortening and margarine. Saturated fat occurs naturally in nearly all fatty foods, but mostly in meats, dairy products, and tropical oils like palm kernel and coconut.

The evidence against both fats is so strong that it's foolish to play one against another.[1] "It's not a question of choosing which artery-clogging fat to avoid," says Meir Stampfer of the Harvard School of Public Health. "People should cut down on both saturated and *trans* fat."

It's easy to see where the confusion started. "Technically, *trans* is worse than saturated fat, because saturated fat raises both LDL ['bad'] cholesterol and HDL ['good'] cholesterol, while *trans* only raises LDL," explains Alice Lichtenstein of the U.S. Department of Agriculture Jean Mayer Human Nutrition Research Center on Aging at Tufts University in Boston.

"But if you have to target one fat for modification, there's a greater potential for change by cutting saturated fat."

That's because only two percent of our calories come from *trans* fat, while sat fat contributes 13 percent. Avoiding sat fat is a tough job because it's in so many popular foods, from pizza and hamburgers to steak, tacos, ice cream, lasagna, and cheese.

What's more, notes Stampfer, *trans* fat is largely dispensable. "We can't get rid of all saturated fat, but most *trans* doesn't have to exist."

"Arguing about whether one fat is worse isn't a practical discussion," says Lichtenstein. "The message needs to be loud, it needs to be clear, and it needs to be unequivocal: Limit your intake of both saturated and *trans* fats."

BETTER FATS: MONOS & POLYS

In the early 1970s, corn oil was king. Researchers had just confirmed that higher *polyunsaturated* fats (Like corn, soy, and sunflower oil) could lower total cholesterol. (We call them polys, but all fats are really a mixture of polys, monos, and sat fat. See "Oil in the Family.")

In contrast, highly *saturated* fats (like butter and beef) raised cholesterol, while highly *monounsaturated* fats (like canola and olive oil) were neutral. (Monos are neutral when researchers compare them to carbohydrates. But if you substitute monos for saturated fats, monos will lower your cholesterol.)

"After corn oil lowered total cholesterol in the Los Angeles Veterans Administration Diet Study, some researchers recommended that everyone take a tablespoon or two a day," says Connor.

But by the 1990s, the pendulum had swung towards monos. In part, the enthusiasm was fueled by lavish conferences for researchers and the media sponsored by the olive oil industry. The science looked promising, too.

"People got very excited about monos because, unlike polys, they didn't cause oxidation of LDL in test-tube studies," explains Lichtenstein. Oxidized LDL is more likely to clog arteries.

"Some researchers also argued that unlike polys, monos don't lower HDL, the so-called good cholesterol," she adds. But those arguments have lost some credence. For one thing, it became clear that polys lowered HDL more than monos only when ingested in huge quantities.

"If you feed people reasonable amounts of polys," Lichtenstein explains, "their HDL is not much different than when you feed them monos. And even though

---

THE BOTTOM LINE

1. **Cut your intake of saturated plus *trans* fat** to less than 10 percent of calories, or about 20 grams a day *of both combined*. Of course, without *trans* numbers on most food labels, that's not easy.
2. **At home, use canola oil as your main oil, with a variety of others for taste.**
3. **Shoot for between 1/2 and 1 gram (500 mg and 1,000 mg) a day of omega-3 fats (DHA plus EPA) from one of the following:**

- Consume seafood two to five times a week.
- If you take fish oil pills, there's no reason to take more than 1 gram a day of EPA and DHA combined. More than 3 grams may increase the risk of bleeding or hemorrhagic stroke.
- If you're a vegetarian, you can get DHA (but not EPA) from supplements made from algae. Or you can get alpha-linolenic acid from walnuts, soybeans, or flaxseed, canola, or soy oils, though the body doesn't convert much of it into EPA and DHA.

---

monos didn't cause oxidation of LDL in test tubes, all bets are off in the body."

Meanwhile, researchers rediscovered that polys have more power to lower cholesterol than monos. And studies found cleaner arteries in monkeys that were fed polys than in those that were fed monos.[2]

"You can't make a decision based on a few animal studies," says Lichtenstein. "But it does look like monos aren't as magical as some people have claimed."

At the same time, some earlier fears about polys have dissipated.

"We've put to rest the theoretical concerns that too much polyunsaturated fat may cause cancer," says Stampfer. "We were wary of recommending too much because a diet high in polys is new for humans. But the concerns haven't really panned out."

Does that mean that people should spill out all their olive or canola oil and rush to the store for soy oil? Not quite. First of all, some dishes taste better with certain oils.

"At home, we use olive oil for salad dressing because the taste matters," says Stampfer. "We bake with canola. And we also use sesame, peanut, and safflower, depending on the dish."

Taste aside, if you're like most people, the oil you buy is just a small fraction of the fat you eat. What's in your bottled salad dressing and mayonnaise? What's in the spaghetti sauce, muffins, cookies, or other foods in your pantry?

And don't forget restaurants. What oil does your favorite Chinese takeout use? What greases the griddle

FISHING FOR OMEGAS

The simplest advice is to eat at least two servings of seafood a week to lower your risk of sudden cardiac death. But if you want to make sure you're getting enough omega-3 fats, shoot for between 1/2 and 1 gram (500 mg and 1,000 mg) a day.

In general, fattier fish are richer sources, but some—like farmed catfish--are relatively low in omega-3s. Farmed fish are higher in fat than their wild cousins, but most of the extra fat is unsaturated, so it's not a real threat to your heart.

For most species, our serving size is six ounces of cooked fish because that's a typical portion served at seafood restaurants. To get that much when you're cooking at home, start with about eight ounces raw.

Fish (6-oz. cooked, unless noted)	Total Fat (grams)	Omega-3 Fats* (grams)
Salmon, Atlantic, farmed	21#	3.7
Salmon, Atlantic, wild	14	3.1
Sardines, in sardine oil (3 oz.)	13	2.8
Salmon, coho, farmed	14#	2.2
Trout, rainbow, farmed	12#	2.0
Salmon, coho, wild	7	1.8
Herring, kippered (3 oz.)	11	1.8
Trout, rainbow, wild	10#	1.7
Swordfish	9	1.4
Sardines, in tomato sauce (3 oz.)	10	1.4
Herring, pickled (3 oz.)	15	1.2
Oysters (3 oz.)	4	1.1
Mackerel, canned (3 oz.)	5	1.0
Pollock	2	0.9
Flounder or sole	3	0.9
Whiting	3	0.9
Rockfish	3	0.8
Halibut	5	0.8
Sardines, in vegetable oil (3 oz.)	10	0.8
Tuna, white, canned (3 oz.)[1]	3	0.7
Scallops	1	0.6
Perch, ocean	4	0.6
Cod, Pacific	1	0.5
Tuna, fresh	2	0.5
Crab, blue (3 oz.)	2	0.4
Haddock	2	0.4
Catfish, wild	5	0.4
Fish sticks (6)	21#	0.4
Cod, Atlantic	1	0.3
Crab, Dungeness (3 oz.)	1	0.3
Shrimp (3 oz.)	1	0.3
Catfish, farmed	14#	0.3
Tuna, light, canned (3 oz.)[1]	1	0.2
Clams (3 oz.)	2	0.2
Crayfish, farmed (3 oz.)	1	0.1
Lobster (3 oz.)	1	0.1

* Includes EPA and DHA only. [1] canned in water.

Includes 3 to 5 grams of saturated fat (most other fish are lower).

Sources: USDA and (for sardines in sardine oil) *Amer. J. Clin. Nutr.* 66: 1029S, 1997.

IF YOU DON'T EAT FISH

Experts recommend that people eat seafood at least twice a week to get the omega-3 fats that can protect against sudden cardiac death. But what if you eat little or no seafood? While the U.S. government has no advice, it's reasonable to shoot for a combined 1/2 to 1 gram (500 mg to 1,000 mg) of EPA plus DHA a day. Here's what will—and won't—get you there.

Fish oil pills. "The best alternative to seafood is to get both DHA and EPA from fish oil pills or from fish oil that's been added to other foods," says omega-3 expert Bruce Holub of the University of Guelph in Canada. But be careful.

Fish oil pills can cause side effects like belching and nausea. And getting more than a combined three grams (3,000 mg) of EPA and DHA a day from foods *and* supplements may raise the risk of hemorrhagic stroke, says the Food and Drug Administration. Most fish oil pills contain only 0.18 grams (180 mg) of EPA and 0.12 grams (120 mg) of DHA, so it would take more than ten capsules a day to exceed three grams.

Designer eggs. Some companies now feed fish oil, algae, or flaxseed to their hens to raise the omega-3s in their eggs. But most brands of "omega-3 eggs" have very little DHA. Eggland's Best eggs, for example, have only 0.05 grams (50 mg) apiece, while Gold Circle Farms eggs have just 0.15 grams (150 mg) each. Neither has EPA, which may be essential to protect against sudden cardiac death. And the eggs still contain cholesterol and saturated fat, both of which can raise your risk of heart disease.

DHA supplements. "You can take DHA supplements that are made from algae, though they're rather costly," says Holub. Each capsule has 0.1 grams (100 mg), and a bottle of 30 capsules can cost $10 or more. Another problem: DHA supplements made from algae have no EPA.

"There is internal conversion between EPA and DHA, so eating one may mean you get both," explains William Connor of the Oregon Health & Science University. "But we don't have evidence from studies on people that taking DHA is as good as taking both."

Alpha-linolenic acid. Alpha-linolenic acid (found in canola, soy, and flaxseed oils) is an omega-3 fat that our bodies can convert into EPA and DHA. But it's difficult to measure how much gets converted. In some studies, people convert almost none. In others, they convert more (though not necessarily as much as they'd get from eating fish).

Still, says Holub, if you eat no fish or fish oil, getting alpha-linolenic acid by using an oil like canola is better than nothing. "Your cardiovascular protection may go up, though not nearly as much as with fish oils or fish."

—David Schardt

---

when you order chicken or shrimp fajitas? What went into that spicy peanut sauce, vinaigrette, or clam sauce?

Odds are it's soy. More than 80 percent of the oil used in the U.S. is soy, though half gets partially hydrogenated in order to make margarine or shortening. A growing body of evidence suggests that it makes sense to balance all that soy by using mostly canola at home.

"I buy about three bottles of canola for every bottle of soy," says Lichtenstein. Why?

The soy oil adds cholesterol-lowering polys. But canola is the mainstay because it's very low in saturated fat and has a good dose of polys (more than olive oil). What's more, canola's omega-3 fats may help protect your heart, though the evidence is stronger for the omega-3 fats that come from fish.

BEST FATS: OMEGA-3S

Unlike polyunsaturated *vegetable* oils, polyunsaturated *fish* oils have always had a stellar reputation. And last April, the news got even better.

"Three new studies showed that the omega-3 fats in fish oil protected people from sudden death," says Stampfer, who co-authored two of them. (In "sudden cardiac death," which causes half of all heart disease deaths, the heartbeat goes awry and then stops. Most victims have clogged coronary arteries.)

- Healthy men who had more omega-3 fats in their blood were less likely to die of sudden death over the next 17 years than healthy men with lower blood levels of omega-3s.[3]

- Healthy women who reported eating fish at least five times a week had a 45 percent lower risk of dying of heart disease over the next 16 years than healthy women who ate fish less than once a month.[4]

- Men who had survived a heart attack and were randomly assigned to take fish oil supplements (1 gram, or 1,000 mg, a day) were 53 percent less likely to die of sudden death than survivors who were given a placebo.[5]

Oil in the Family

All fats are a mixture of saturated, monounsaturated, and polyunsaturated fatty acids (though we usually call them by the name of the fatty acid they have the most of). Look for the least saturated (gray), and a good mixture of everything else. Polys (white and lighter gray) lower cholesterol, while monos (darker gray) only lower cholesterol if you eat them in place of saturated fats. Alpha-linolenic acid (lighter gray) is an omega-3 polyunsaturated fat that may protect the heart. Canola, soy, and flaxseed oil are good sources. Many researchers recommend a mix of alpha-linolenic acid and linoleic acid (white). (Linoleic is a polyunsaturated omega-6 fat.) *If you don't want the details, just stick with canola for cooking. It's among the lowest in saturated fat and it has a good mix of alpha-linolenic and linoleic acids.*

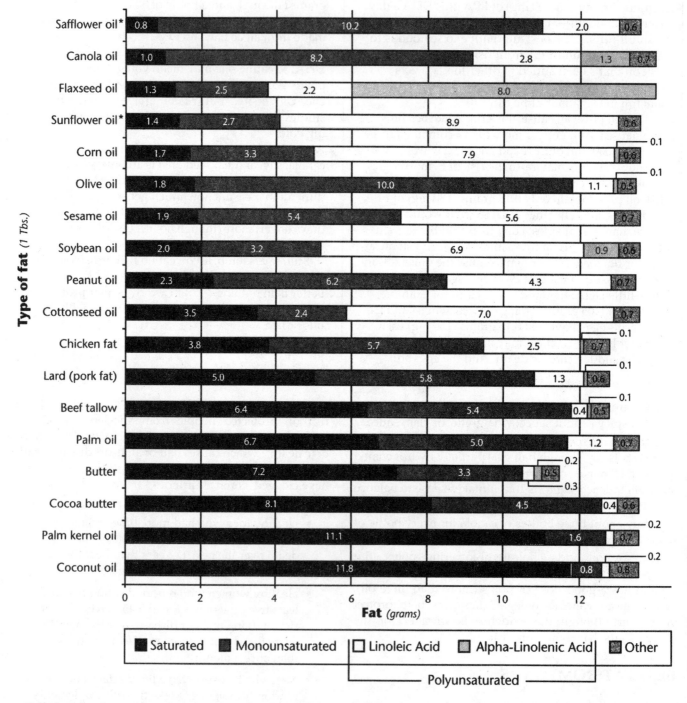

*Safflower and sunflower oils can be high in polys or monos. Most safflower oil sold in bottles is the high-oleic (high-mono) variety shown here, but some brands that are sold in health food stores are the high-linoleic (high-poly) variety. The sunflower oil sold in bottles is usually high in polys (as shown here), but most chips and other packaged foods that are made with sunflower oil use the high-mono variety.

Sources: USDA Nutrient Database for Standard Reference (Release 14), the National Sunflower Association, and the Flax Council of Canada.

The last study is the most powerful because it's a clinical trial, says Stampfer. "Add that to earlier studies on humans, animals, and cell cultures and we can now say that fish oils prevent arrythmias and sudden death."

Exactly how fish oils work isn't certain. The leading theory: When the heart is under severe stress, a key fish fat stabilizes heart cells, which allows the heart to maintain its regular beat. (That fat is likely to be eicosapentaenoic acid, or EPA. DHA, or docosahexaenoic acid, is the other key fish fat.)

"When there's trouble, EPA is released from the cell membrane and it suppresses the extra heartbeats," says Oregon's William Connor.

At higher doses, omega-3 fats may also protect the heart by lowering triglyceride levels and preventing blood clots, though that wouldn't explain why they stave off sudden deaths.

In any case, the take-home message is to eat more seafood. The American Heart Association now recommends at least two servings per week, preferably of fatty fish (see "Fishing for Omegas.")

If you don't eat seafood, there are other options (see "If You Don't Eat Fish"). Among them: alpha-linolenic acid, an omega-3 that's largely found in flaxseed, canola, and soy oils as well as flaxseeds, walnuts, and soybeans.

In some animal studies, alpha-linolenic acid prevents irregular heartbeats as well as fish oils do.[6] And most studies find that people who consume more alpha-linolenic acid have a lower risk of heart disease than people who consume less.[7-9]

"The evidence for alpha-linolenic acid isn't as compelling as it is for fish oils," says Bruce Holub of the University of Guelph in Canada. "But alpha-linolenic may have a beneficial effect, so why take chances by using an oil that has none?"

Both soy and canola are good sources of alpha-linolenic acid, but soy has more *linoleic* acid (an omega-6 polyunsaturated fat). And too much linoleic may keep omega-3 fats from doing their job. "That makes canola a better source of omega-3s than soy or other oils," says Connor.

So far, though, too much linoleic acid doesn't seem to be a problem. "In our study of women, fish oils were protective regardless of how much linoleic acid the women consumed," says Stampfer.

Just keep in mind that researchers are still waiting for final answers.

"I use canola and soy to get a balance of monos and polys and a balance of alpha-linolenic and linoleic acid, rather than put all my eggs in one basket," says Tufts University's Alice Lichtenstein. "That's my best guess until things are sorted out."

Notes

1. *Circulation 102*: 2284, 2000.
2. *Arterioscler. Thromb. Vasc. Biol. 15*: 2101, 1995.
3. *New Eng. J. Med. 346*: 1102, 1113, 2002.
4. *J. Amer. Med. Assoc. 287*: 1815, 2002.
5. *Circulation 105*: 1897, 2002.
6. *Circulation 99*: 2452, 1999.
7. *Am. J. Clin. Nutr. 74*: 612, 2001.
8. *Am. J. Clin. Nutr. 69*: 890, 1999.
9. *Brit. Med. J. 313*: 84, 1996.

From *Nutrition Action Healthletter*, July/August 2002, pp. 3-6. © 2002 by Center for Science in the Public Interest. Reprinted by permission.

Revealing Trans Fats

Scientific evidence shows that consumption of saturated fat, trans fat, and dietary cholesterol raises low-density lipoprotein (LDL), or "bad" cholesterol, levels that increase the risk of coronary heart disease (CHD). According to the National Heart, Lung, and Blood Institute of the National Institutes of Health, more than 12.5 million Americans have CHD, and more than 500,000 die each year. That makes CHD one of the leading causes of death in the United States.

The Food and Drug Administration has required that saturated fat and dietary cholesterol be listed on food labels since 1993. With trans fat added to the Nutrition Facts panel, you know how much of all three—saturated fat, *trans* fat, and cholesterol—are in the foods you choose. Identifying saturated fat, *trans* fat, and cholesterol on the food label gives you information you need to make food choices that help reduce the risk of CHD. This revised label is of particular interest to people concerned about high blood cholesterol and heart disease.

However, everyone should be aware of the risk posed by consuming too much saturated fat, *trans* fat, and cholesterol. But what is *trans* fat, and how can you limit the amount of this fat in your diet?

What is *Trans* Fat?

Basically, *trans* fat is made when manufacturers add hydrogen to vegetable oil—a process called hydrogenation. Hydrogenation increases the shelf life and flavor stability of foods containing these fats.

Trans fat can be found in vegetable shortenings, some margarines, crackers, cookies, snack foods, and other foods made with or fried in partially hydrogenated oils. Unlike other fats, the majority of *trans* fat is formed when food manufacturers turn liquid oils into solid fats like shortening and hard margarine. A small amount of *trans* fat is found naturally, primarily in dairy products, some meat, and other animal-based foods.

Trans fat, like saturated fat and dietary cholesterol, raises the LDL cholesterol that increases your risk for CHD. Americans consume on average 4 to 5 times as much saturated fat as *trans* fat in their diets.

Although saturated fat is the main dietary culprit that raises LDL, *trans* fat and dietary cholesterol also contribute significantly.

Are All Fats the Same?

Simply put: No. Fat is a major source of energy for the body and aids in the absorption of vitamins A, D, E, and K, and caro-tenoids. Both animal- and plant-derived food products contain fat, and when eaten in moderation, fat is important for proper growth, development, and maintenance of good health. As a food ingredient, fat provides taste, consistency, and stability and helps you feel full. In addition, parents should be aware that fats are an especially important source of calories and nutrients for infants and toddlers (up to 2 years of age), who have the highest energy needs per unit of body weight of any age group.

While unsaturated fats (monounsaturated and polyunsaturated) are beneficial when consumed in moderation, saturated and *trans* fats are not. Saturated fat and *trans* fat raise LDL cholesterol levels in the blood. Dietary cholesterol also raises LDL cholesterol and may contribute to heart disease even without raising LDL. Therefore, it is advisable to choose foods low in saturated fat, *trans* fat, and cholesterol as part of a healthful diet.

What Can You Do About Saturated Fat, *Trans* Fat, and Cholesterol?

When comparing foods, look at the Nutrition Facts panel, and choose the food with the lower amounts of saturated fat, *trans* fat, and cholesterol. Health experts recommend that you keep your intake of saturated fat, *trans* fat, and cholesterol as low as possible while consuming a nutritionally adequate diet. However, these experts recognize that eliminating these three components entirely from your diet is not practical because they are unavoidable in ordinary diets.

Where Can You Find *Trans* Fat on the Food Label?

Although some food products already have *trans* fat on the label, food manufacturers have until January 2006 to list it on all their products.

You will find *trans* fat listed on the Nutrition Facts panel directly under the line for saturated fat.

How Do Your Choices Stack Up?

With the addition of *trans* fat to the Nutrition Facts panel, you can review your food choices and see how they stack up.

Don't assume similar products are the same. Be sure to check the Nutrition Facts panel because even similar foods can vary in calories, ingredients, nutrients, and the size and number of servings in a package.

How Can You Use the Label to Make Heart-Healthy Food Choices?

The Nutrition Facts panel can help you choose foods lower in saturated fat, *trans* fat, and cholesterol. Compare similar foods and choose the food with the lower combined saturated and *trans* fats and the lower amount of cholesterol.

Although the updated Nutrition Facts panel will list the amount of *trans* fat in a product, it will not show a Percent Daily Value (%DV). While scientific reports have confirmed the relationship between *trans* fat and an increased risk of CHD, none has provided a reference value for *trans* fat or any other information that the FDA believes is sufficient to establish a Daily Reference Value or a %DV.

Saturated fat and cholesterol, however, do have a %DV. To choose foods low in saturated fat and cholesterol, use the general rule of thumb that 5 percent of the Daily Value or less is low and 20 percent or more is high.

You can also use the %DV to make dietary trade-offs with other foods throughout the day. You don't have to give up a favorite food to eat a healthy diet. When a food you like is high in saturated fat or cholesterol, balance it with foods that are low in saturated fat and cholesterol at other times of the day.

The FDA's *trans* fat labeling regulations don't take effect until Jan. 1, 2006, but some manufacturers are already listing the amount of *trans* fat in their products.

Do Dietary Supplements Contain *Trans* Fat?

Would it surprise you to know that some dietary supplements contain *trans* fat from partially hydrogenated vegetable oil as well as saturated fat or cholesterol? It's true. As a result of the FDA's new label requirement, if a dietary supplement contains a reportable amount of *trans* or saturated fat, which is 0.5 gram or more, dietary supplement manufacturers must list the amounts on the Supplement Facts panel. Some dietary supplements that may contain saturated fat, *trans* fat, and cholesterol include energy and nutrition bars.

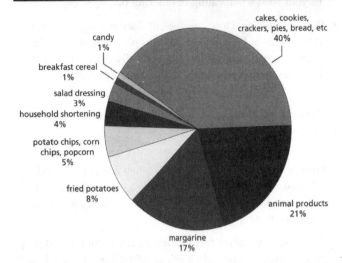

Major Food Sources of Trans Fat for American Adults
(Average Daily Trans Fat Intake is 5.8 Grams or 2.6 Percent of Calories)

cakes, cookies, crackers, pies, bread, etc 40%
candy 1%
breakfast cereal 1%
salad dressing 3%
household shortening 4%
potato chips, corn chips, popcorn 5%
fried potatoes 8%
margarine 17%
animal products 21%

Data based on FDA's economic analysis for the final *trans* fatty acid labeling rule, "*Trans* Fatty Acids in Nutrition Labeling, Nutrient Content Claims, and Health Claims" (July 11, 2003)

Fat Tips

Here are some practical tips you can use every day to keep your consumption of saturated fat, *trans* fat, and cholesterol low while consuming a nutritionally adequate diet.

- **Check the Nutrition Facts panel** to compare foods because the serving sizes are generally consistent in similar types of foods. Choose foods lower in saturated fat, *trans* fat, and cholesterol. For saturated fat and cholesterol, keep in mind that 5 percent of the daily value (%DV) or less is low and 20 percent or more is high. (There is no %DV for *trans* fat.)

- **Choose alternative fats.** Replace saturated and *trans* fats in your diet with monounsaturated and polyunsaturated fats. These fats do not raise LDL cholesterol levels and have health benefits when eaten in moderation. Sources of monounsaturated fats include olive and canola oils. Sources of polyunsaturated fats include soybean oil, corn oil, sunflower oil and foods like nuts and fish.

- **Choose vegetable oils** (except coconut and palm kernel oils) and soft margarines (liquid, tub, or spray) more often because the amounts of saturated fat, *trans* fat, and cholesterol are lower than the amounts in solid shortenings, hard margarines, and animal fats, including butter.

- **Consider fish.** Most fish are lower in saturated fat than meat. Some fish, such as mackerel, sardines, and salmon, contain omega-3 fatty acids that are being studied to determine if they offer protection against heart disease.

• **Ask before you order when eating out**. A good tip to remember is to ask which fats are being used in the preparation of your food when eating or ordering out.

• **Watch calories**. Don't be fooled! Fats are high in calories. All sources of fat contain 9 calories per gram, making fat the most concentrated source of calories. By comparison, carbohydrates and protein have only 4 calories per gram.

To keep your intake of saturated fat, *trans* fat, and cholesterol low:

• Look at the Nutrition Facts panel when comparing products. Choose foods low in the combined amount of saturated fat and *trans* fat and low in cholesterol as part of a nutritionally adequate diet.

• Substitute alternative fats that are higher in mono- and poly-unsaturated fats like olive oil, canola oil, soybean oil, corn oil, and sunflower oil.

Highlights of the Final Rule on *Trans* Fat

• Manufacturers of conventional foods and some dietary supplements will be required to list *trans* fat on a separate line, immediately under saturated fat on the nutrition label.

• Food manufacturers have until Jan. 1, 2006, to list *trans* fat on the nutrition label. The phase-in period minimizes the need for multiple labeling changes, allows small businesses to use current label inventories, and provides economic savings.

• FDA's regulatory chemical definition for *trans* fatty acids is all unsaturated fatty acids that contain one or more isolated (i.e., nonconjugated) double bonds in a *trans* configuration. Under the agency's definition, conjugated linoleic acid would be excluded from the definition of *trans* fat.

• Dietary supplement manufacturers must also list *trans* fat on the Supplement Facts panel when their products contain reportable amounts (0.5 gram or more) of *trans* fat. Examples of dietary supplements with *trans* fat are energy and nutrition bars.

From *FDA Consumer*, September/October 2003. U.S. Food and Drug Administration.

Building Healthy
BONES

Every **dietician** knows that calcium intake is essential to **bone** health, but there are other **nutrients** that affect bone health and aid in osteoporosis **prevention**

BY CAROL M. COUGHLIN, RD

As dietetics professionals, we are aware that osteoporosis is a skeletal disorder characterized by compromised bone strength which leads to an increased risk of fracture. It is estimated that in the United States 10 million people have osteoporosis and 18 million more have low bone mass, placing them at risk for developing this disease. Every dietitian knows that calcium intake is essential to bone health, but there are also other nutrients that affect bone health and aid in osteoporosis prevention.

Although calcium takes center stage in the fight against osteoporosis, bone health clearly requires adequate overall nutrition. This was illustrated in a recent one-year, double-blind, placebo-controlled study of Gambian children, whose mean dietary calcium intake was 300 milligrams daily. The researchers examined the effects of supplementing 1,000 milligrams of calcium carbonate daily for a year. This supplementation resulted in a substantial increase in bone mineral density, but there was no effect on overall skeletal growth (ie, the calcium increased the amount of minerals present within a given bone vol-

ume but did not promote bone growth). This suggests that simply supplementing a diet with calcium is not sufficient if the overall diet is nutritionally inadequate in several nutrients.

Dietetics professionals are aware that vitamin D is needed for calcium absorption. Recently, it has been recognized that vitamin D insufficiency, not just extreme deficiency, contributes to osteoporosis. A study at Massachusetts General Hospital of 290 patients in a general medical ward revealed that 57% were vitamin D-deficient and 22% were severely deficient. It takes about 20 to 30 minutes of sunshine daily on the hands and face to manufacture sufficient levels of vitamin D, but many people get nowhere near that amount of time in the sun. They go from their houses to their cars to their offices and back to their homes. People live, work, and even exercise indoors.

Foods that are natural sources of vitamin D such as eel, liver, and egg yolk, probably aren't most people's favorite foods. One study found vitamin D deficiency in 43% of the patients whose intake of dietary vitamin D reached the recom-

mended daily allowance (RDA). Therefore, it's best to suggest that clients consume fortified foods such as fluid milk or fortified soy and rice milk. Some breakfast cereals are also fortified with vitamin D.

An inadequate amount of vitamin D results in a subtle decrease in the ionized calcium concentration in blood, which triggers parathyroid hormone (PTH) secretion. PTH is a potent bone resorbing agent so even a subtle increase results in measurable bone loss.

Scientific research indicates that moderate protein intake (1 to 1 1/2 grams per kilogram body weight) is associated with normal calcium metabolism and, presumably, bone health. Using this definition, only 40% to 50% of adults in the United States consume diets moderate in protein.

When people don't get enough protein, intestinal calcium absorption is reduced, resulting in a rise in serum PTH and calcitriol that persists at least for two weeks. The long-term implications are not yet proven, but epidemiologic data suggest increased rates of bone loss in people on very low protein diets. In addition, protein undernutrition has been shown to affect sex hormone status in animal studies.

The flip side is that people with high protein intake, particularly from animal sources, have hypercalciuria and negative calcium balance. The epidemiologic evidence shows that diets high in animal protein are associated with an increased rate of fractures. This relationship does not hold true for vegetable protein. The greater concentration of sulfur-containing amino acids in meat creates a high acid load. This acid is buffered by the release of basic ions from the bone, leading to a loss of skeletal mass. Research from the United Kingdom indicates that women with the most acidic diets have the poorest bone density (both in axial and peripheral skeleton) and the highest levels of bone resorption. Acid-base homeostasis disruption in adults has been suggested as a reason behind the progressive decline in bone mass with aging. Bone loss may, therefore, be attributable to the life-long mobilization of skeletal salts to balance the acid generated from foods that produce acid.

This acid/base relationship may also explain why recent population-based studies have suggested a positive association between high intakes of fruits and vegetables in the diet and bone mass and metabolism in premenopausal, perimenopausal, and postmenopausal elderly women and elderly men. The mechanism may be the beneficial effect of the alkaline environment induced by a diet rich in fruits and vegetables and the potassium content of these foods. Supplementation with potassium results in a reduction of urinary calcium, and inadequate potassium stimulates bone resorption. Supplementation of potassium bicarbonate in postmenopausal women improves calcium and phosphorus balance, reduces bone resorption, and increases the rate of bone formation. Researchers are currently calculating the protein-to-potassium ratio in the diet and are finding that it predicts net acid excretion via the urine and that, in turn, net acid excretion predicts calcium excretion.

The positive link between fruit and vegetable consumption and bone health was also shown in the Dietary Approaches to Stopping Hypertension (DASH) trial. Increasing fruit and vegetable intake from 3 3/5 to 9 1/2 daily servings resulted in a reduction of urinary calcium excretion from 157 milligrams to 110 milligrams per day. It is generally accepted that salt increases urinary calcium. The reabsorption of calcium and sodium in the proximal tubule of the kidney and loop of Henle are linked. A

reduction in renal sodium reabsorption leads to a reduction in calcium absorption and increased calcium urinary losses.

Interestingly, there are minimal data available on the effect of high sodium intake on bone health over the long term; most studies show little or no association. This may simply be due to the lack of long-term follow-up, but further research in this area clearly is warranted.

In addition to vitamin D, other vitamins play a role in bone health and osteoporosis prevention. Low levels of vitamin K are associated with low bone density and bone fractures. The principal noncollagenous protein of bone, osteocalcin (also known as gamma-carboxglutamic acid or bone Gla), and matrix Gla protein are dependent on vitamin K for synthesis. The Nurses Health Study found that women who had the lowest intake of vitamin K had the highest rate of hip fractures.

Clearly, we all know that if **people** would obtain and maintain an intake of **calcium** meeting the dietary **reference** guidelines, our nation's bone **health** would be greatly **enhanced**.

Dietitians can remind clients that, previously, those on anticoagulant medications such as Coumadin were advised to restrict their intake of vitamin K; now most dietitians recommend keeping intake at a steady level. An adequate supply of this nutrient can be obtained from green leafy vegetables, which are also good sources of readily absorbable calcium. The friendly bacteria that live in the digestive system also produce vitamin K. Clients who are on repeated courses of antibiotics may get less vitamin K since antibiotics kill the good bacteria that live in the intestines in addition to killing bacteria responsible for illness and infections. Therefore, dietitians

may suggest to clients taking antibiotics that they also take a probiotic supplement of good bacteria, such as acidophilus, or eat food with active cultures, such as yogurt.

Alternately, they could take a prebiotic supplement. Prebiotics are substances that feed the good bacteria that live in the intestines, just as fertilizers promote plant growth. The most common prebiotic is fructooligosaccharide (FOS), which is a naturally-occurring substance consisting of short chains of fructose. The common suggestion is a dosage of 1 to 4 grams daily. Supplementing with FOS not only helps feed the good bacteria that make vitamin K but also helps the absorption of more calcium by lowering the pH of the intestine.

Appropriate gut flora also aid in bone health because of their effect on dietary phytoestrogens. These compounds produce estrogen-like effects in the body only after being converted to the active form by bacteria in the gut. Women who eat higher-carbohydrate diets tend to have healthier gut flora and are, therefore, able to convert more phytoestrogens into the active form. Phytoestrogens, particularly isoflavones, may aid in prevention of bone loss because they act in a fashion similar to estrogen.

Another fat-soluble vitamin with a link to bone health is vitamin A, but its relationship is an opposing one. A recent study showed that women with higher blood levels of vitamin A had a higher risk for hip fracture. For every milligram increase in daily intake of preformed vitamin A, the risk for hip fracture increased by 68%. Aging reduces the ability to rid the body of extra vitamin A, a problem compounded by the fact that vitamin A is one nutrient that is absorbed more readily with aging. Clients should be advised to get adequate amounts of vitamin A, but supplements of preformed vitamin A are generally discouraged.

At a presentation at the World Congress on Osteoporosis 2000 in Chicago, Ill., J. Beynon from the United Kingdom presented the results of his investigation on the role vitamin B_{12} may play in osteoporosis. A total of 263 osteoporotic patients were studied (244 women; 19 men). Of the 44 subjects with low blood vitamin B_{12} levels, 22 had suffered a fracture. (Beynon J, Murray C, Vasishta S. B_{12} deficiency—its role in the development of osteoporosis. *Osteoporos Int.* 2000;11 (suppl 2):S153.) There is some evidence in the literature to suggest that vitamin B_{12} suppresses osteoblastic activity. Further research in this area is required; since it is now recommended that all people over age 50 consume B_{12}-fortified foods or take a supplement, this simply reinforces the importance of vitamin B_{12}.

In addition to calcium, phosphorus, and magnesium, boron may enhance bone health. There is evidence that adequate intake of boron can decrease the amount of calcium lost in urine. Boron deficiency results in osteoporosis-like symptoms such as thin, brittle bones. Because fruits and vegetables are the best source of boron, this adds to the recommendation of eating a DASH-type diet for bone health.

Fluoride may also have a role in keeping bones strong. Just as fluoride is incorporated into teeth, it is also added to the structure of bones. One study of women found that a fluoride supplement of 40 to 60 milligrams a day increased the bone density of the spine. However, a three-year study found that fluoride supplements did nothing to reduce the rate of bone fracture in women. There simply is not enough evidence yet to recommend supplementing with fluoride as a strategy to prevent or treat osteoporosis or bone fractures.

Clearly, we all know that if people would obtain and maintain an intake of calcium meeting the dietary reference guidelines, our nation's bone health would be greatly enhanced. In addition, if everyone's intake of the recommended nutrients—each playing a small role in slowing bone loss—was optimized, the overall rate of fractures could be reduced and health-care costs could be lowered substantially.

With surveys indicating that the public is fatigued with conflicting messages about nutrition, dietitians can use this information to offer a consistent nutrition message. We can tell people that an overall diet adequate in protein, vitamins, and minerals and rich in fruits and vegetables is the one eating pattern that seems to be optimal not only for bone health but also for reducing the risk of hypertension, diabetes, heart disease, and cancer.

Carol M. Coughlin, RD, is a freelance writer in Maine and the executive director of the Massachusetts Dietetic Association.

SOAKING UP THE D'S

Q: *Why do so many people get too little vitamin D?*
A: Very few foods contain it, and most people get too little sun to make it. Your skin can make vitamin D when it's exposed to sunlight. When the highest energy ultra-violet light, called UVB, penetrates the skin, it converts a precursor into Vitamin D, which becomes 25-hydroxyvitamin D in the liver, and is then activated to 1,25-dihydroxyvitamin D in the kidneys.

But if you live north of Los Angeles on the West Coast or Atlanta in the East, you don't get enough UVB from the sun in the winter to make adequate vitamin D (see "The Winter Sun," p. 5).

And even in the summer, many people are so concerned about getting too much sun that they always use sun protection, which blocks the UV light that makes vitamin D in your skin. The message used to be "don't burn" and "get some safe sun," which I totally agree with. But now the recommendation is to get no direct sun exposure. That has put many more people at high risk of vitamin D deficiency.

Q: *What harm does vitamin D deficiency do?*
A: It increases the risk of bone fracture. Vitamin D increases the efficiency of your intestine to absorb calcium and phosphorus from food, so you can mineralize your skeleton. It also increases the activity of bone cells that make and lay down bone matrix.

Q: *The matrix is like the frame of a building?*
A: Yes. If you have an adequate amount of calcium and phosphorus, it gets incorporated into the bone matrix and you have good, healthy bone. Young children who are deficient in calcium and vitamin D are unable to properly mineralize the rubbery matrix. Gravity pushes on the skeleton and causes the typical bowing of the legs that you see in a child with rickets.

By the time you're an adult, your long bones have stopped growing and you have enough calcium in your bones to prevent skeletal deformities. Instead, if an adult is deficient in vitamin D and not getting enough calcium, calcium is drawn out from the bones, which causes osteoporosis.

Q: *The bones break down?*
A: Yes. Bone cells called osteoclasts dissolve the matrix and release the calcium out of the bones and into the bloodstream. So a vitamin D deficiency will precipitate and exacerbate osteoporosis because it's increasing the number of holes in your bones.

In addition, bone cells called osteoblasts continue to produce new matrix, just like they do in children. However, when you are deficient in vitamin D, the matrix cannot be properly mineralized. The result is osteomalacia, the bone disease that's caused by vitamin D deficiency.

Q: *How does osteomalacia differ from osteoporosis?*
A: Osteoporosis isn't painful unless you have an acute fracture. Holes in your bones don't hurt.

In contrast, osteomalacia can cause muscle weakness as well as bone ache and bone pain. Until you have it, you can't really appreciate this gnawing sensation. Many patients are diagnosed with some kind of arthritis or collagen-vascular disease or fibromyalgia. In my clinic, I find that patients with aching bones are often suffering from vitamin D deficiency.

Q: *Why does the body take calcium from the bones?*
A: We evolved from the ocean, which is a high-calcium bath. Early in evolution, calcium became critically important for most metabolic functions—for example, to keep your heart beating and your muscles contracting. So the body makes sure that your blood calcium is in the normal range, even if it means removing calcium from your bones.

Q: *Do people who get more vitamin D have stronger bones?*
A: Yes. For example, postmenopausal women in Boston who were given 700 International Units of vitamin D a day for two years lost less bone than women who got 100 IU a day in addition to the 100 IU from their usual diets. All the women also received 500 milligrams of calcium a day.

Q: *Does vitamin D reduce fracture rates?*
A: Absolutely. For example, in 1992, French researchers showed that by giving nursing home residents 800 IU of vitamin D and 800 mg of calcium a day, they could markedly reduce the risk of fractures. Multiple studies done in the U.S. show the same in men and women.

Q: *Why give both vitamin D and calcium?*
A: You need the vitamin D to increase the efficiency of calcium absorption. If you're deficient in vitamin D, you only absorb about 10 to 15 percent of the calcium you

consume. So if you just take calcium it may not do you any good.

Every day you lose about 100 to 200 milligrams of calcium in your urine and about 100 to 200 mg from the gastrointestinal tract. So if you had 1,000 mg of calcium in your diet and you absorb 15 percent, that's 150 mg. But if you've lost 100 mg in urine and 100 mg from the gastrointestinal tract, you have a 50-milligram deficit.

Where does that come from? It's not like the federal government, which can just forget about the deficit. Your body takes those 50 milligrams out of your skeleton to make sure your blood calcium remains normal.

Q: Are women at greater risk of osteomalacia?
A: No. But women start out with lower bone density so they begin to fracture earlier in life due to both osteoporosis and vitamin D deficiency.

BEYOND BONES

Q: *Could vitamin D deficiency cause other problems?*
A: It may rise the risk of Type 1 diabetes, multiple sclerosis, congestive heart failure, and some cancers.

We also have preliminary evidence that vitamin D may lower blood pressure. When we exposed vitamin-D-deficient people with mild hypertension to just enough UVB light to raise their blood levels of vitamin D to normal, their blood pressures became normal. We were able to maintain them at a normal blood pressure for nine months by continuing that therapy. But the results need to be confirmed.

Q: *How might vitamin D affect blood pressure?*
A: If your kidneys produce more of a hormone called renin, you have a higher risk of hypertension. And the active form of vitamin D—1,25-dihydroxyvitamin D—decreases renin production.

Q: *What's the evidence on vitamin D and diabetes?*
A: It's intriguing. The NOD mouse, which is used to study diabetes, gets Type 1 diabetes when it's about 200 days old. If you treat the mice with activated vitamin D throughout their lives, it reduces their chances of getting diabetes by 80 percent. And a study in Finland—where vitamin D deficiency is common—followed 10,000 children for 30 years. Those who took at least 2,000 IU of vitamin D a day during the first year of life had an 80 percent lower risk of diabetes than those who took no vitamin D.

Q: *How is vitamin D linked to multiple sclerosis?*
A: In MS, the body's antibodies attack the myelin sheath that covers nerves. To study the disease, researchers inject myelin into mice. The mice develop antibodies to it and the antibodies start destroying myelin on the animals' nerves. That doesn't happen if the animals get activated vitamin D first.

Q: *Any evidence in people?*
A: So far, it's just circumstantial. For example, we know

GETTING YOUR D's

Most of the vitamin D in food is put there by the manufacturers. The FDA allows only a few kinds of food to contain added D, but not all brands do. All milks and most cold cereals are fortified, but only a few orange juices, yogurts, margarines, and hot cereals are. The vitamin D in fish occurs naturally. Food labels list their vitamin D content as a "%DV." The DV, or Daily Value, is 400 International Units (IU). So a food with 15% of the DV for vitamin D contains 60 IU.

Food	VitaminD *(IU)*
Halibut *(3 oz. cooked)*	680
Catfish *(3 oz. cooked)*	570
Pink salmon, canned *(1/4 cup)*	400
Quaker Nutrition for Women Instant Oatmeal *(1 packet)*	140
Tuna, canned *(1/4 cup)*	130
Milk *(1 cup)*	100
Minute Maid Calcium + Vit D Orange Juice *(8 oz.)*	100
Tropicana Calcium + Vit D Orange Juice *(8 oz.)*	100
Viactiv Soft Calcium Chews *(1 chew)*	100
Yoplait Light Yogurt *(6 oz.)*	80
Dannon Light'n Fit Yogurt *(6 oz.)*	60
Fleishmann's Original Margarine *(1 Tbs.)*	60
Parkay Calcium Plus *(1 Tbs.)*	60
Breakfast cereal, fortified *(3/4-1 cup)*	40

Sources: U.S. Department of Agriculture and manufacturers.

that the further you live from the equator, the higher the risk of multiple sclerosis.

Q: *What's the link between vitamin D and cancer?*
A: We know that almost every tissue in your body—brain, breast, bone, colon, intestine, heart, kidneys, and prostate—has a receptor for the active form of vitamin D. The question is: why?

It turns out that the active form of vitamin D is one of the most potent hormones to inhibit cell proliferation. So if you have a cancer cell that's proliferating out of control, activated vitamin D could inhibit its growth. That's what happens when activated vitamin D is added to breast, colon, lung, or prostate cancer cells.

Q: *In test tubes?*
A: Yes. And researchers are getting excited about using vitamin D-like compounds called analogs to treat cancer. The analogs are designed to suppress proliferation more—and raise calcium levels less—than activated vitamin D. The problem is that the cells can become resistant.

Q: *Are there any human studies?*
A: Researchers are investigating a vitamin D analog on liver cancer—hepatoma. The preliminary data look spectacular. Liver cancer isn't a big problem in the U.S. But it's a major problem in Asia, because many Asians have hepatitis C, a viral infection that markedly increases their risk of developing hepatoma later in life.

Q: *What about other cancers?*
A: The results haven't been as good. Early studies showed that leukemia patients who were given activated vitamin D went into remission, but then they all died. Researchers think that some of the cells became resistant and more aggressive in their growth. But a recent study found that giving a vitamin D analog with chemotherapy may be effective in treating prostate cancer, so that's another possibility.

> In most of the U.S., you can't make vitamin D from sunlight for four months of the year.

SUN SHY

Q: *So sunscreens can be a problem?*
A: Yes. If you use a sunscreen rated SPF 8 properly, it reduces your ability to make vitamin D by more than 90 percent. The same happens if you use an SPF 15 improperly—if you use too little or don't reapply it every two hours. And that's a shame, because there are clear benefits to sensible exposure to sunlight, and essentially no evidence that it will increase your risk of skin cancer.

Q: *What's sensible?*
A: If the sun's UVB rays are reaching you, we're talking about no more than maybe five to ten minutes of sun exposure on the arms and legs or face and arms two to three times a week. I recommend going out sometime between the hours of 11 a.m. and 2 p.m., because that's when your skin makes the most vitamin D. You could make vitamin D at 10 a.m., but then you'd have to be out for a longer period of time. In Boston, you wouldn't make any vitamin D at 8 a.m., even if it's a sunny summer day.

Q: *Because the sun's UVB rays aren't reaching you?*
A: Yes. Just like in the wintertime, the UV rays come in at an angle. That means that the rays—or photons—have to pass through more ozone in the atmosphere, and UVB rays are efficiently absorbed by ozone. Even if the sun is directly above you at noontime at the equator, only one tenth of one percent of the UVB photons, which are responsible for making vitamin D, actually penetrate to the earth's surface. So if the sun comes in at an angle, essentially none of those photons reach the Earth.

Q: *You'd need less time in Florida than Boston?*
A: Yes. Five to ten minutes is for a light-skinned Caucasian in Boston in June between 11 a.m. and 2 p.m. In Florida, it may be only two to three minutes.

Q: *And Floridians can make vitamin D year-round?*
A: Yes, even as far north as Los Angeles or Atlanta. But you may need to stay out a little longer because the sun isn't as strong. North of that latitude—above 35 degrees—you can't make any vitamin D in your skin in the winter, even at noon. In fact, Canadians can't make vitamin D in their skin for four to seven months of the year. They're at high risk of vitamin D deficiency.

Q: *Why not get vitamin D from foods?*
A: It's not easy. Many experts now agree that, on average, you need 1,000 IU a day if you're not exposed to sunlight. Only a few foods contain vitamin D (see "Getting Your D's"). And a typical multivitamin-mineral supplement has only 400 IU.

Q: *Why did the National Academy of Sciences recommend only 400 IU for people over 50 and 600 IU for people over 70?*
A: I was on the committee that issued the recommendations. Many committee members believed that the levels were inadequate, but we were obligated to base our recommendations on published studies. We had evidence that much higher levels were needed, but it hadn't yet been published.

For example, in the study we just published, we gave healthy young and middle-aged adults 1,000 units of vitamin D a day at the end of the winter and the beginning of the spring. That raised and maintained their blood levels of 25-hydroxyvitamin D right where you want them—between 30 and 40 nanograms per milliliter. In the absence of sun, that's what you need to maintain a healthy vitamin D status all year round.

Q: *What level is deficient?*
A: A 25-hydroxyvitamin D below 20 nanograms per milliliter. From 20 to 30 is borderline adequate. A healthy level is between 30 and 50.

Q: *Do older people absorb less vitamin D?*
A: Aging has no impact on how much vitamin D you absorb from food or pills. How much you make from the sun is a different story. If you're 70, your skin can make only a quarter of the vitamin D that a 20-year-old can make when exposed to the same amount of sun. But a 70-year-old can make enough.

Studies have shown that if elders are out in the sunlight for 15 to 20 minutes a couple times a week, they'll maintain their vitamin D levels. In Britain, researchers showed that if you put a UVB light source in the ceiling in a nursing home, you can maintain adequate vitamin D levels in residents.

TOXIC LEVELS

Q: *Why is milk fortified with only 100 IU of vitamin D per cup?*
A: Because of the risk of toxicity. That's been the limit since the 1930's, even though it takes huge amounts to

cause toxicity. We got a call from a doctor in Florida whose patient bought a powdered vitamin D supplement from a company in Canada. The patient started taking two teaspoons a day, which was supposed to have 2,000 IU.

But the company forgot to dilute the powder, so the patient was actually ingesting up to a million units a day. And he ended up with vitamin D toxicity. But most experts agree that even if you take 5,000 to 10,000 IU a day, you won't get vitamin D toxicity.

Q: *Why did the National Academy say that people shouldn't exceed 2,000 IU a day?*
A: Our committee recommended an upper safe limit of 2,000 IU because we had to rely only on published studies. Other studies suggest that at least 5,000 IU and maybe 10,000 IU a day is safe. It's virtually impossible to get that much from diet and supplements. And there's never been a reported case of vitamin D toxicity because of too much sun. Nature has cleverly programmed into the system that any excess from the sun is destroyed.

Q: *What happens if you consume too much vitamin D from food or pills?*
A: You absorb too much calcium, so you can get high blood calcium, kidney stones, kidney calcification, kidney failure, soft-tissue calcification, and calcification of your blood vessels that can ultimately lead to death. But you're talking about huge amounts. Remember the Florida patient who was taking a million units a day? Once he stopped taking the vitamin D, his levels fell gradually over three years and now he's perfectly fine.

Q: *So you have to take high levels for a long time?*
A: Exactly. Typically, I'll give my patients who are deficient in vitamin D 50,000 IU once a week for eight weeks to fill up their vitamin D tank because it's on empty. That works extremely well. Then I put them on 50,000 units once or twice a month. And I've never seen any toxicity.

TESTING

Q: *Should people get their vitamin D levels checked?*
A: Yes, just like you get your cholesterol checked at least once a year. The best time is around November, because if you're deficient then, you'll be severely deficient at the end of winter. And make sure that your doctor orders a test for 25-hydroxyvitamin D, not 1,25-dihydroxyvitamin D, which is the active form. That can be misleading.

Q: *How?*
A: Your 1,25-dihydroxyvitamin D levels are a thousand-fold less than your 25-hydroxyvitamin D levels. As you become deficient, the body tries to compensate by increasing the kidneys' production of 1,25-dihydroxyvitamin D. So those levels are normal or even elevated. In 50 percent of all assays done worldwide, doctors order a 1,25-dihydroxyvitamin D assay. I don't have a clue what they do with that information.

Q: *They may misinterpret it?*
A: Yes. It comes back normal or high, so they think the patient has more than enough vitamin D, when it's really a sign that the patient is becoming deficient.

Q: *Do you recommend taking a supplement?*
A: Yes. If you get enough sun in the summer and fall, it will carry you through the winter, because you store vitamin D in your body fat. But most people don't get enough.

To give you an example, my mother recently went into a nursing home. While she lived at home, I made sure she wasn't deficient by prescribing 50,000 IU of vitamin D twice a month. I urged her primary care doctor to make sure she didn't become deficient. He finally tested her blood level and she was severely deficient. He's now treating her, as I would, with 50,000 IU of vitamin D once a week for eight weeks followed by 50,000 IU twice a month.

Michael F. Holick is director of the Vitamin D, Skin and Bone Research Laboratory and Professor of Medicine, Dermatology, Physiology, and Biophysics at Boston University Medical Center. His book, *The UV Advantage,* will be published by iBooks and distributed by Simon & Schuster in May. He spoke to *Nutrition Action's* Bonnie Liebman by phone.

Feast For Your Eyes

Nutrients That May Help Save Your Sight

Research is uncovering yet another reason to eat with health in mind—our eyes. Going beyond the vitamin A in carrots that help us to see well in the dark, other nutrients may protect vision, particularly for aging eyes, including vitamins C and E, beta-carotene, two related carotenoids (lutein and zeaxanthin), zinc, and even certain types of fats.

Age-Related Eye Diseases

Age brings about changes that can lead to two common sight-robbing disorders, cataracts and age-related macular degeneration (AMD).

A cataract is a cloudy area in a part of the eye lens or the entire eye lens that keeps light from passing through the lens. As a cataract develops, it can cause blurred vision, sensitivity to light, increased nearsightedness, and distorted images, eventually causing partial or full loss of eyesight. Cataracts are also associated with diabetes, other systemic diseases, alcoholism, premature birth or birth defects, heredity, smoking, eye injuries, exposure to ultraviolet (UV) rays, and certain medications.

Macular degeneration involves damage to the macula; an area of the retina in the back of the eye responsible for the sharp central vision needed to read, drive, and perform other daily activities. Although the causes of macular degeneration are not known, risk factors include family history, smoking, high blood pressure, high blood cholesterol, and exposure to sunlight.

Visionary Research

Research is shedding rays of hope for individuals suffering from age-related eye disease, and for those at

---

Focus on Food

Although nutrients from supplements may help slow the progression of AMD—mainly for people with intermediate and advanced stages of AMD—data on the benefits of supplementation of these nutrients is still preliminary. A strong body of evidence, however, points to foods that can be consumed to reduce the risk of both AMD and cataracts.

In a study that looked at the intakes of carotenoids and antioxidants from food, people who ate the most antioxidant-rich dark, leafy greens, particularly those rich in lutein and zeaxanthin, had about a 40 percent lower risk of macular degeneration than those who ate the least amount of these vegetables.

The project examined food records and cataract development in women between 50 and 70 years old. The results confirm that antioxidant nutrients, particularly vitamin C, at daily intakes of about three times the Daily Value for vitamin C (60 mg/day), reduced the odds for the development of cataracts by nearly half. With higher intakes, easily attained by five to nine daily servings of fruits and vegetables, the odds were reduced even more.

---

risk of eye disease. Emerging evidence suggests that risk of certain eye changes associated with aging may be reduced by dietary components.

Antioxidant Vitamins and Zinc

The Age-Related Eye Disease Study (AREDS), launched by the National

---

Institutes of Health's National Eye Institute, is an ongoing study aimed at evaluating various combinations of high-dose antioxidant vitamins (beta-carotene and vitamins C and E) and zinc supplements on eye health. One published analysis of a 6-year period in the double-blind study examined these effects on nearly 3,600 people between the ages of 55 and 80. Subjects included men and women with varying macular status ranging from no evidence of AMD in either eye to relatively severe disease in one eye.

Study results related to AMD were impressive, although somewhat limiting. Only individuals with the intermediate and advanced stages of AMD appeared to benefit. Nevertheless, the benefit was such that the study's authors urged high risk individuals with no contraindications such as smoking, to consider taking daily supplements similar to those used in the study: 500 mg vitamin C, 400 International Units vitamin E, 15 mg beta carotene, 80 mg zinc, and 2 mg copper (copper needs are increased with high doses of zinc). The effectiveness and safety of routine use of this regimen by individuals with early AMD or persons at risk for developing AMD remain unclear. It is also important to note that this is a single study and further research is needed.

The high-dose formulations used in the AREDs study had no significant effect on the development or progression of age-related cataracts. Nevertheless, other studies have found that antioxidants have favorable effects, especially vitamin C in larger amounts and for a longer duration (>10 years).

Lutein and Zeaxanthin

The yellow-colored carotenoids, lutein and zeaxanthin, are found in a variety of vegetables, including leafy greens, broccoli, zucchini, corn, peas, and brussels sprouts to name a few. Highly concentrated deposits of lutein and zeaxanthin are also present in the macula. Here they are referred to as macular pigment.

Research has shown that the macular pigment density, or the amount of lutein and zeaxanthin in the macula, appears to be associated with AMD. Dr. Richard Bone, a professor of biophysics at Florida International University, has been studying macular pigments for more than 20 years. In a postmortem study of the eyes of people who had AMD and those who did not, Bone found that those with the highest concentrations of lutein and zeaxanthin had an 82 percent lower incidence of AMD.

Bone and colleagues also studied how lutein and zeaxanthin in the diet affect macular pigment density. "These results suggest an association between dietary intake of lutein and zeaxanthin and macular pigment density," said Bone. "But we don't know yet how much lutein and zeaxanthin are needed to raise the macular pigment density to a protective level." Currently Bone is conducting a dose-response study to determine the appropriate doses.

Dietary Fats

Several studies have hinted at an association between the amount and type of dietary fats consumed and the risk for AMD. Findings from the ongoing Beaver Dam Eye Study suggest that higher intakes of saturated fats and cholesterol may confer an increased risk for AMD.

The high level of polyunsaturated fatty acids in the retina supports the possibility that certain fats may have a protective effect against the development of AMD. Although some results have linked higher intakes of omega-3 fatty acids and fish with a decreased risk for advanced AMD, the majority of population studies have failed to establish a clear connection.

More recently, a case-control population study led by Dr. Johanna Seddon, an eye expert at Harvard University, found that diets high in vegetable (mono- and polyunsaturated) fats were associated with a higher risk for advanced AMD. Although polyunsaturated fats are considered protective against cardiovascular disease, the study's authors suggest that consumption of high levels of unsaturated fats may increase the susceptibility of the macula to oxidative damage. However, an optimal balance of high levels of omega-3 fatty acids (found in fatty fish such as salmon and mackerel) and lower levels of linoleic acid (an omega-6 fatty acid found in various vegetable fats) in the diet appeared to offer a protective effect.

Seeing is Believing

Although some of the results of studies related to the maintenance of eye health through diet are compelling for specific populations, it is too early in the study of nutrition and eye disease to draw general conclusions, advises Julie Mares-Perlman, PhD, associate professor in the Department of Ophthalmology and Visual Sciences at the University of Wisconsin-Madison.

"There are holes in the evidence that need further study," contends Mares-Perlman. As with any research, one or two studies showing a tendency are not enough. "What we do know is that a large body of evidence supports the fact that diet is important in maintaining eye health. How specific nutrients from food or supplements affect the types and stages of eye disease is yet to be defined," she said.

The Vitamin That Does Almost Everything

Folate—also called folacin or, when used in supplements or fortified foods, folic acid—is one of the B vitamins. It is not as well known as vitamin C, but it deserves to be just as famous. Abundant in green vegetables, beans, some fruits, and wheat germ, folate is essential to the healthy division of cells and thus to fertility and healthy offspring. It is also an important factor in heart health, and may play a role in the prevention of colon, cervical, and possibly even breast cancer.

Folate = healthy mothers and babies

One folate success story started with the discovery that low blood levels of this vitamin in pregnant women can lead to neural tube birth defects, such an spina bifida and anencephaly (failure of the spine and brain to form normally), which can be disabling or fatal for the infant. These defects occur in the first days or weeks of pregnancy, *before* a woman can know she is pregnant. So women should start building folate stores at least several weeks before becoming pregnant. Adequate folate levels may also reduce the risk of early miscarriages. *Another benefit*: Pregnant women who take folic acid supplements are less likely to develop high blood pressure during pregnancy.

In 1992 the U.S. Public Health Service urged all women of childbearing age to consume at least 400 micrograms of folate daily; and in 1998 the government began to require food makers to fortify refined grain products to help meet this goal. Since then the number of neural tube defects in the U.S. has fallen by almost 25%, and about 4,000 children have been spared. And the picture will certainly continue to improve. This is a worldwide effort, not just an American one.

To be sure they're getting enough folate, all women of childbearing age should take a multivitamin containing 400 micrograms of folic acid or eat a highly fortified cereal (a few supply 400 micrograms), as well as foods rich in folate. The folic acid from supplements and fortified foods is better absorbed than the folate that occurs naturally in foods.

Folate = healthy hearts?

Homocysteine is an interesting chemical in the ongoing puzzle of heart disease. Our bodies manufacture it, and high levels are now thought to be a risk factor for heart disease. In the normal course of things, three B vitamins (B_6, B_{12}, and folate) convert homocysteine into amino acids. If you are deficient in these vitamins, especially folate, homocysteine may build up and damage blood vessels, starting the cascade of events that lead to a heart attack. As we've reported (*Wellness Letter*, March 2001), the homocysteine theory of heart disease is still only a theory; but there's every reason to increase your consumption of folate and other B vitamins. It might save your life.

Other news: Several small studies have shown that boosting folate intake improves blood vessel function in people who already have heart disease. And a large government study in 2002 found that people who consume the most folate have a lower risk of stroke and heart disease than those consuming little folate.

Folate = protection against cancer?

Since folate is so important in healthy cell division, it makes sense that it might prevent the unhealthy cell divisions characteristic of cancer. A high folate intake appears to play a role in reducing the risk of colon cancer, according to a recent Dutch study and other research. Diets rich in fruits and vegetables go along with a lower risk of colon cancer, and the folate in these foods may be one reason for this. There's also some evidence that folate may help prevent cervical cancer.

As for breast cancer, the evidence for a protective effect is less convincing, but some studies have suggested that a high intake of folate may reduce the risk—but only in certain groups of women, such as heavy drinkers.

Complicating factors

Folate has some enemies. One of these is alcohol. Heavy drinking lowers your stores of B vitamins, especially folate. Thus, heavy drinking and a poor diet may increase cancer risk synergistically—that is, more than either factor would alone.

Another complicating factor for folate may be sunlight. A recent article in *Scientific American* cited evidence that ultraviolet radiation can actually penetrate the skin and destroy folate in the bloodstream, especially in fair-skinned people. This is another reason to avoid sunbathing.

Bottom line: *The adult RDA for folate is 400 micrograms daily (600 micrograms for pregnant women). A diet rich in veg-*

etables, fruits, and grains should supply ample amounts. Particularly good sources are leafy greens, broccoli, beans, wheat germ, whole grains, peanuts, corn, oranges, and orange juice. A cup of cooked spinach or asparagus has 260 milligrams, a cup of beans anywhere from 160 to 350. And, as we've said, the folic acid in supplements and fortified grain products is even better absorbed. Most multivitamins have 400 micrograms; many breakfast cereals are fortified with high levels of folic acid.

And by the way: The government has set an upper limit for folic acid from pills or fortified foods at 1,000 micrograms a day, since higher levels can worsen the neurological damage of a vitamin B_{12} deficiency. This is especially a problem in older people. Such high levels can also "mask" a B_{12} deficiency and thus delay its diagnosis and treatment.

UNIT 3

Diet and Disease Through the Life Span

Unit Selections

Key Points to Consider

- What do you need to know for early detection of diabetes?

- What interventions are helpful in the management of arthritis?

- How can individuals lessen their risk of heart attack through dietary choices?

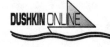 **Links: www.dushkin.com/online/**
These sites are annotated in the World Wide Web pages.

American Cancer Society
http://www.cancer.org

American Heart Association (AHA)
http://www.americanheart.org

The Food Allergy and Anaphylaxis Network
http://www.foodallergy.org

Heinz Infant & Toddler Nutrition
http://www.heinzbaby.com

LaLeche League International
http://www.lalecheleague.org

Vegetarian Pages
http://www.veg.org

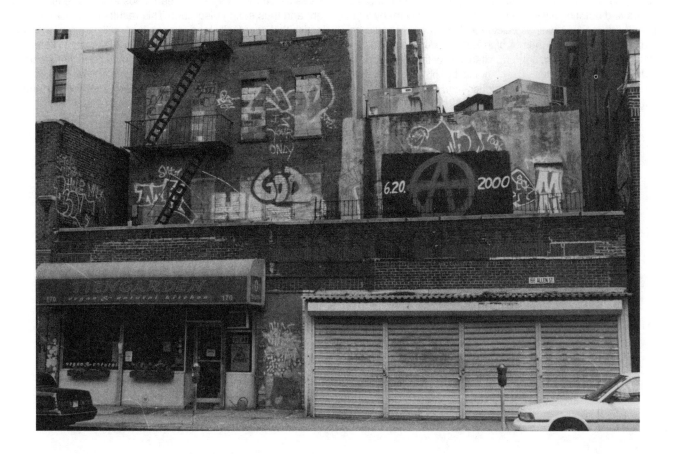

In Ancient Greece, Hippocrates, the father of medicine, stated in his oath to serve humanity that the physician should use diet as part of his "arsenal" to fight disease. In ancient times, the healing arts included diet, exercise, and the power of the mind to cure disease.

Since those times, research that focuses on the connection between diet and disease has unraveled the role of many nutrients in degenerative disease prevention or reversal, but, frequently, results are controversial and need to be interpreted cautiously before a population-wide health message is mandated. We have also come to better understand the role of genetics in the expression of disease and its importance in how we respond to dietary change. The decoding of the Human Genome has heralded one of the most crucial medical projects of all time and has improved our understanding of the genetics behind certain diseases. It will help "fingerprint" people, this identifying the exact gene that makes a person susceptible to a certain disease. The emerging science of Nutrigenomics will help screening, detecting, and treating disease at early stages and will help nutritionists prescribe "individualized" diets for high risk persons.

Research about diet and disease has enabled us to understand the importance and uniqueness of the individual (age, gender, ethnicity, and genetics) and his or her particular relation to diet. With the recent advances in research in the area of phytochemicals such as flavonoids, carotenoids, saponins, indoles, and others in foods, especially fruits and vegetables, and their potential to prevent disease, thereby increasing both quality of life and life expectancy, we are at the zenith of a nutrition revolution. The most prevalent degenerative diseases in industrial countries, which are quickly spreading in developing countries, re cancer, cardiovascular disease, diabetes, obesity, and osteoporosis. Phytochemicals have been reported to lower the risk of certain types of cancer and to decrease cholesterol in blood and prevent oxidation of the LDL lipoprotein-risk factors for developing cardiovascular disease. Furthermore, phytochemicals may protect against the development of diabetes and help prevent obesity.

Hypertension is a disease that plagues one out of five Americans. Until recently, health professionals advised reducing body weight and dietary sodium as a non-drug approach to reducing high blood pressure. The Dietary Approach to Stop Hypertension (DASH) diet, which emphasizes low-fat dairy products rich in calcium for every meal, and fruits and vegetables rich in potassium and many minerals and vitamins, will not only help you reduce high blood pressure but also decrease your risk for heart attack and osteoporosis. Another risk factor for heart disease is obesity. Eating an excessive number of calories leads to obesity. Animal studies have shown that restricting calories prevents disease and prolongs life. If that also supplies to humans, radical changes need to be instituted in American life styles to change food-related behaviors to achieve the above.

Twenty-two percent of the U.S. population by the year 2030 will be composed of people 65 years old and older. The elderly are at higher nutritional risk due to high prevalence of chronic diseases and nutritionally inadequate diets lacking in many vitamins and minerals as well as calcium. Older people should be encouraged to choose foods of high nutrient density and adequate amounts of protein, calcium, vitamin D, vitamin B12, fiber and drink plenty of water. They should be physically active, avoid smoking, limit alcohol consumption, and choose nutritional supplements carefully. To reduce malnutrition and food insecurity, and to prolong independence of the elderly, establishment of effective governmental policies is warranted.

A widespread problem among women athletes is the triad of eating disorders, menstrual irregularities, and osteoporosis. Pressure on athletes to look lean leads to erratic eating behaviors and thus eating disorders. This results in menstrual irregularities that eventually lead to bone loss, with women in their 20s having fragile bones resembling those of women in their 70s. The typical groups at risk are not only high school students and intercollegiate athletes but also active girls and women. Nutrition education to emphasize prevention and teach good nutrition habits will support high levels of performance and reduce the incidence of this triad.

NUTRIGENOMICS

IT'S IN THE GENES

*Scientists are working toward a future in which
dietitians will provide individual nutrition advice
based on their clients' specific genetic profiles.*

BY KATE JACKSON

We're all aware that the food we eat influences our health. We try to follow recommendations and keep up with emerging science, but it's clear that not all of us respond to the recommendations in the same way. One person may show no ill-effect from a diet heavy on hot dogs and burgers, while another may have high cholesterol levels despite a vegetarian diet.

Many people take vitamins and supplements, but to a large extent, this practice is based upon guesswork and, as with food, supplementation appears to influence health in a somewhat unpredictable manner. The science of nutrigenomics—which acknowledges not only that nutrition influences health, but also that food may influence expression of genetic makeup—promises to take the guesswork out of nutrition for optimal health through personalized genetic profiles that may make across-the-board nutrition recommendations obsolete and usher in the age of individualized nutrition. Soon prescriptions for food may be as common, if not more common, than those for drugs.

On April 14, the International Human Genome Sequencing Consortium, led in the United States by the National Human Genome Research Institute and the Department of Energy, acknowledged the completion of the Human Genome Project more than two years ahead of schedule. This international cooperative undertaking sequenced 3 billion DNA letters in the human genome, advancing the possibility of strides in a new field of nutrigenomics—a discipline through which dietitians enter a realm where their expertise will be invaluable and in which their responsibility will be heightened and highlighted.

The emerging science of nutrigenomics explores the ways in which nutrition impacts health by influencing genes. It looks at the effect of nutrition upon health at the molecular level and explores the manner in which nutritional components directly or indirectly affect the human genome by changing an individual's genetic structure or altering the expression of genes. By understanding more about the molecular basis of nutrition's effect upon the human genome, scientists hope that diet-influenced diseases can be prevented, ameliorated, or eradicated. Nutrigenomics will lead the way to allowing individuals to tailor their diets according to the dictates of their genetic makeup to reduce their risks of developing diet-related diseases or to actually treat existing conditions.

It is well-known that diet is a factor in a wide variety of diseases, including diabetes, cancer, heart disease, and birth defects. To a large extent, the effect of diet upon disease development or upon the alteration of the course of disease has not been well-understood, and the degree to which that effect is individually based upon one's genetic makeup has not been well-appreciated.

Information gleaned from the Human Genome Project has shed light upon these connections and made it clear that diet does not affect individuals equally with respect to disease prevention or development. A diet that is healthful for one individual may not be healthful for another. Nutrigenomics investigates these differences and explores the genetic variation among individuals that influences how nutrition influences health, an endeavor that calls into question a "one-size-fits-all" approach to nutrition.

It's well-known, for example, that certain minority populations have increased risks of chronic diseases such as diabetes, obesity, cardiovascular disease, and some cancers. Nutrigenomics is revealing the ways in which certain genotypes, shared by minority populations, respond differently to nutrition, honing in on these diet-influenced conditions and exploring the ways in which nutrition can be targeted more specifically to these specific genotypes and their unique reactions to dietary chemicals.

Researchers have found, for example, that individuals with a particular variant gene show less increase in cholesterol and low-density lipoproteins in response to a diet rich in eggs. They theorize that the variant gene changes the way in which cholesterol is absorbed in the intestines. Other researchers have revealed that a genetic variation results in an increase in homocysteine levels and have suggested that genetic testing for this variant will help individuals determine their risk for cardiovascular disease and use nutrition prophylactically.

A research team led by Jose M. Ordovas, PhD, of the Jean Mayer USDA Human Nutrition Research Center on Aging at Tufts University, Boston, Mass., has studied 40 of the genes known to influence cardiovascular health. Ordovas theorizes that genetic testing early in life will allow individuals to get a jump-start on eating to prevent disease and avoiding foods that increase risk. Another Tufts researcher, Joel B. Mason, MD, is examining how certain individuals may require more folate than others to help protect them against colon cancer. In addition, researchers are looking at a host of diseases, including breast cancer, autism, and schizophrenia, and using genomic information to tease out risk factors and prevention possibilities.

The science of nutrigenomics promises to take the guesswork out of nutrition for optimal health through personalized genetic profiles that may make across-the-board nutrition recommendations obsolete and usher in the age of individualized nutrition.

Genomic information will be used to understand these individual differences in diet-gene interactions and the mechanisms by which they lead to the development or suppression of disease in some individuals. As genetic research leads to the creation of more precise and more widespread genetic testing, it will become easier for scientists and, ultimately, healthcare providers to determine individuals' precise nutritional needs and develop strategies to more effectively use food as a weapon against disease.

YOU ARE WHAT YOU EAT

The promise of nutrigenomics, say experts, is not a distant possibility, but rather a certainty that's just around the bend. The most likely scenario, suggest many researchers, is that within 10 years, individuals will be able to visit their doctors and undergo a battery of genetic tests merely by providing a blood sample that will be analyzed to reveal their particular susceptibility to disease. Once these genetic profiles are available, an individualized eating plan can be developed.

The most likely scenario, suggest many researchers, is that within 10 years, individuals will be able to visit their doctors and undergo a battery of genetic tests merely by providing a blood sample that will be analyzed to reveal their particular susceptibility to disease.

Food, at this point, truly will be used as medicine. Furthermore, foods and supplements are likely to be developed with the particular needs of certain genotypes in mind. Products will be targeted to subgroups of people with similar genetic variations and thus similar risks. "To some extent," says Jim Kaput, PhD,

president and CSO of NutraGenomics, "Nutrigenomics is already here. We as scientists could easily develop a test for lactose intolerance, and we have been testing for phenylketonuria [PKU] for years." Certain gene variants, he says, have been shown to alter the link between diet and health. "That means some individuals with certain gene variants can already be told to alter intake of specific foods. The best example of this is lactose intolerance. However, we do not currently have enough data to tell an individual exactly what to eat to prevent complex diseases, such as obesity, diabetes, or other chronic disease."

HEALTH DISPARITIES

The National Center of Excellence for Nutritional Genomics at the University of California, Davis was launched in January under a five-year grant to explore the interactions between diet, genome, and disease, according to director Ray Rodriquez, molecular biologist, geneticist, and professor of molecular and cellular biology at the university. The center is looking at the role of genes and diet in health disparities, a subject Rodriquez calls a hot-button issue in medicine, science, and politics. "After 50 years of wonderful advancement, there are still pockets of health disparities by which individuals have either a higher rate or a higher frequency of a particualr disease, or they have an early onset or greater severity of a particular disease." He points, for example, to increased cardiovascular disease in Alaskan natives, type 2 diabetes in specific Native American populations, and prostate cancer in African Americans.

As a geneticist who works with people who are interested in populations and population differences, Rodriquez began contemplating the interaction between diet and the human genome and speculating whether or not some of these health disparities are due to genetic differences. These might be slight genetic differences called *common genetic variances* (not mutations), he explains.

Rodriquez speculated that the effect of these variances might manifest in various subpopulations under conditions of nutritional stress, which might be malnutrition or overconsumption. He mentions the Alaskan Eskimo, who often spent most of the day in cold climates, burning tremendous amounts of calories to find fish and blubber—high-calorie food that, because of the Eskimos' active lifestyle, had no ill effect. Now, however, when encouraged to lead a sedentary lifestyle in heated homes as opposed to igloos, Eskimos experience a rise in obesity and cardiovascular disease. This, he says, is an example of a conflict between diet and genome.

Rodriquez believes that nutrigenomics will lead to personalized nutrition that will address nutritional stress and its impact upon diet-gene interaction. "It won't be dramatically different. You won't have some people eating all carbs while other people eat all proteins and still others eat a lot of fats or oils," he suggests. "It will be subtle but important adjustments to the diet that, if practiced over a long period of time, will increase the likelihood and maintenance of optimal health."

The promise, he says, is close at hand. "I believe that in five to 10 years we will have a situation in which people can customize their diets. Eventually, they will go to their physicians and get genotypes of diet-regulated genes—those genes that are dramatically controlled and influenced by diet—and get assessed to see if they have a predisposition." He says this screening is already done with infants with galactosemia and PKU—the most common and best known examples of adverse diet-genome interactions.

"What we're talking about," says Rodriquez, "are the fruits of the human genome revolution that are trickling up from the laboratory into the clinical setting, into the hospital wards and doctors' offices." He says that technology is being developed that will lead to point-of-care diagnostic tests that are genome-based.

It's likely that this will be an area of great interest to healthcare consumers who do not have serious acute disease but who are interested in optimizing their long-term health. People are thinking this way now, he observes, but without knowledge of genetic components. Dietary chemicals, he says, have drug effects, so when we eat, we are basically medicating ourselves. "Sometimes we do it successfully, and sometimes we do it unsuccessfully. I take multivitamin and dietary supplements," he says. "I'm making an educated guess that higher levels of vitamins C and E at the end of the day are going to be good for me. I'm only making decisions based on hunches. And, it could be that with my genotype, I might not need so much vitamin C, but I need more folic acid. Perhaps I could do with less than 400 units of vitamin E because I have enzymes that are efficient at metabolizing vitamin E and translating it to membranes. We're all taking educated guesses, but genomic science will be providing a scientific basis upon which these dietary recommendations can be made."

Rodriquez likes to tell his students that what he calls nutritional genomics is basically hundreds of thousands of years of folk wisdom based upon thousands of genes and billions of base pairs of DNA. "People have known for many years from trial and error and to a certain extent from many clinical and dietary studies what is probably good for you and what is probably not good for you, and now we can take that one step further and say that a person will benefit from a particular diet."

As a result of this emerging knowledge, suggests Rodriquez, the Food Guide Pyramid is being questioned and the idea of a one-size-fits-all nutritional recommendation is being revised. "What we'll find when we look at the genetic factors is a way of tweaking the Food Guide Pyramid so that we get the maximum impact of those recommendations."

Caveat Emptor

The emergence of nutrigenomics will likely be accompanied by a wave of food product and testing service introductions—all of which, says Rodriquez, must be approached with caution. There's a high degree of public interest and acceptance in the idea of personal nutrition or nutrigenomics, and as a consequence, a number of companies have sprung up, some Internet-based, he says, that promise to give individuals precise dietary recommendations based upon urine samples or buccal swab. "People have been scrambling to get products out on the market, so it's important to be careful and determine if there's a scientific basis for these products."

The Role of Dietitians

The explosion of information that nutrigenomics is likely to bring forth will increase the need for nutrition education and guidance and will highlight the expertise of dietitians who are well-versed in genetics. Dietitians are likely to play a role in the development of foods targeted to specific genetic profiles, to counsel clients on genetic testing, and to help clients devise nutritional models geared toward their specific genotypes and resulting needs. As the field develops, dietitians should lead the way in helping the medical profession define nutrient requirements and create individuals' nutrition plans and plans targeted to subgroups of individuals that will address their unique needs and ensure optimal wellness.

"I believe dietitians are going to emerge as an important link in this chain between optimal health and disease prevention," says Rodriquez. "As a result, he says, they will bear the burden of being knowledgeable and cognizant of all the breakthroughs in genomics." Dietitians are already the experts in food, but to be at the forefront of this emerging field, he suggests, they will need to become more knowledgeable about all of the other genetic components and become devoted students of genomics.

—Kate Jackson is a staff writer
at *Today's Dietitian.*

Curtains for Heart Disease?

"**W**e can end the heart disease epidemic in the U.S.," says epidemiologist and world-renowned cardiovascular disease expert Jeremiah Stamler. Stamler's work, which spans more than half a century, has homed in on the causes of cardiovascular disease and the strategies to prevent it. His latest findings demonstrate that diet, exercise, and not smoking can head off most heart attacks and strokes.

Diet is like tobacco, Stamler suggests. "The science is no longer in doubt."

Q: You say that we can now end the heart disease epidemic. What's changed?

A: We've had two major advances. For decades, we've known that three major risk factors for heart disease are smoking, high cholesterol, and high blood pressure. And we've addressed two of the three. Advice to the public on not smoking and on diets that lower cholesterol has had a big impact. Smoking has dropped, and average adult cholesterol levels have declined from about 240 to about 200. We've achieved a national health goal.

But now we know how to solve the third piece of the puzzle—how to lower blood pressure with population-wide improvements in diet and exercise.

Furthermore, we now have, for the first time, data on what happens to people who have none of these three major risk factors. With that knowledge, we can end heart disease as an epidemic. It's that simple.

Q: Haven't researchers estimated the risks of high cholesterol, high blood pressure, and smoking before?

A: Yes. And we learned that the more risk factors you've got, the worse off you are. But the earlier comparisons focused on unfavorable or adverse levels. For example, we compared people with cholesterol of 240 and higher to those who were below 240. But below 240 is not favorable. Below 200 is. And optimal is below 180.

We did the same thing with blood pressure. We compared people with blood pressure of 140 over 90 and above to those whose blood pressures were below. But below 140 over 90 isn't favorable—120 over 80 and lower is. We never looked at people with favorable levels.

Q: Why not?

A: There were just too few people who were low-risk. We wanted men and women who had none of the three major risk factors when our studies began in the late 1960s—people who didn't smoke and who had total cholesterol levels below 200 and blood pressures of 120 over 80 or below. And we wanted people who had no history of diabetes or heart attack.

Those people made up less than ten percent of every group of men we looked at, and about 20 percent of younger women. It wasn't until we screened roughly 400,000 people in two major studies that we could identify enough low-risk people. Our latest studies have tracked them for at least 25 years.

Q: Did they live longer?

A: Yes. The findings were all that we could hope for. For example, for two

groups of men who were under age 40 when the study began—about 82,000 men altogether—the long-term death rate from coronary heart disease was reduced by 90 percent for low-risk men compared to all others.

We estimated that these low-risk younger men—freed of the burden of epidemic coronary disease—lived six to ten years longer than the other men. The results were similar for low-risk women. For these people, there was no heart disease epidemic.

Q: How about people who were middle-aged when the study began?

A: We estimated that low-risk middle-aged people would live six years longer than all others. Our results probably also apply to older low-risk people, but we didn't have enough of them to say for sure.

Q: Are you just talking about heart disease?

A: No. The low-risk people also had lower death rates from stroke and cancer. And people who were low-risk in middle age were more likely to sail into older age with a better quality of life, less chronic illness, lower Medicare costs, and no evidence of advanced atherosclerosis in their coronary arteries.

Q: What about other risk factors?

A: Diet is a risk factor, but it isn't readily measured. Overweight is a risk factor beyond its impact on blood cholesterol, blood pressure, and diabetes, but we were unsure of that in the late 1960s. And we measured total instead of LDL—so-called bad—cholesterol because when these large studies started, it was cheaper, easier, and less error-prone to measure. But that's not a problem because total cholesterol mirrors LDL, and it predicts heart disease risk.

Q: Why are so few Americans at low risk?

A: It's interesting—in young adults, average levels are still favorable. Blood pressure averages about 116 over 70 and cholesterol averages about 180. But as people age, their blood pressure and cholesterol rise. In part, that's because we eat too much salt, sugar, and fatty baked goods, red meat, and dairy products. And we eat too many calories and exercise too little.

Now we have a diet that can lower blood pressure and cholesterol and keep both from rising with age. It's called DASH, or Dietary Approaches to Stop Hypertension (see "A DASH-ing Pyramid,").

The DASH Diet

Q: What is the DASH diet?

A: Six years ago, in a study of about 450 people, researchers found that a diet rich in fruits, vegetables, and low-fat dairy foods lowered blood pressure by an average of 6 points over 3 points. That's a significant drop. Blood pressures on the DASH diet were lower than pressures on a typical American diet, or even on a typical American diet with fruits and vegetables replacing some snacks and sweets.

Three years later, the researchers reported that blood pressure fell even more dramatically—about 9 points over 5 points—in people who ate the DASH diet and cut salt by two-thirds. The DASH diet lowered blood pressure whether or not blood pressure was high to begin with. And it also cut LDL cholesterol by an average of 11 points.

Is DASH a low-fat diet? No, but the DASH diet is low in cholesterol. It's also low in saturated fat—only six percent of calories. That's about half the level of the typical American diet. DASH also has a modest increase in protein and carbohydrates. We're talking about more fruits, vegetables, whole grains, beans, and low-fat dairy products, and fewer sweets, fatty meats, and egg yolks.

*T*he people with low risk of heart disease also had lower death rates from stroke and cancer.

Q: Is DASH the healthiest diet?

A: We know that it's a very good diet, but there may be others that are equally good. Two of the DASH investigators—Lawrence Appel of Johns Hopkins and Frank Sacks of Harvard—are testing DASH diets that are higher in protein or in monounsaturated fats.

Q: Are diet and exercise enough to cut risk?

A: Yes, along with not smoking, of course. How many people are on statin drugs and blood pressure pills now? Tens of millions? Americans are pushed to solve problems with pills—for cholesterol, for diabetes, for blood pressure. But pills often fail to lower risk to optimal levels. They're costly and have side effects. They ameliorate—but don't cure—the underlying problem.

Heart disease is caused by adverse lifestyles. If you want to get rid of the disease, get rid of these lifestyles.

Q: Don't some people need those medications?

A: Yes. The risk of high blood pressure, high cholesterol, and high blood sugar outweighs any risk of taking medications to lower them. And many people already have levels that are too high to control with diet and exercise. I'm not talking about individual patients. I'm addressing the public health challenge.

On a mass scale there never was a need for estrogen therapy to prevent coronaries in women. On a mass scale there never was a need for aspirin to prevent coronaries in people who had never had a heart attack. Drugs can't end the epidemic.

Q: Why don't Americans eat healthier diets?

A: The government doesn't spend enough money to counter the marketing, advertising, and politicking that industry uses to promote products. The tobacco, drink, and food industries create a lot of noise in the system. For example, the salt industry propagandizes that salt is not a public health problem—it says that salt is only a problem for a limited number of patients.

The meat, egg, dairy, fast food, and soft drink industries have abandoned a head-on assault on the science. Instead they weave and bob, throwing sand in the machinery. For example, instead of claiming that saturated fat is harmless, the pork industry calls pork the 'other white meat.' That implies that it's as lean and low in saturated fat as poultry.

Q: Some experts argue that it's impossible to change what Americans eat.

A: Not true. Remember that in the 1950s, Americans got 17 percent of their calories from saturated fat, and cholesterol intakes averaged 700 milligrams a day. We began to recommend changes, and some people at first said we were hopelessly optimistic. They said you're not going to influence the way Americans eat. But we did. And average blood cholesterol dropped despite the increase in obesity.

Americans are health-conscious. Communicate with them—consistently, repeatedly, and without a lot of noise—and they move in the right direction.

Jeremiah Stamler was the first chair of the Department of Preventive Medicine of Northwestern University Medical School in Chicago, where he is now professor emeritus. He has published more than 1,000 scientific papers on the prevention of cardiovascular diseases. He has served on numerous expert panels and editorial boards and has chaired the American Heart Association's Council on Arteriosclerosis and its Council on Epidemiology. Stamler, who is a member of *Nutrition Action Healthletter*'s Scientific Advisory Board, spoke with *NAH*'s Bonnie Liebman.

A DASHING PYRAMID

Pyramids are everywhere these days. The U.S. Department of Agriculture and the Mayo Clinic each has one. Harvard has several. Pyramids (or other graphics) make it easier for people to visualize *how much of what* to eat. So we've taken the DASH diet and, with a few tweaks (like recommending whole grains), turned it into a pyramid. The only missing advice: A DASH diet should be low in salt (sodium chloride), even though the pyramid can't show it.

A DASH diet may not be the only healthy way to eat. But it's one of the few diets that have been tested and shown to lower blood pressure and cholesterol. Just remember that what we call a serving may be much smaller than you expect. For example:

- **Grains.** An order of spaghetti at a typical Italian restaurant is three cups. That would be six of the half-cup servings in the DASH diet. A typical bagel, which weighs four or five ounces, would be four or five servings.

- **Meat & poultry.** DASH says that a serving of chicken or meat is three ounces. Most restaurants serve six to nine ounces of chicken (two to three servings) and seven to 16 ounces of steak (two to five servings).

- **Vegetables.** A DASH serving is one cup of lettuce and half a cup of most other vegetables. At a restaurant, a side Caesar salad is two cups (two servings).

- **Oils, salad dressings, mayo.** A DASH serving is only one *tea*spoon of full-fat mayo or oil. (Food labels list one *table*spoon for both.) A DASH serving of full-fat salad dressing is one tablespoon. It's two tablespoons for light dressing only.

If you think you'd starve on this diet, keep in mind that it's for someone who eats 2,000 calories a day. It applies to most women, but not to the average man, who needs 2,900 calories (if he's 50 or under) and 2,300 calories (if he's over 50). Any man or woman who is fairly active will need more.

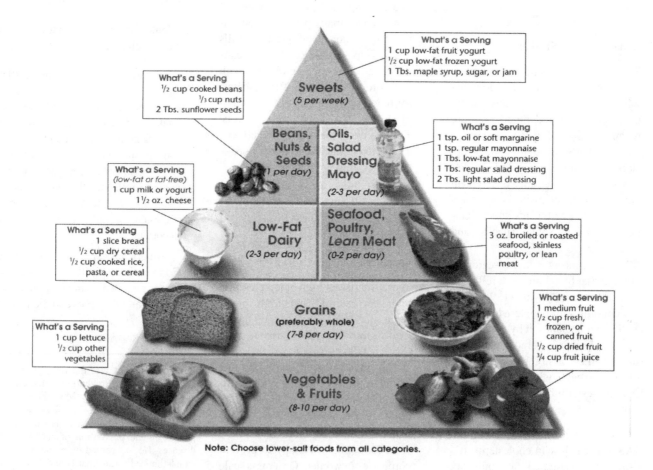

What's a Serving
1 cup low-fat fruit yogurt
½ cup low-fat frozen yogurt
1 Tbs. maple syrup, sugar, or jam

What's a Serving
½ cup cooked beans
⅓ cup nuts
2 Tbs. sunflower seeds

Sweets
(5 per week)

Beans, Nuts & Seeds
(1 per day)

Oils, Salad Dressing, Mayo
(2-3 per day)

What's a Serving
1 tsp. oil or soft margarine
1 tsp. regular mayonnaise
1 Tbs. low-fat mayonnaise
1 Tbs. regular salad dressing
2 Tbs. light salad dressing

What's a Serving
(low-fat or fat-free)
1 cup milk or yogurt
1½ oz. cheese

Low-Fat Dairy
(2-3 per day)

Seafood, Poultry, Lean Meat
(0-2 per day)

What's a Serving
3 oz. broiled or roasted seafood, skinless poultry, or lean meat

What's a Serving
1 slice bread
½ cup dry cereal
½ cup cooked rice, pasta, or cereal

Grains
(preferably whole)
(7-8 per day)

What's a Serving
1 medium fruit
½ cup fresh, frozen, or canned fruit
½ cup dried fruit
¾ cup fruit juice

What's a Serving
1 cup lettuce
½ cup other vegetables

Vegetables & Fruits
(8-10 per day)

Note: Choose lower-salt foods from all categories.

Eat less live longer?
Does calorie restriction work?

David Schardt

If you're a worm or a spider, a guppie or a hamster, or a mouse, a rat, or a dog the evidence is clear: Cut calories by 25 to 30 percent and you'll increase your lifespan by 10, 25, maybe even 40 percent. It helps if you haven't hit puberty when you start, though you'll also get some benefit if you begin in middle age.

The promise of calorie restriction (CR) is so intriguing that the National Institutes of Health is launching $20 million worth of research over seven years to study CR's effect on metabolism in humans. And pharmaceutical and gene therapy companies are scrambling to find out how people can get the benefits of calorie restriction without having to go hungry.

A few brave souls like Mark Cummins can't wait. They're willing to tinker with one of life's great pleasures now on the chance that it might pay off later.

Low (Cal) Society

Mark Cummins says that he has been eating from 1,500 to 1,900 calories a day for most of the last 14 years. That's 850 to 1,250 fewer calories than what most men his size should eat (he's 6'2" and weighs 175 pounds).

Cummins is not alone. He serves on the board of directors of the Calorie Restriction Society (www.calorierestriction.org), a small group of (mostly) men who hope to live far longer by eating far less.

Using a computer program, Cummins and his fellow members have each calculated exactly how much food they need to consume every day to get all the protein, vitamins, and minerals to stay healthy, while cutting back on their recommended calorie intake by 25 percent or more. (Most take a multivitamin for insurance.)

"The only way you can do this is by eating lots of fruits and vegetables," says Cummins. "I have it easier than many CR people, who spend one to three hours a day preparing their food. I eat pretty much the same food each day and I buy it ready-made."

One of Cummins's two main meals is a large salad that he assembles from the fixings he buys from local salad bars and tops off with pieces of fish, chicken, or tofu. "For the other one, I buy a 650-calorie vegetarian burrito that contains rice, beans, and vegetables, but no cheese or sour cream." That's pretty much all he eats. Every day.

Cummins and the others in the Calorie Restriction Society will never know whether their diets prolong their lives. Even so, they see some short-term benefits.

"My LDL [bad cholesterol] and my blood pressure are low, and my HDL [good cholesterol] is high," Cummins says. "And I know this is only anecdotal, but I feel full of energy and I think my mind and my memory are sharper than they've ever been."

Isn't he always hungry? "Hunger can be an issue," concedes Cummins. "But I'm not tempted by food all the time like some other CR people are." A survey of calorie restriction followers a few years ago found that all were hungry to some degree. Roy Walford, the University of California at Los Angeles pathologist whose pioneering research launched the CR movement, has acknowledged that it's not a diet for everyone.

"Walford is a kind of patron saint of CR," says George Roth, a senior guest scientist at the National Institute on Aging (NIA) in Baltimore. "He's the guy we credit with sparking today's interest in calorie restriction and in how it might apply to people."

The 79-year-old Walford now suffers from amyotrophic lateral sclerosis (ALS), or Lou Gehrig's disease, and no longer expects to come close to the age of 120 that he once predicted for himself. He blames his disease on a poisonous gas he was exposed to in Biosphere 2—the two-year experiment in the Arizona desert in the early 1990s that was supposed to simulate conditions in a space colony.

When the Biosphere environment couldn't produce enough food to give each of the eight inhabitants who were sealed in the colony 2,500 calories a day, Walford put them all, including himself, on an 1,800-to-2,200-calorie diet.

Six months on the calorie-restricted regimen produced dramatic results: Average cholesterol plummeted from 191 to 123, fasting blood sugar dropped from 92 to 74, blood pressure went from 109/74 to 89/58, and weight fell from 163 to 136 pounds (for the men) and from 134 to 119 pounds (for the women).[1]

That's not all the diet did. Contemporary news accounts based on interviews with the participants described them as obsessed with food and meals.

"Hunger was an almost constant companion," said one. At mealtimes they would stare at each others' plates to make sure no one took a morsel more than his or her share. Dessert became a time to fantasize about the sweets they were missing. And the food in the movies they watched held them mesmerized.

OF MICE AND DOGS

Where did Walford get the idea to restrict calories? In the mid-1970s, he and his co-workers at UCLA found that laboratory mice and rats deprived of a full food ration, but not vitamins, minerals, or other essential nutrients, lived longer and aged more slowly than similar animals who weren't calorie deprived.

In the 25 years since then, "moderate calorie restriction has proven beneficial for prolonging life or slowing the progression of disease in essentially every species of animal that's been tested," says Roth.

For example, Labrador retrievers fed 25 percent fewer calories than other Labs throughout their lives lived about 15 percent longer and were in better health, according to research published last year by the Purina Pet Institute in St. Louis. [2]

"It's the first study completed in an animal larger than laboratory rodents that proves the significant power that diet restriction wields in extending life," says Richard Weindruch, who studied under Roy Walford at UCLA before setting up a CR research program at the University of Wisconsin in Madison.

Longer life isn't the only benefit researchers have seen in calorie-restricted animals:

Cancer

"Caloric restriction inhibits the growth of tumors in virtually every study done in rats or mice," says researcher David Kritchevsky of the Wistar Institute in Philadelphia. In one study, mice destined to develop tumors because of a genetic defect got fewer tumors when they were on a CR diet or a one-day-a-week fast—even when the restriction started late in life. [3]

"Calorie restriction is the most potent, broadly acting cancer-prevention regimen in experimental cancer models," concludes Stephen Hursting of the National Cancer Institute.

One possible explanation: Calorie restricted animals have lower body temperatures than non-CR animals. And "at lower temperatures, the body may be more efficient at repairing damaged DNA," speculates Donald Ingram, acting chief of the Laboratory of Experimental Gerontology at the Gerontology Research Center of the National Institute on Aging (NIA).

In the Baltimore Longitudinal Study of Aging, a lower body temperature is one of the characteristics of men who live longer. [4] (Some members of the Calorie

Restriction Society report typical body temperatures of 97°F.)

Insulin Sensitivity

Calorie-restricted animals have lower levels of insulin and blood sugar and greater insulin sensitivity, which means that their bodies need less insulin to control the sugar in their blood. And that reduces their risk of diabetes and cardiovascular disease. "Lower insulin levels are also characteristic of the men who are living the longest in the Baltimore Study of Aging," says George Roth.

Brain Cells

Mice susceptible to Alzheimer's or Parkinson's disease are slower to develop those conditions if they've been put on a CR diet. What's more, "If you restrict the calories of rodents, they'll perform better at learning and memory tasks later in life than rodents eating a normal diet," says Ingram.

But healthier rats and dogs with an extra couple of years to chase the postman aren't exactly proof that people who slash their calories will live longer. Evidence in monkeys would be more impressive.

MONKEYING AROUND

"Rhesus monkeys are the next best thing we have to doing a long-term human study," says Roth. "If you go by the DNA, they're 90 to 95 percent human, and they certainly have brains and patterns of disease more similar to people than rodents have."

In the late 1980s, both the NIA and the University of Wisconsin started studying calorie restriction in large colonies of rhesus monkeys.

National Institute on Aging (NIA)

Researchers are feeding about 60 control monkeys a normal diet that maintains a healthy body weight. "We took pains to make sure that they're not fat or pre-diabetic," says Roth. Sixty similar monkeys are being fed the same food, but with 30 percent fewer calories than are recommended for their age and body weight.

"Both groups are supplemented with vitamins, minerals, and trace elements to make sure they don't get short changed on micronutrients," says Roth. So far, the results are tantalizing. "Two control monkeys are dying for every one calorie-restricted monkey," says Roth. "Even the monkeys who started CR later in life are tending to out-survive the con-

trol monkeys, though this isn't statistically significant." (So it's possible that the longer lifespan of the monkeys who started calorie restriction in middle age is due to chance.)

"We're also seeing that they have about half the rates of diseases like cancer, cardiovascular disease, and diabetes," Roth adds.

Both groups of monkeys look and behave the same, according to Roth, with two exceptions: The calorie restricted monkeys tend to be shorter and thinner (especially if they started cutting calories before puberty)…and they get more excited at mealtimes.

University of Wisconsin

In 1989, researchers started feeding young adult rhesus monkeys 30 percent fewer calories than they were eating before the study began.

"Our restricted monkeys are healthier than the conventionally fed controls," says researcher Richard Weindruch. "They're much leaner, have lower levels of circulating glucose and insulin, and have greater insulin sensitivity."

Researchers caution that the monkey studies aren't complete, and that the promising results could change. The 25-year average lifespan of normal rhesus monkeys will be up for both the NIA and University of Wisconsin colonies during the next five years, so we should have some answers by then, notes Ingram.

MONKEY DO, PEOPLE SEE

"Calorie restriction has worked in every species it's been tried in, and it would probably work in people, too," says the National Institute on Aging's George Roth. But is "probably" enough to embark on a difficult and demanding experiment for the rest of a person's life? "No," says the NIA's Donald Ingram. "We don't know for certain whether this kind of severe diet will have the same effect in humans. We differ from small animals in our metabolism and in how we develop and reproduce."

He points out that the rhesus monkeys at NIA don't go outside, play with other monkeys, or reproduce. "Who knows what would happen to them in the real world that has bugs, environmental dangers, and other animals?"

"Until we know more, it's just too soon for us to say that we'll respond to calorie restriction in the same way with the same benefits."

The first step in finding out: "We're trying to see if CR is feasible for motivated people to do in a controlled scientific experiment," says Eric Ravussin of the Pennington Biomedical Research Center in Baton Rouge, Louisiana, the site for one of the upcoming human studies.

It hasn't been easy. After nine months of recruiting, Ravussin has found only 26 willing participants of the 48 he will need. And he's only looking for overweight people who are willing to cut a quarter of their calories, not normal-weight people who are willing to become underweight.

At Tufts University in Boston, researchers will also take overweight people and cut 30 percent of the calories "that they are currently eating to maintain their unhealthy weight," according to researcher Susan Roberts.

But by starting with overweight people, these first human studies may not be a true test of calorie restriction. Why not use volunteers who are normal weight? "We wanted to avoid any risks from excessive weight loss in skinny people as well as people with possible eating disorders," explains Ravussin.

"CR is going to be a struggle for people to do in our food-rich environment that's so unconducive to eating less," he says. "It may be possible for people to do on their own, but they would have to be very, very motivated."

That describes the members of the Calorie Restriction Society. Yet just 34 people have registered member profiles on the society's Web site.

An informal survey six years ago found that half the members thought their alertness had increased, and two thirds thought they didn't need as much sleep as before. But about half also reported suffering low moods or depression and half thought that their sex drive had diminished. All reported occasional hunger and sensitivity to cold weather.

"The society attracts a certain kind of person," says member Mark Cummins. "They have very high IQs and they're introverted problem-solvers who can carry out intellectual tasks with a high degree of self-discipline and persistence." He adds that many work out of their homes, which gives them extra time to prepare meals.

THE FAST LANE?

Is it possible to reap the gains of calorie restriction without the pain? Perhaps.

"Intermittent fasting may become an effective alternative to cutting back on calories every day," says Donald Ingram. His research group at the National Institute on Aging found that out by trying to make their lives a little easier. "Our lab workers didn't want to go into work every Saturday and Sunday to feed the animals, so they started going in only once and giving the mice two days' worth of food at a time," he recalls

Eventually, Ingram and his co-workers discovered that an every-other-day feeding produced the same drops in cholesterol and blood pressure, and the same other health benefits as calorie restriction. It also prolonged the animals' lives.

"After some interval of no food, the body apparently switches on some protective defenses that produce the benefits we see from calorie restriction," Ingram explains. The National Institutes of Health is so intrigued by the discovery that it's considering a study of fasting in older people, he adds.

The other potential alternative to calorie restriction: a drug or other chemical that can trigger the same changes.

"It's clear from the research in animals that CR extends the lifespan through several major metabolic pathways in the body," says Pennington's Eric Ravussin. "If that's the case, then we should be able to develop drugs that produce the same effects."

"It's a very competitive field," adds the NIA's George Roth. "A number of companies are trying to develop drugs of substances derived from food that will mimic calorie restriction. Most of the research is proprietary right now, so we'll have to wait a few more years to find out if they've been successful."

Notes

1. *Proc. Nat. Acad. Sci.* 89: 11533, 1992.

2. *J. Amer. Vet. Med. Assoc.* 220: 1315, 2002.

3. *Carcinogenesis 23*: 817, 2002.

4. *Science 297*: 811, 2002.

NUTRITION IN THE LIFE CYCLE

Healthy Eating in Later Years

The growing population of older adults in the United States presents challenges for health professionals, such as nutrition educators and dietitians, to provide nutrition services that best meet older adults' diverse needs. The National Dairy Council sponsored an expert panel to learn more about older adults' eating habits and nutritional status, their nutrient needs, and dietary guidance and policies directed to this population. This article highlights and updates information presented by the panel.

LOIS D. McBEAN, MS, RD; SUSAN M. GROZIAK, PhD, RD;
GREGORY D. MILLER, PhD, FACN; JUDITH K. JARVIS, MS, RD, LD

INTRODUCTION

One in 8 Americans, or about 13% of the US population, is 65 years of age and older.[1] By 2030 as many as 1 in 5 Americans (ie, 20% of the US population) is estimated to be 65 years and older.[1] As shown in Figure 1, the most rapidly growing age group of older adults is the 85 years and older population, which is expected to double its current size by 2025 and increase fivefold by 2050.[1] These changing demographics have profound effects on our healthcare system. Older adults comprise 13 % of the US population, yet they account for at least 30% of all healthcare expenditures.[2]

WHO ARE OLDER ADULTS?

Older adults are clearly a heterogeneous group.[3] Although they belong to the same age category (65 years and older), older adults differ widely from one another in their age, socioeconomic status, ethnicity, education, health status, perception of health status, functional ability, access to health/nutrition care, food security, and food choices.[4]

Compared to the general population, older adults consist of more women than men. There are also fewer older African Americans, Hispanics, Asian or Pacific Islanders, and American Indians or Native Alaskans than older non-Hispanic whites.[4] In addition, a greater proportion of older adults have limited incomes, especially women.[4] In 1997, 10% of older adults lived in a family at or below the poverty level.[4] In general, the majority of older adults in the United States rate their health as excellent to good.[4] Nevertheless, many older adults exhibit one or more chronic diseases (eg, hypertension, heart disease, arthritis).[1,2,4] In terms of their functional ability, 38% of older adults are limited in activity, 4% live in nursing homes, and 12% experience difficulty with one or more aspects of daily living, such as mobility.[5] Hip fractures are a major contributor to immobility among older adults, especially those 85 years of age and older.[6] Because many older adults are living longer, there are more frail older adults today than in the past.

OLDER ADULTS' OVERALL NUTRITIONAL STATUS

Only recently have national surveys provided information on older adults' food consumption patterns and nutrient intakes.[7-11] In general, the quality of older adults' diets needs to be improved.[11] Only 1% of older adults have a food intake pattern consistent with the US Department of Agriculture's (USDA) Food Guide Pyramid.[12] As shown in Figure 2, older adults' Healthy Eating Score (ie,

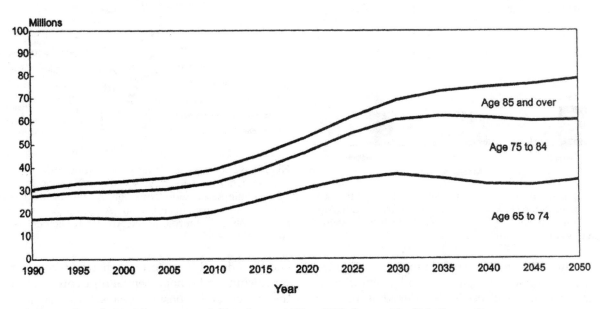

FIGURE 1. Population of persons aged 65 and over: 1990 to 2050. Source: The U.S. Census Bureau.

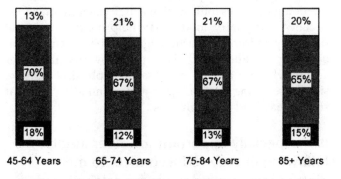

■ Poor (HEI < 51) ■ Needs Improvement (HEI 51-80) □ Good (HEI > 80)

FIGURE 2. Older adults' overall diet quality based on the Healthy Eating Index (HEI). Source: USDA Center for Nutrition Policy and Promotion, *Nutrition Insights,* July 1999, p. 1.

a summary measure of people's overall diet quality) is 67.2 out of a possible 100.[7] Median fruit and milk scores are particularly low for older adults.[7] In terms of specific nutrients, dietary intakes of calcium, vitamin D, vitamin B[12], riboflavin, and zinc, among other nutrients, are low for many older adults.[4] A recent investigation of healthy free-living older adults in Arizona found that more than 60% of those surveyed reported consuming fewer than the recommended intakes of vitamin D, vitamin E, folate, and calcium.[13] Fewer than than half of the study participants consumed recommended daily servings of dairy, grains, vegetables, or fruits.[13] In fact, fewer than 5% of the older adults consumed recommended daily servings of dairy foods.[13] Older adults' low calcium intake, especially among women (Figure 3), is attributed to their low intake of calcium-rich foods, such as dairy products.[11,14] The declining use of fluid milk products, along with older adults' increased intake of soft drinks and fruit drinks,

adversely affects the overall nutritional quality of their diets.[11] Although national surveys provide general information about older adults' food behaviors and nutritional status, it is important to remember that diversity exists among older adults' eating habits and dietary intakes.

FACTORS INFLUENCING OLDER ADULTS' NUTRITIONAL STATUS

Numerous factors, both genetic and environmental, influence older adults' nutritional status. These factors include hunger, poverty, inadequate food and nutrient intake, social isolation, poor dentition and oral health, difficulty chewing and swallowing, diet-related diseases/disorders, polypharmacy, advanced age, and living alone (Figure 4).[4] Difficulty related to walking, shopping for groceries, preparing food, and eating food may place older adults at increased risk of nutritional deficiencies.[15] The Boston Health Study found that 22% of older adults studied exhibited a medical condition that adversely affected their ability to eat, 17% experienced chewing problems, 45% took more than 3 medications a day, and 20% had a medical condition that limited their ability to shop for food.[16]

Older adults frequently experience an increased prevalence of a number of diseases and disabilities, such as arthritis, coronary heart disease, cancer, osteoporosis, and visual impairment.[17,18] These diseases influence older adults' nutritional status, and nutritional status, in turn, can affect a number of major chronic diseases of aging. Older adults with limited access to food are particularly vulnerable to low dietary variety, nutrient deficiencies, weight loss, and poor health.[19]

Many older adults experience a decrease in appetite (ie, so-called "anorexia of aging") and consume less food than

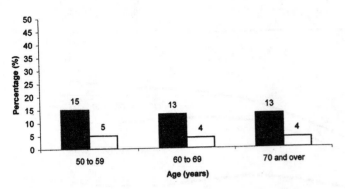

FIGURE 3. Percentage of older adults meeting 100% of the calcium recommendation (1200 mg/day). Data source: USDA, Agricultural Research Service, 1997. Available at http://www. barc.usda.gov/bhnrc/foodsurvey/home.htm.

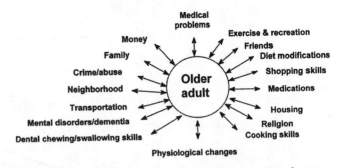

FIGURE 4. Factors affecting older adults' nutritional status. Source: American Dietetic Association, "Position of the American Dietetic Association: Nutrition, Aging and the Continuum of Care," The American Dietetic Association. Reprinted with permission from Journal of the American Dietetic Association 2000; 100:580-595.

younger adults. This, in turn, can lead to decreased nutrient intake, involuntary weight loss, and malnutrition.[4] Taste, and especially smell, decline in older adults because of normal aging.[20] Studies indicate that the rate of gastric emptying slows in older adults compared with younger adults, at least in response to large meals, resulting in longer periods of distention and a feeling of satiety.[21] The reduced rate of gastric emptying that occurs with age may result from high post-prandial levels of the satiating hormone cholecystokinin that are found in older adults. However, no studies have directly examined the effectiveness of this hormone in decreasing food intake in older adults. Depression is a major cause of weight loss and undernutrition for many older adults.[4,22] A reduction in dietary variety and social isolation may also contribute to reduced food intake and unintentional weight loss in older adults.[23] Regular monitoring of older adults' body weight may help to detect unintentional weight loss.[23]

WEIGHT CONTROL

Many older adults are trying to lose weight, including approximately 20% who are at normal weight.[8,24] Although food (energy) intake generally decreases with age, body fat and obesity increase in later years.[21,22,24] Obesity in older adults has adverse health and psychosocial consequences.[4] Decreased physical activity, age-related changes in resting metabolic rate, or an increased efficiency of body fat storage are likely contributors to obesity among older adults.[24] Overweight and obesity need not be an inevitable consequence of the aging process. Although there are no obesity guidelines specifically designed for older adults, health professionals recommend small changes in lifestyles, such as increasing physical activity, and following a healthful diet moderately reduced in energy (eg, 1,200 to 1,500 kcal for women and 1,500 to 1,800 kcal for men), low in fat (30% of energy or less), and high in fiber.[24,25] Weight loss has been linked to decreased bone loss and increased risk of osteoporosis,[26,27] a disease prevalent among older adults. Therefore, it is especially important for older adults following

energy-reduced diets to meet dietary recommendations for calcium and other essential nutrients. A study found that when obese postmenopausal women following a moderate energy-restricted diet consumed about 1,500 mg calcium/day, the increase in bone turnover rate caused by a 10% loss in body weight was prevented.[27] New findings from experimental animal and human epidemiologic studies indicate that a high calcium intake, especially from dairy foods, may help control body fat, thereby providing protection against obesity and/or facilitating weight loss.[28] For many overweight older adults who are able to increase their physical activity, simply reducing serving sizes and eliminating high-fat snacks may lead to weight loss.[24]

> It is especially important for older adults following energy-reduced diets to meet dietary recommendations for calcium and other essential nutrients.

PHYSICAL ACTIVITY

Physical activity influences older adults' nutrient needs, risks for chronic diseases, and overall quality of life.[4] Advancing age is accompanied by a decrease in lean body mass and increase in body fat.[3,22] The decrease in lean body mass occurs mainly as a result of a loss in skeletal muscle mass called sarcopenia. Sarcopenia accounts for age-associated decreases in muscle strength, basal metabolic rate, energy requirements, and aerobic capacity, as well as increased body fatness and frailty.[29] Indirectly, sarcopenia reduces insulin activity and contributes to older adults' risk for non-insulin dependent diabetes. Older adults' diminished muscle strength heightens their risk for falls and bone fractures.

Older adults' decreased energy needs may be explained by a decline in physical activity and not to the aging process per se. A study found that participating in moderate-intensity aerobic exercise 3 times a week for 6 months increased older adults' energy needs by 5% to 8%

per day.[30] Strength or resistance exercise can also increase older adults' energy needs.[29,31] Participating in strength training for 3 days/week for 12 weeks increased older adults' energy needs by about 15%.[31] A study involving frail older adults aged 72 to 98 years found that high-intensity resistance (strength) exercise training for 10 weeks effectively counteracted muscle weakness and frailty in this population.[32] The exercise not only increased muscle strength and size but also improved gait speed, stair climbing power, balance, and spontaneous activity levels.[32] Staying physically active helps older adults maintain muscle mass and bone strength.[25]

The *Dietary Guidelines for Americans* recommend that older adults engage in moderate physical activity for at least 30 minutes most days of the week, preferably daily, and participate in activities to strengthen muscles and improve flexibility.[25] Older adults should consult their healthcare provider before starting a vigorous physical activity program.[25] Unfortunately, two thirds of older adults do not exercise regularly.[4] According to a recent survey, older adults avoid leisure time physical activity because of fatigue, arthritis, past injury, concern about falling, other health problems, no interest, and lack of an exercise companion.[33] Recognition of these barriers to exercise can help health professionals to develop strategies to encourage older adults to be more physically active. Suggestions to help older adults increase their activity levels can be found in the American Dietetic Association's "The Nutrition and Health Campaign for Older Americans Toolkit."[34]

DIETARY RECOMMENDATIONS

In recent years, new knowledge has accumulated that indicates that nutrient needs for persons 51 years and older are not necessarily the same as those for persons older than 70 years. This new knowledge has led to more defined nutrient recommendations for older adults. In contrast to the 1989 Recommended Dietary Allowances (RDAs), which grouped all older adults 51 years and older into one category,[35] separate Dietary Reference Intakes (DRIs) are being issued for adults aged 51 through 70 years and those older than 70 years.[36-38]

PROTEIN

Meeting protein needs is especially important for older adults to help preserve muscle mass and bone health. Some research indicates that protein recommendations for older adults should be increased to 1.0 to 1.25 g/kg/day, which exceeds the 1989 RDA[35] of 0.8 g/kg/day.[29,39] Older adults' low physical activity may contribute to their higher needs for dietary protein, although different types of physical activity have unique influences on protein metabolism.[29,40] The DRIs for macronutrients, including protein, are being considered by a committee of the Food and Nutrition Board. Recommendations should be issued this year or in early 2002.

RIBOFLAVIN

The 1989 RDA for riboflavin for adults was based, in large part, on studies conducted in the 1950s on young adults.[35,41] These studies measured urinary excretion of riboflavin and determined a "critical" point at which tissue stores of riboflavin become saturated with riboflavin. For young adults, this critical point was about 1.1 mg riboflavin per day, and the RDA was increased slightly to account for individual variation. The 1989 RDA for riboflavin for older adults (51 years and older) was decreased slightly lower than that for younger adults because of older adults' reduced energy expenditures. However, researchers in Guatemala found that the critical intake point for riboflavin for older adults was 1.1 mg/day, the same as for younger adults.[42] Despite older adults' lower energy expenditure, riboflavin needs are constant throughout life. The DRIs for riboflavin (1.3 mg/day for men and 1.1 mg/day for women) are currently the same for everyone older than 19 years.[36]

VITAMIN B$_{12}$

Vitamin B$_{12}$ is interesting because a deficiency of this vitamin may be more prevalent among older adults than previously believed and because a vitamin B$_{12}$ deficiency may lead to problems with dementia in older adults.[43,44] In the 1989 RDAs,[35] the recommendation for vitamin B$_{12}$ was lowered from the previous (1980) edition. It is now recognized that the requirement for vitamin B$_{12}$ does not change with age. However, many older adults malabsorb protein-bound vitamin B$_{12}$ as a result of atrophic gastritis or loss of stomach acid with aging.[36] This condition affects about 25% of adults aged 50 to 69 years and up to 40% of adults older than 80 years. To ensure that older adults with atrophic gastritis receive the required amount of vitamin B$_{12}$, the DRIs for vitamin B$_{12}$ (2.4 µg/day) include the advice to meet needs for this vitamin by either taking a supplement containing vitamin B$_{12}$ and/or consuming foods fortified with vitamin B$_{12}$.[36] Relatively little information is available regarding the bioavailability of vitamin B$_{12}$ from various foods, including dairy foods.[3] However, a recent investigation, including more than 500 older adults, found that vitamin B$_{12}$ was absorbed more efficiently from dairy products than it was from meat, poultry, or fish.[44]

In recent years, new knowledge has accumulated indicating that nutrient needs for persons 51 years of age and older are not necessarily the same as those for persons older than 70 years old.

VITAMIN A

Although new dietary recommendations have not yet been issued for vitamin A, vitamin A requirements for older adults are lower than the 1989 RDAs of 1,000 µg retinol equivalents/day for men and 800 µg retinol equivalents for women and are more likely in the range of 600 to 700 µg retinol equivalents/day.[3,41] Older adults generally consume lower intakes of vitamin A than recommended; however, liver stores of this vitamin appear to be preserved. Studies in experimental animals and humans indicate that the absorption of vitamin A increases with advancing age.[41] When a meal high in fat and vitamin A was fed to both young and older adults, clearance of vitamin A (retinyl esters) from the blood was found to be lower in older persons than in younger persons. These findings indicate that high-dose vitamin A supplements may be more harmful to older adults than to young adults.[41]

CALCIUM

New dietary intake recommendations for calcium call for increased intakes of calcium for older adults.[37] The DRI for calcium for all adults aged 51 years and older is 1,200 mg/day,[37] 400 mg/day higher than previously recommended for older adults[35] and 200 mg/day higher than for adults aged 31 through 50 years. Adequate calcium intake throughout life helps to protect bones from osteoporosis, a disease affecting 28 million people, mostly women and older adults.[25,45,46] This disease is estimated to cost $10 to $15 billion a year,[45] with an expected rise to $50 billion a year by 2040 because of growth of the older population.[4]

It is well recognized that adequate calcium intake throughout life helps to protect bones from osteoporosis, a disease affecting 28 million people, mostly women and older adults.

Bone loss leading to fractures is no longer considered a normal consequence of aging.[45] Rather, osteoporosis is largely preventable.[45] According to a recent National Institutes of Health Expert Panel, "calcium is the nutrient most important for attaining peak bone mass and for preventing and treating osteoporosis."[45(pp788-789)] This panel adds that a low intake of dairy products, fruits, and vegetables increases the risk for osteoporosis.[45] Increasing older adults' intake of calcium helps to reduce their risk of bone loss and fractures. Several recent studies indicate that calcium intakes in the range of 1,200 to 2,000 mg/day may be necessary to protect older adults' bones.[45-49] Calcium's bone-sparing effect has recently been demonstrated in adults aged 60 years and older whose median calcium intake was 546 mg/day.[49] Increasing calcium intake by 759 mg/day prevented loss of bone mineral density and reduced bone turnover.[49] Another investigation found that when older adults whose diets contained fewer than 1.5 servings of dairy foods a day consumed 3 servings of fat-free or lowfat milk for 12 weeks as part of their daily diets, bone resorption significantly de-

creased.[47] The increased need for calcium in later years may be explained by older adults' lower reserve capacity with advancing age and their reduced ability to adapt to short periods of inadequate calcium intake. Younger adults can adapt to brief periods of low calcium intake by several mechanisms, including increasing calcium absorption and renal conservation. This ability to adapt decreases with age, peaking during youth and falling close to zero by age 80.[50,51] Low calcium absorption in older adults, particularly those with a low dietary intake of calcium, is a risk factor for hip fractures.[52]

Failure to adapt to a low calcium intake means loss of bone. In fact, relatively small changes in the calcium economy can exert a relatively large effect on bone health. Loss of estrogen at menopause and the age-related decrease in the ability to adapt to reduced calcium intake contribute to older adults' increased need for calcium.[37] Intake of other nutrients, such as protein and sodium, may slightly increase the requirement for calcium by increasing urinary calcium losses. However, at optimal calcium intakes, these effects disappear.[45,53,54] Meeting protein needs is particularly important for older adults to protect their skeleton and decrease their risk for bone fractures.[53]

Calcium is only one component of skeletal health and fracture risk. Vitamin D helps the body absorb calcium.[37,45] Many older adults are at risk of vitamin D deficiency as a result of reduced exposure to sunlight, decreased capacity of the skin to produce vitamin D, and low dietary intake of vitamin D.[3,25,37,49] Vitamin D fortified milk is one of the few food sources of vitamin D, providing 400 international units (IU) (10 µg) per quart. The authors of a recent study state that providing vitamin D-fortified milk to older adults is a "safe, effective, and acceptable method of administering vitamin D."[55(p300)] Numerous studies indicate that increasing older adults' intake of calcium and vitamin D improves their bone health and/or reduces bone fractures.[37,56,57] However, continuous intake of calcium and vitamin D is necessary to maintain improvements in bone mineral density in older adults.[58]

Policy makers and health professionals agree that adequate calcium intake is important for bone health throughout life.[45,46,59] However, the public may be unaware of this consensus, in large part because of media attention to opposition expressed by calcium critics.[59] Robert Heaney, MD, of Creighton University in Omaha, Neb, urges health communicators to convey to the general public the message that "there are effectively no true experimental data in humans that have failed to find a skeletal benefit of added calcium above prevailing intakes."[59(p3010)] A recent analysis of 139 papers relating to calcium intake and bone health published since 1975 provides convincing evidence of the beneficial role of calcium and calcium-rich foods in skeletal health.[46] In 39 randomized controlled trials of calcium with a skeletal end point, all but two found a beneficial effect of calcium

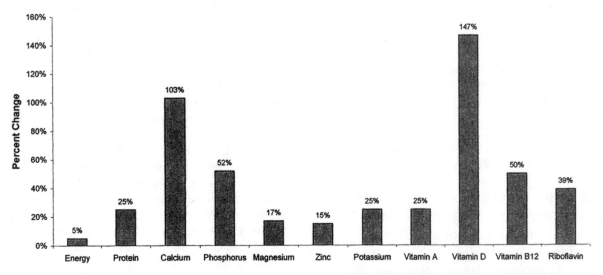

FIGURE 5. Increasing intake of milk by 3 servings/day for 12 weeks improves older women's diet quality.

(eg, fewer osteoporotic fractures).[46] The two exceptions could be readily explained. Each of the studies that used dairy sources of calcium was positive.[46] The findings led the author to conclude that "a high dairy food intake is cost-efficient as well as cost-effective" in terms of bone health.[46(p91S)]

Another review article examining the evidence between dairy food intake and bone health was less positive.[60] However, a critical analysis of the evidence cited in this review[60] reveals several methodologic limitations, including combining fundamentally different types of studies.[61] For example, equal weight was incorrectly given to randomized controlled trials (ie, the gold standard) and inherently weaker large-scale long-term prospective cohort studies.[61] Combining these different types of studies dilutes the overwhelmingly positive evidence found that dairy foods protect against bone health in randomized controlled trials.[46,61]

In addition to reducing older adults' risk of osteoporosis, consuming a diet containing calcium-rich foods helps to protect against hypertension and colon cancer, two chronic diseases affecting older adults.[62-64] According to the Dietary Approaches to Stop Hypertension (DASH) study, intake of a diet reduced in fat and high in low-fat dairy foods (3 servings/day) and fruits and vegetables (8 to 10 servings/day) not only reduced blood pressure in non-hypertensive and hypertensive adults but also decreased blood pressure to levels that rival those achieved with antihypertensive medication.[62] The DASH diet is endorsed by federal government and health professional organizations, including the National Heart, Lung and Blood Institute and the American Heart Association.[63,65] Increasing intake of low-fat dairy foods to reach 1,500 mg calcium/day is associated with reduced risk of colon cancer in adults at risk of this disease.[64] Also, calcium intake, particularly from dairy products, may have a beneficial role in controlling body fat, according to recent experimental animal and human epidemiologic studies.[28]

Considering calcium's many health benefits and older adults' generally low calcium intake, considerable interest centers on how best to meet calcium needs. Foods are the preferred source of calcium.[37,46,47,66] Milk and other dairy foods are the major dietary sources of calcium in the US diet.[67] Also, because these foods provide other essential nutrients, their intake improves the overall nutritional quality of the diet, with little or no effect on calorie or fat intake, body weight, or percent body fat.[47,67] As shown in Figure 5, when older adult women increased their intake of fluid milk (fat-free or 1%) by three 8-ounce servings/day for 12 weeks, their intake of several nutrients, especially vitamin D, calcium, vitamin B_{12}, and riboflavin substantially increased.[66]

In addition to dairy foods, other foods, such as some green leafy vegetables, legumes, and cereals provide calcium, although generally in lower amounts per serving than dairy foods. Also, some components, such as phytates in cereals and oxalates in spinach, reduce the bioavailability of calcium.[37] Calcium-fortified foods and calcium supplements are another option for older adults who cannot meet their calcium needs from foods naturally containing this mineral. However, their intake cannot correct poor dietary patterns of food selection, which underlie many older adults' low calcium intake.

DIETARY GUIDANCE AND POLICIES DIRECTED TO OLDER ADULTS

The Dietary Guidelines for Americans[25] targets all healthy Americans across a wide range age (ie, two years of age and older). However, older adults' unique nutrient needs and their increased risk for nutrient deficiencies and chronic diseases support consideration of separate dietary guidelines. Recently, a modification of USDA's

Food Guide Pyramid has been published to help adults 70 years of age and older meet their unique nutrient needs.[68] This modified Pyramid emphasizes nutrient-dense foods, fiber, and water. Because older adults have decreased energy needs and constant or higher nutrient needs than their younger counterparts, intake of nutrient-dense foods (ie, a high ratio of nutrients to energy) within each food group category is recommended,[68] Older adults are advised to consume a diet low in saturated fat (<10% of calories) and cholesterol (< 300 mg/day) and moderate in total fat (30% or less of calories).[25,65]

Effective policies must be put in place to reduce malnutrition and food insecurity among older adults, to prolong their independence, and to decrease nursing home admissions and hospitalizations.

Although dietary fat (saturated, mono- and polyunsaturated, trans fat) has received the most attention in relation to risk of heart disease in later years, several other dietary factors are being investigated for their role in this disease.[65] These include energy balance, dietary antioxidants, homocysteine, fiber, alcohol, and phytoestrogens.[65] An elevated blood cholesterol level is a risk factor for heart disease. However, some research indicates that cholesterol levels may be less predictive of heart disease in older adults than they are in younger adults.[69] Also, when subsets of older adults were examined, very low blood cholesterol levels were associated with increased morbidity and mortality.[4] Therefore, efforts to lower blood cholesterol levels may not be equally beneficial or without risk for all older adults. Intake of the DASH diet, a low-fat diet rich in low-fat dairy products, fruits, and vegetables, has recently been demonstrated to reduce risk for heart disease by 7% to 9% by lowering blood homocysteine levels.[70]

Fluid intake is a highly important, but often overlooked, consideration for older adults.[3,4,71,72] The 70+ Food Pyramid recommends that older adults consume at least 2 quarts (8 cups) of water per day.[68] A number of factors, including physical activity, medications, renal function, ambient temperature, and an age-related decrease in thirst sensation, influence older adults' fluid needs.[22,71] Dehydration can increase older adults' risk of infections, constipation, pneumonia, pressure ulcers, and confusion/disorientation.[71]

With the aging of the US population, policy issues related to not only dietary guidance but also to delivering health and other services to this population are at the forefront. Because nutrition is critical to health, functioning, and quality of life, it is an important component of policies to improve older adults' health status and prolong their functional independence.[4] Many older adults are at nutritional risk, particularly the frail homebound elderly, and many participate in congregate meal programs or receive home-delivered meals often following a hospital or nursing stay.[4,15] Effective policies must be put in place to reduce malnutrition and food insecurity among older adults, to prolong their independence, and to decrease nursing home admissions and hospitalizations.

Recent advances have been made in policies related to determining the nutritional status of older adults. Previously, national nutrition surveys rarely, if at all, included adults older than 74 years. Now, surveys such as USDA's Continuing Survey of Food Intakes by Individuals (CSFII), 1994-1996,[10] and the Third National Health and Nutrition Examination Survey (NHANES), Phase I,[9] among others, include adults in their 70s and older. Despite these advances, there is still room for improvement. The US Department of Health and Human Services' *Healthy People 2010 National Health Promotion and Disease Prevention Objectives for the Nation* do not include a separate aging or nutrition section.[73]

After age 65, quality of life can change dramatically. Basically, there are two seasons of aging: independence and dependence. Obviously, the goal is to maintain independence for as long as possible. To maintain older adults' independence, various programs and policies are in place, including nutrient recommendations for older adults and managed care with access to nutrition services. The current emphasis of managed care is on health maintenance and disease prevention. For dependent older adults, the quality and cost effectiveness of care need to be improved. More attention should be given to meeting the nutritional and hydration needs of dependent older adults with chronic diseases such as diabetes mellitus. The quality of nursing home care, especially in preventing malnutrition, dehydration, urinary tract infections, and bedsores, is of primary concern. Recently, a Senate Select Committee on Aging hearing and a Government Accounting Office report in California identified deficiencies in nursing homes that were contributing to residents' malnutrition and dehydration. Efforts are underway to amend legislation that would provide coverage for the nutrition therapy services of registered dietitians and health professionals under the Medicare Program (Medical Nutrition Therapy Act). Recent studies document the cost-effectiveness of medical nutrition therapy.[74-76] According to a study carried out by the Lewin Group, providing medical nutrition therapy to the Medicare population would pay for itself with savings in use of other services after a 3-year period.[76] Health professional organizations such as the American Dietetic Association recognize the importance of meeting the nutritional needs of both independent and dependent older adults.[4,34]

CONCLUSION

Older adults are a diverse, heterogeneous group with unique nutritional needs and health risks. Health professionals, such as nutrition educators and dietitians, can provide practical dietary and lifestyle advice tailored to individuals in this growing segment of the population to help them age successfully and ensure their quality of life. Healthful food choices, including high-quality, nutrient-dense foods, adequate hydration, and regular physical activity, are critical components of successful aging.

Lifestyle choices such as food, nutrition, and exercise determine how well we age, regardless of how late in life they are initiated, according to Drs Rowe and Kahn in their book, *Successful Aging.*[77] What does successful aging mean? According to these authors, it means avoiding disease and disability, maintaining high cognitive and physical functioning, and being engaged with life.[77] In this era of accountability, the challenge facing health professionals is to demonstrate that effective interventions produce long-term outcomes and that there is an opportunity to age successfully.

ACKNOWLEDGMENT

The authors thank the following expert panel members: Carole Suitor, ScD, RD; John E. Morley, MB, BCh; Philip J. Garry, PhD; William Evans, PhD; Robert Russell, MD; Robert P. Heaney, MD; Stephen Kritchevsky, PhD; Nancy S. Wellman, PhD, RD; Sandra Raymond; Ronnie Chernoff, PhD; and Connie W. Bales, PhD, RD.

REFERENCES

1. US Census Bureau, Population Division, Population Projections Branch, Population Projections. Available at: www.census.gov/population/www/ projections/ popproj.html. Accessed October 12, 2000.
2. American Association of Retired Persons, Resource Services Group. *A profile of older Americans: 1997.* Washington, DC: AARP Fulfillment; 1997.
3. Russell RM, Rasmussen H. The impact of nutritional needs of older adults on recommended food intakes. *Nutr Clin Care.* 1999;2:164–176.
4. American Dietetic Association. Position of the American Dietetic Association: nutrition, aging, and the continuum of care. *J Am Diet Assoc.* 2000;100:580–595.
5. Guralnik JM, Fried LP, Salive ME. Disability as a public health outcome in the aging population. *Annu Rev Public Health.* 1996;17:25–46.
6. Sattin RW. Falls among older persons: a public health perspective. *Annu Rev Public Health.* 1992;13:489–508.
7. Gaston NW, Mardis A, Gerrior S, Sahyoun N, Anand RS. A focus on nutrition for the elderly: it's time to take a closer look. *Nutrition Insight.* 1999;14:1–2.
8. FASEB (Federation of American Societies for Experimental Biology), Life Sciences Research Office. Prepared for the Interagency Board for Nutrition Monitoring and Related Research. *Third Report on Nutrition Monitoring in the United States: Volumes 1 and 2.* Washington, DC: US Government Printing Office; 1995.
9. Alaimo K, McDowell MA, Briefel RR, Bischof AM, Gaughman, CR, Loria CM, et al. *Dietary intake of vitamins, minerals, and fiber of persons ages 2 months and over in the United States: Third National Health and Nutrition Examination Survey, Phase I, 1988–91. Advance Data from Vital and Health Statistics; No. 258.* Hyattsville, MD: US Department of Health and Human Services, National Center for Health Statistics; 1994.
10. US Department of Agriculture, Agricultural Research Service, 1997. Data tables: Results from USDA's 1994–96 Continuing Survey of Food Intakes by Individuals and 1994–96 Diet and Health Knowledge Survey [Online]. ARS Food Surveys Research Group. Available at: http:// www.barc.usda.gov/bhnrc/ foodsurvey/home.htm. Accessed November 2000.
11. Gerrior SA. Dietary changes in older Americans from 1977 to 1996: implications for dietary quality. *Family Economics and Nutrition Review.* 1999;12:3–14.
12. Krebs-Smith SM, Cleveland LE, Ballard-Barbash R, Cook DA, Kahle LL. Characterizing food intake patterns of American adults. *Am J Clin Nutr.* 1997;65(suppl 4):1264s–1268s.
13. Foote JA, Giuliano AR, Harris RB. Older adults need guidance to meet nutritional recommendations. *J Am Coll Nutr.* 2000;19:628–640.
14. Fischer JG, Johnson MA, Poon LW, Martin P. Dairy product intake of the oldest old. *J Am Diet Assoc.* 1995;95:918–920.
15. Wellman NS, Weddle DO, Kranz S, Brain CT. Elder insecurities: poverty, hunger, and malnutrition. *J Am Diet Assoc.* 1997;97(suppl 2):120s–122s.
16. Hartz SC, Russell RM, Rosenberg IH, eds. *Nutrition in the Elderly. The Boston Nutritional Status Survey.* London: Smith-Gordon; 1992.
17. Anderson RN, Kochanek KD, Murphy SL. Report of final mortality statistics, 1995. *Monthly Vital Stat Rep.* 1997;45(suppl 2):1–80.
18. Fried LP, Kronmal RA, Newman AB, Bild DE, Mittelmark MB, Polak JF, et al. Risk factors for 5-year mortality in older adults. *JAMA.* 1998;279:585–592.
19. Sahyoun N, Basiotis PP. Food insufficiency and the nutritional status of the elderly population. *Nutrition Insights.* 2000;18:1–2.
20. Schiffman SS. Taste and smell losses in normal aging and disease. *JAMA.* 1997;278:1357–1362.
21. Morley JE. Anorexia of aging: physiologic and pathologic. *Am J Clin Nutr.* 1997;66:760–773.
22. Morley JE, Glick Z, Rubenstein LZ, eds. *Geriatric Nutrition. A Comprehensive Review.* 2nd ed. New York: Raven Press; 1995.
23. Roberts SB. Energy regulation and aging: recent findings and their implications. *Nutr Rev.* 2000;58:91–97.
24. Jensen GL, Rogers J. Obesity in older persons. *J Am Diet Assoc.* 1998;98:1308–1311.
25. US Department of Agriculture, US Department of Health and Human Services. *Nutrition and Your Health: Dietary Guidelines for Americans.* 5th ed. Home and Garden Bulletin No. 232. Washington, DC: US Departments of Agriculture and Health and Human Services; 2000.
26. Mussolino ME, Looker AC, Madans JH, Langlois JA, Orwall ES. Risk factors for hip fracture in white men: The NHANES I epidemiologic follow-up study. *J Bone Miner Res.* 1998;13:918–924.
27. Ricci TA, Chowdhury HA, Heymsfield SB, Stahl T, Pierson RN Jr, Shapes SA. Calcium supplementation suppresses bone turnover during weight reduction in postmenopausal women. *J Bone Miner Res.* 1998;13:1045–1050.
28. Zemel MB, Shi H, Greer B, DiRienzo D, Zemel PC. Regulation of adiposity by dietary calcium. *FASEB J.* 2000;14:1132–1138.
29. Evans WJ, Cyr-Campbell D. Nutrition, exercise, and healthy aging. *J Am Diet Assoc.* 1997;97:632–638.
30. Bunyard LB, Katzel LI, Busby-Whitehead MJ, Wu Z, Goldberg AP. Energy requirements of middle-aged men are modifiable by physical activity. *Am J Clin Nutr.* 1998;68:1136–1142.
31. Campbell WW, Crim MC, Young VR, Evans WJ. Increased energy requirements and body composition changes with

resistance training in older adults. *Am J Clin Nutr.* 1994;60:167–175.

32. Fiatarone MA, O'Neill EF, Ryan ND, Clements KM, Solares GR, Nelson ME, et al. Exercise training and nutritional supplementation for physical frailty in very elderly people. *N Engl J Med.* 1994;330:1769–1775.

33. Satariano WA, Haight T-J, Tager IB. Reasons given by older people for limitations or avoidance of leisure time physical activity. *J Am Geriatr Soc.* 2000;48:505–512.

34. Expert Committee of Nutrition and Health for Older Americans. *The Nutrition and Health Campaign for Older Americans Toolkit.* Chicago, Ill: American Dietetic Association; 1998.

35. National Research Council, Subcommittee on the 10th Edition of the RDAs, Commission on Life Sciences. *Dietary Allowances.* 10th ed. Washington, DC: National Academy Press; 1989.

36. Institute of Medicine, Food and Nutrition Board. *Dietary Reference Intakes for Thiamin, Riboflavin, Niacin, Vitamin B6, Folate, Vitamin B_{12}, Pantothenic Acid, Biotin, and Choline.* Washington, DC: National Academy Press; 1998.

37. Institute of Medicine, Food and Nutrition Board. *Dietary Reference Intakes for Calcium, Phosphorus, Magnesium, Vitamin D, and Fluoride.* Washington, DC: National Academy Press; 1997.

38. Institute of Medicine, Food and Nutrition Board. *Dietary Reference Intakes for Vitamin C, Vitamin E, Selenium, and Carotenoids.* Washington, DC: National Academy Press; 2000.

39. Campbell WW. Dietary protein requirements of older people: is the RDA adequate? *Nutr Today.* 1996;31:192–197.

40. Campbell WW, Crim MC, Young VR, Joseph LJ, Evans WJ. Effects of resistance training and dietary protein intake on protein metabolism in older adults. Part 1. *Am J Physiol.* 1995;268(6):E1143–E1153.

41. Russell RM. New views on the RDAs for older adults. *J Am Diet Assoc.* 1997;97:515–518.

42. Boisvert WA, Mendoza I, Castaneda C, de Portocarrero L, Solomons NW, Gershoff SN, et al. Riboflavin requirement of healthy elderly humans and its relationship to macronutrient composition of the diet. *J Nutr.* 1993;123:915–924.

43. Selhub J, Bagley LC, Miller J, Rosenberg IH. B vitamins, homocysteine, and neurocognitive function in the elderly. *Am J Clin Nutr.* 2000;71(suppl): 614s–620s.

44. Tucker KL, Rich S, Rosenberg I, Jacques P, Dallal G, Wilson PWF, et al. Plasma vitamin B^{12} concentrations relate to intake source in the Framingham Offspring Study. *Am J Clin Nutr.* 2000;71:514–522.

45. NIH Consensus Development Panel on Osteoporosis prevention, diagnosis, and therapy. JAMA. 2001; 285:785–795.

46. Heaney RP. Calcium, dairy products and osteoporosis. *J Am Coll Nutr.* 2000;19(suppl):83s–99s.

47. Heaney RP, McCarron DA, Dawson-Hughes B, Oparil S, Berga SL, Stern JS, et al. Dietary changes favorably affect bone remodeling in older adults. *J Am Diet Assoc.* 1999;99:1228–1233.

48. Recker RR, Hinders S, Davies KM, Heaney RP, Stegman MR, Lappe JM, et al. Correcting calcium nutritional deficiency prevents spine fractures in elderly women. *J Bone Miner Res.* 1996;11:1961–1966.

49. Peacock M, Liu G, Carey M, McClintock R, Ambrosius W, Hui S, et al. Effect of calcium or 25 OH Vitamin D3 dietary supplementation on bone loss at the hip in men and women over the age of 60. *J Clin Endocrinol Metab.* 2000;95:3011–3019.

50. Heaney RP, Recker PR, Stegmen MR, Moy AJ. Calcium absorption in women: relationships to calcium intake, estrogen status, and age. *J Bone Miner Res.* 1989;4: 469–475.

51. Heaney RP. The bone remodeling transient: implications for the interpretation of clinical studies of bone mass change. *J Bone Miner Res.* 1994;9:1515–1523.

52. Ensrud KE, Duong T, Cauley JA, Heaney RP, Wolf RL, Harris E, Cummings SR for the Study of Osteoporotic Fractures Research Group. Low fractional calcium absorption increases the risk for hip fractures in women with low calcium intake. *Ann Intern Med.* 2000;132:345–353.

53. Heaney RP Excess dietary protein may not adversely affect bone. *J Nutr.* 1998;128:1054–1057.

54. Heaney RP Dietary protein and phosphorus do not affect calcium absorption. *Am J Clin Nutr.* 2000;72:758–761.

55. Keane EM, Healy M, O'Moore R, Coakley D, Walsh JB. Vitamin D-fortified liquid milk: benefits for the elderly community-based population. *Calcif Tissue Int.* 1998;62:300–302.

56. Chapuy MC, Arlot ME, Duboeuf F, Brun J, Crouzet B, Arnaud S, et al. Vitamin D and calcium to prevent hip fractures in elderly women. *N Engl J Med.* 1992;327:1637–1642.

57. Dawson-Hughes B, Harris SS, Krall EA, Dallal GE. A controlled calcium and vitamin D supplementation trial in men and women age 65 and older. *N Engl J Med.* 1997;337:670–676.

58. Dawson-Hughes B, Harris SS, Krall EA, Dallal GE. Effect of withdrawal of calcium and vitamin D on bone mass in elderly men and women. *Am J Clin Nutr.* 2000;72:745–750.

59. Heaney RP More evidence and still no action[editorial]. *J Clin Endocrinol Metab.* 2000;86:3009–3010.

60. Weinsier RL, Krumdieck CL. Dairy foods and bone health: examination of the evidence. *Am J Clin Nutr.* 2000;72:681–689.

61. Weaver CM, Heaney RP. Letter to the editor. *Am J Clin Nutr.* 2001;73:600.

62. Appel LJ, Moore TJ, Obarzanek E, Vollmer WM, Svetkey LP, Sacks FM, et al. A clinical trial of the effects of dietary patterns on blood pressure. *N Engl J Med.* 1997;336:1117–1124.

63. Miller GD, DiRienzo DD, Reusser ME, McCarron DA. Benefits of dairy product consumption on blood pressure in humans: a summary of the biomedical literature. *J Am Coll Nutr.* 2000;19(suppl):147s–164s.

64. Holt PR, Atillasoy EO, Gilman J, Guss J, Moss SF, Newmark H, et al. Modulation of abnormal colonic epithelial cell proliferation and differentiation by low-fat dairy foods. *JAMA.* 1998;280:1074–1079.

65. Krauss RM, Eckel RH, Howard B, et. al. AHA dietary guidelines. Revision 2000: a statement for healthcare professionals from the Nutrition Committee of the American Heart Association. *Circulation.* 2000;102:2284–2299.

66. Barr SI, McCarron DA, Heaney RP, Dawson-Hughes B, Berga SL, Stern JS, et al. Effects of increased consumption of fluid milk on energy and nutrient intake, body weight, and cardiovascular risk factors in healthy older adults. *J Am Diet Assoc.* 2000;100:810–817.

67. Gerrior S, Bente L. *Nutrient Content of the US Food Supply 1909–97. Home Economics Research Report No. 54.* Washington, DC: US Department of Agriculture, Center for Nutrition Policy and Promotion; 2001.

68. Russell RM, Rasmussen H, Lichtenstein AH. Modified Food Guide Pyramid for people over seventy years of age. *J Nutr.* 1999;129:751–753.

69. Kronmal RA, Cain KC, Ye Z, Omenn GS. Total serum cholesterol levels and mortality risk as a function of age. A report based on the Framingham data. *Arch Intern Med.* 1993;153:1065–1073.

70. Appel LJ, Miller ER III, Jee SH, Stolzenberg-Solomon R, Lin P-H, Erlinger T, et al. Effect of dietary patterns on serum homocysteine. Results of a randomized, controlled feeding trial. *Circulation.* 2000;102:852–857.

71. Chidester JC, Spangler AA. Fluid intake in the institutionalized elderly. *J Am Diet Assoc.* 1997;97:23–28.
72. Kleiner SM. Water: an essential but overlooked nutrient. *J Am Diet Assoc.* 1999;99:200–206.
73. US Department of Health and Human Services. *Healthy People 2010 (Conference Edition in Two Volumes).* Washington, DC: US Government Printing Office; 2000.
74. Barents Group. *The clinical and cost-effectiveness of medical nutrition therapy: evidence and estimates of potential Medicare savings from the use of selected nutrition interventions.* Washington DC: Nutrition Screening Initiative; 1996.
75. Johnson RK. The Lewin Group study—what does it tell us and why does it matter? *J Am Diet Assoc.* 1999;99:426–427.
76. Sheils JF, Rubin R, Stapleton DC. The estimated costs and savings of medical nutrition therapy: the Medicare population. *J Am Diet Assoc.* 1999;99:428–435.
77. Rowe JW, Kahn RL. *Successful Aging.* New York: Pantheon Books; 1998.

Lois D. McBean, MS, RD, Ann Arbor, Mich, is a consultant for the National Dairy Council.

Susan M. Groziak, PhD, RD, is an assistant professor, Finch University School of Related Health Sciences, The Chicago Medical School, North Chicago, Ill.

Gregory D. Miller, PhD, FACN, is vice-president, Nutrition Research and Technology Transfer, National Dairy Council, Rosemont, Ill.

Judith K. Jarvis, MS, RD, LD, is manager, Nutrition and Health Information, National Dairy Council, Rosemont, Ill.

From the National Dairy Council, Rosemont, Ill (Ms McBean, Dr Miller, and Ms Jarvis), and the Finch University School of Related Health Sciences, The Chicago Medical School, North Chicago, Ill (Dr Groziak).

Address correspondence and reprint requests to: Judith K. Jarvis, MS, RD, LD, Manager, Nutrition and Health Information, National Dairy Council, 10255 West Higgins Rd, Suite 900, Rosemont, IL 60018–5616 (e-mail: judithj@rosedmi.com).

From *Nutrition Today,* Vol. 38, July/August 2001, pp. 192-201. © 2001 by Lippincott Williams & Wilkins, a Wolters Kluwer Company. Reprinted by permission.

The Female Athlete Triad: Nutrition, Menstrual Disturbances, and Low Bone Mass

The female athlete triad represents the combination of disordered eating, amenorrhea, and osteopenia or osteoporosis. Women who otherwise consider themselves to be in exceptional condition may be most vulnerable to these complications. This manuscript provides a review of literature pertaining to the female athlete triad and examines the related nutritional risks.

LEE E. THRASH, BS, AND JOHN J.B. ANDERSON, PhD

INTRODUCTION

The female athlete triad—disordered eating behaviors, oligomenorrhea/amenorrhea, and osteopenia/osteoporosis (Fig. 1)—is an area of immense concern for women who otherwise consider themselves to be in superior physical condition. Highly competitive women in sports or other activities that emphasize endurance (long-distance running, rowing, etc.) or physical conformation and appearance (gymnastics, ballet dancing, figure skating, diving, etc.) may be at greatest risk of succumbing to the triad.[1] One study, for example, performed on a group of lean, college female gymnasts revealed that the majority were not satisfied with their current body weight and appearance.[2] These results suggest the presence of underlying issues, such as psychological factors and societal pressures, that may negatively affect the women's perspective of themselves.

The triad of disordered eating, menstrual irregularity, and osteopenia afflicts too many female athletes.

The first manifestation of the triad is usually erratic eating behaviors to control body weight, including poor food choices and meal skipping, which are typically combined with high-intensity exercise.[2] In order to enhance performance or to comply with society's view of the ideal for thinness, many females further reduce their caloric consumption to lose pounds or to maintain a low body weight. This decreased caloric intake by athletes may lead to deficiencies in numerous micronutrients, including calcium, and the rates of peak performance may decline because of reduced intakes of both energy and nutrients. Amenorrhea or oligomenorrhea in female athletes may result from the subsequent exercise stress and low energy availability.[3] Consequently, lower circulating plasma estrogen levels may reduce calcium retention by bone and lead to osteopenia (low bone mass) and premature osteoporosis.[2] The lack of menstruation for extended periods of time (more than six months) may cause a decrease in bone density that is potentially irreversible. Low bone mineral density (BMD) heightens the risk of stress fractures, especially of the spine and hip.[2] The combined strain of these factors may also lead to future complications. Singly, or in combination, the components of the female athlete triad may contribute to decreased physical performance, morbidity, and the deterioration of health. The aim of this manuscript is to provide a review of current information relating to these aspects of the female athlete triad.

EATING DISORDERS

Some female athletes, especially gymnasts and dancers, begin training as young as the age of three. By the time they reach adolescence, an ideal "body image" for their sport pressures them to look lean and perfectly fit. In addition, some females want to obtain an optimally thin

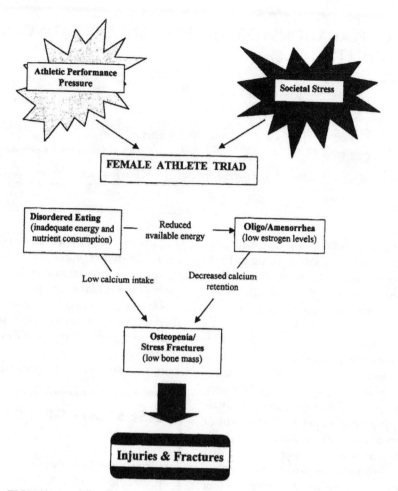

FIGURE 1. The female athlete triad.

body weight to enhance athletic performance. These pressures on many female athletes to be thin may lead to disordered eating behaviors, including, but not limited to, anorexia nervosa (a psychiatric disorder consisting of an unwillingness or inability to consume enough calories to maintain a healthy weight), bulimia nervosa (binge eating followed by purging, vomiting, or excessive laxative use), anorexia or bulimia with excessive exercise, and/or normal food intake with excessive exercise patterns. Any of these behaviors creating low energy availability may be associated with the cessation of menstruation. In turn, amenorrhea leads to inadequate production of estrogen, especially during the critical adolescent period. These problems are most commonly observed in activities that are judged in part on appearance (such as gymnastics, ballet, diving, and figure skating), and a fear of losing one's level of athletic performance may contribute to one of the above practices. However, in actuality, the women are depriving their own bodies of essential nutrients and ultimately harming their performance and encouraging potential injuries.

Further ramifications of disordered eating by female athletes, other than poor performance and deficient nutrient intakes, include fatigue, decreased immunity, cogni-

tive losses, decreased concentration, and risk of depression, suicide, and other psychological problems related to low self-esteem.[4] If a severe eating disorder such as anorexia nervosa ensues, an athletic woman may experience seizures, cardiac arrhythmia, myocardial infarction, or other critical complications—possibly leading to morbidity and chronic disease.

Osteopenia is a known complication of anorexia nervosa. In a retrospective investigation measuring BMD of the hip and lumbar spine in 18 recovered anorexic women, an unexpectedly high incidence of osteopenia was found, with 14 of the 18 women affected. The previous duration of amenorrhea and the duration of anorexia nervosa of the subjects were both highly correlated with reduced BMD.[5]

Female athletes too frequently make poor food choices that do not adequately meet the energy needs of their active lifestyles because of peer and societal pressures to be thin. For example, some vegetarian choices may deprive these women of energy and selected micronutrients, such as vitamin B12 and iron. In a vegetarian (vegan) athlete, this potential deprivation may be detrimental to her general health in addition to her performance. A vegetarian diet may, however, be beneficial because of nutrients pro-

Table 1. POSSIBLE EXPLANATIONS FOR THE PREVALENCE OF EATING DISORDERS AMONG FEMALE ATHLETES

- Competitive athletic atmosphere
- Constant pressure to succeed
- Heightened body awareness
- Compulsiveness and perfectionism
- Fluctuation of self-esteem with fluctuation of performance

- Ability to block pain and hunger
- Willingness to take unnecessary risks to win
- Importance of aesthetics in sport or dance
- Belief that body leanness optimizes performance
- Lack of identity beyond the sport or dance

Adapted from Anderson et al.[14]

vided by increased fruit and vegetable consumption and decreased intake of foods high in fat, salt, and sugar. Physicians and nutritionists recommend, nonetheless, that strict vegetarians, ie, those following a vegan diet, may need to be screened for potential disordered eating behaviors.[6]

Risk factors for the development of eating disorders in female collegiate athletes were examined in a correlational study[7] that suggests that symptoms of eating disorders are significantly influenced by the interaction of the sociocultural pressure for thinness, athletic performance anxiety, and negative self-appraisal of athletic achievement. If having these risk factors leads to excessive concern with body size and shape, then the emergence of an eating disorder is more probable.[7] Related critical trigger factors associated with the onset of disordered eating among female athletes include prolonged or erratic periods of dieting, skipping of meals, frequent weight fluctuations, a sudden increase in training volume, and traumatic personal injuries. Table 1 summarizes possible explanations for the prevalence of eating disorders among female athletes.

Athletes with the female athlete triad are strongly advised to obtain nutrition counseling for the wise selection of foods that provide adequate nutrients, especially calcium-containing dairy foods. The goal is to prevent the relapse of eating disorders, a common occurrence,[8] as well as to delay osteoporosis and to prevent other consequences of the triad.

Eating disorders prove to be a continuing concern for female athletes. Body image is drastically emphasized in many sports; some events even incorporate this image into judging and performance. The pressure placed upon young athletes sometimes proves too intense, resulting in abnormal eating behaviors or binge/purge cycles. Society and performance demands greatly contribute to this incredible pressure to be thin, and, for some athletes, eating disorders may become permanent.

MENSTRUAL IRREGULARITIES

Amenorrhea is defined as the absence or suppression of the menstrual period to fewer than four per year, ie, 0 to

3. Primary amenorrhea consists of no menses prior to age 16, while the secondary form is classified as one or more episodes of menstrual bleeding prior to cessation. Oligomenorrhea is classified as a sporadic menstrual cycle (3–9 menses per year). Amenorrhea and especially oligomenorrhea are more common in athletes than in nonathletes, and particularly in endurance performers. Altered menstrual cyclicity approached 70% in strenuously exercising women, according to one study.[9]

CASE STUDY OF A DISTANCE RUNNER

A case study of an 18-year-old cross-country distance runner illustrates the female athlete triad and its applicable treatment.[14] This young athlete experienced aggravated pain in her left thigh and right tibia and she was diagnosed with the following: multiple stress fractures, iron deficiency anemia, exercise-associated oligomenorrhea, and a possible eating disorder. Her eating practices, ie, too little food consumption, were typical of those experiencing the female athlete triad. Consequently, the young woman noted a general decline in energy and complained of feeling lightheaded during intense interval training and a slowing of her usual race times. At her one-month follow-up, the athlete displayed good compliance with iron replacement as manifested by the reappearance of menses and the return of red blood cell indices toward normal. Furthermore, at 10 weeks, she showed satisfactory clinical healing of the stress fractures. This case highlights the great need for, and efficacy of, education among highly competitive athletes concerning diet and osteoporosis.[14]

Blood concentrations of estrogen and progesterone depend on a balance between production, metabolism, and clearance rates. Intensive physical exercise may affect this balance via different mechanisms, such as stress and dieting.[10] Amenorrhea or oligomenorrhea may occur as a result of abnormalities of the female reproductive tract,

Table 2. RECOMMENDED INTAKES OF NUTRIENTS FOR ADULT FEMALE ATHLETES (18 AND OLDER) IN RELATION TO BONE HEALTH

Nutrient Variable	Recommended: RDA or AI	Additional Amounts Needed According to ↑ Energy Expenditure
Energy, kcal	2200 (RDA)	+
Protein, g	50 (RDA)	+
Calcium, mg	1000 (AI)	+
Magnesium, mg	280 (RDA)	+
Vitamin D, IU	400 (AI)[*]	
Vitamin K, mg	70 (RDA)	+

Note: RDA = Recommended Dietary Allowance; AI = adequate intake.

[*]400 IU = µg

Adapted from Anderson et al.[14]

hypothalamus, or pituitary gland; ovarian failure; chromosomal anomalies; steroid use; insufficient body fat stores; or a genetic disorder.[11] Amenorrhea may also be associated with emotional or physical stress; severe dieting, including eating disorders; or increased levels of exercise. Other potential factors that contribute to irregularities are depression, malnutrition, drugs, chronic illness,[12] strict vegetarianism, low caloric intakes, and specific training behaviors.[13]

Although the precise mechanism is unknown, exercise-associated amenorrhea is considered most likely to be a form of hypothalamic amenorrhea.[14] Specifically, amenorrhea is caused by a reduction in the frequency of gonadotrophic releasing hormone (GnRH) secreted from the hypothalamus.[3] Both exercise stress and energy availability are being investigated as potential causes of this disruption.[3] Exercise, in particular, has been shown to activate the hypothalamic-pituitary-adrenal axis acutely.[15] For instance, cortisol levels of amenorrheic athletes remain elevated throughout the day and evening, unlike the normal, ie, eumenorrheic (having regular menses), pattern of cortisol elevation solely in the early morning.[16]

Menstrual disturbances and bone density problems are related.

Optimal treatment for exercise-associated amenorrhea remains controversial, but the following figures from a recent survey reflect physician practices regarding preferred management of female athletes: 92%—sex steroid replacement, 87%—calcium supplementation, 64%—increased caloric intake, 57%—decreased exercise intensity, 43%—weight gain, and 26%—vitamin supplementation.[17] These findings suggest that increasing circulating levels of estrogens and progestins and incorporating elevated calcium in-

takes may prove to be the most effective methods of treatment. Usually these will promote the resumption of menses. However, the inconsistent treatment practices evident in this survey show the need for further research as well as education of physicians in treatment options.

OSTEOPENIA/OSTEOPOROSIS

The nutritional needs of female athletes are principally determined by their size (weight and height), training load (frequency and duration), and lean body mass. Table 2 lists general dietary recommendations for the optimal bone health of athletes, as well as necessary increases in particular nutrients when energy expenditure is high. Peak bone mass, which is defined as the greatest amount of bone at any time of life, is typically attained by the age of 30 years or even earlier. Before this age, bone modeling, or the development of this dynamic tissue, predominates; skeletal growth (height) of girls is normally completed by 16 to 18 years, depending on the age of menarche. Bone remodeling is the process through which bone is lost and reformed; this occurs throughout life. Osteopenia is defined as low BMD, while the accepted definition of osteoporosis is BMD greater than 2.5 standard deviations below the mean values for healthy young adults.[18]

Stress fractures occur in a small percentage of athletes, especially runners, but they may account for as much as 10% of all sports-related injuries. A stress fracture (minimal or traumatic) is a partial or complete fracture of bone resulting in the inability of the athlete to withstand rhythmic, nonviolent stress applied repeatedly in a submaximal manner.[19] Stress fractures are a major concern for athletes, not only because of the physical consequences but also because of the temporary (or permanent) cessation from training. Female athletes, especially those women with decreased BMD and menstrual disturbances, experience these fractures much more often than

Table 3. CROSS-SECTIONAL STUDIES OF BMD IN FEMALE ATHLETES

Study	Subjects	Bone Mineral Density
Alfredson et al.[32]	Volleyball players	Total body, lumbar spine, femoral neck, Ward's triangle, trochanter, non-dominant femur, humerus are all significantly higher in athletes than in controls.
Kirchner et al.[33]	Gymnasts	Athletes maintained higher BMD than controls.
Robinson et al.[22]	Runners and gymnasts	Eumenorrheics maintained slightly higher BMDs than amenorrheics. Runner's whole body BMD lower than gymnasts or controls.
Young et al.[34]	Dancers	BMD was elevated at weight-bearing sites. BMD deficits similar to those found in anorexics in non-weight-bearing sites.
Haenggi et al.[35]	Nonathletes	BMD is lower in amenorrheic women than in eumenorrheic controls. Hormone-replacement therapy resulted in increased BMD.
Rutherford[36]	Triathletes and runners	Lumbar spine, arm, trunk, total spine—Amenorrheics less than eumenorrheics. Lumbar and total spine—Amenorrheics less than controls.
Myerson et al.[37]	Runners	Amenorrheics less than eumenorrheics, but not significantly different from controls.
Wolman et al.[38]	Elite athletes	Amenorrheics less than eumenorrheics and OCA users.
Snead et al.[39]	Runners	Lumbar spine--oligomenorrheics and amenorrheics less than eumenorrheics.

BMD = Bone Mineral Density

men.[20,21] As a result, low BMDs in athletic women may serve as a signal of potential risk for future bone injury.

Female military populations have been shown to be at risk of stress fracture 1.2 to 10 times that of men. This increased rate persists even when training loads are gradually increased to moderate levels. Possible reasons for these findings include lower BMD, differences in gait, slender bones, unfavorable biomechanical conditions, greater percentage of body fat, endocrine factors, and/or lower initial physical fitness.[20]

Low concentrations of ovarian hormones in amenorrhea and oligomenorrhea are associated with reduced bone mass and increased rates of bone loss.[3] Many studies have been performed on female athletes to examine the beneficial and adverse effects of menstruation status and certain activities on their BMD. Eumenorrheic women and those participating in weight-bearing exercises seem to maintain higher BMDs. Table 3 provides a summary of important cross-sectional research findings concerning the BMDs of female athletes in relation to specific sports and menstruation.

In one investigation of forty-four 20-year-old female gymnasts and runners, approximately one third of each group exhibited amenorrhea and oligomenorrhea; all control subjects were eumenorrheic.[22] Percent change of BMD was measured over an eight-month period, and it was shown that menstrual cycle status had a significant effect on percent change, which varied depending on skeletal site and type of sport. The decrease in BMD was greater in those athletes with irregular menstrual cycles. Initially higher BMD measurements in gymnasts, and continued improvement over time while active, suggest that the skeletal benefit results from both higher impact loads on the skeleton during training and greater calcium consumption.[22] A second study on gymnasts and runners confirmed the results of the previous study.[23]

Unfortunately, the effects on vertebral bone loss in oligomenorrheic/amenorrheic athletes seem to be irreversible and, therefore, intervention is necessary to prevent further bone loss. Keen et al.[24] suggested that in spite of several years of normal menses and/or the use of contraceptives, former oligomenorrheic/amenorrheic athletes continued to have a significantly lower BMD of the lumbar spine in comparison with athletes who had always had regular cycles. Their lumbar vertebral BMD was approximately 85% of that of the eumenorrheic athletes. Although resumption of regular menses for several months between episodes of amenorrhea or oligomenorrhea may exert a protective effect on bone, this study suggests that complete normalization of the vertebral BMD in former amenorrheic athletes is not likely.[24]

In other studies of female gymnasts, Lewis et al.[25,26] found that some athletes may be at risk for osteoporosis because of the combination of restrictive eating, intense exercise, and irregular menstruation. They compared the lumbar spine, hip bone, and whole body BMD of 26 female college gymnasts to a group of nonathletes of similar size, age, and weight. They also studied 18 former college gymnasts, aged 29–45 years, and compared them to another control group of women who had never competed in sports. Despite the gymnasts' restricted diets (especially inadequate dietary calcium) and high prevalence of menstrual irregularities, the younger gymnasts consistently had higher BMDs than their nonathlete counterparts.[25] Even the former gymnasts, whose lifestyles had since been altered to a more normal diet and exercise regimen, maintained elevated BMDs compared to other women their own age.[26] The critical skeletal sites that retained greater BMDs in both groups of gymnasts included the vertebrae, hip, and whole body. The main conclusion from these studies is that participation in gymnastics, and possibly other weight-bearing sports, actually helps to maintain BMD of vertebrae, hips, and whole body and might even protect these athletes from developing osteopenia and osteoporosis,[27] despite abnormal menstrual status during participation.

The prevention of osteoporosis and the subsequent reduction in fracture risk rests on the identification of those modifiable lifestyle factors that increase peak bone mass and, then, the optimization of behaviors that promote health. A threshold level of weight bearing (from exercise and body weight) is necessary to stimulate bone growth (osteogenesis), according to one study.[28] An understanding of the relationship between weight-bearing exercise and BMD is important in devising strategies to maximize

the skeletal strength of females. Other research has revealed that women who participate regularly in high-impact physical activity during the premenopausal years have higher BMDs at most skeletal sites than nonathletic control subjects.[29]

The triad of problems is best dealt with by prevention

Cyclic hormone therapy with conjugated estrogens (essential for maintaining normal bone density) and progesterone, or oral contraceptives, may also be beneficial, as may daily supplements of 1.5 grams of elemental calcium. Decreased intensity of training until menstruation resumes may be necessary as well.[19] Many young female athletes have low concentrations of circulating estrogens, which may lead to decreases in BMD, and these athletes would appear to benefit from hormone and diet therapy.

SUMMARY

Data on the prevalence of the triad do not exist. The prevalence of eating disorders in female athletes, however, has been determined to range from approximately 15% to 62%, while the prevalence of amenorrhea has been estimated to be 3.4% to 66%.[30] The broad ranges of values seem to overlap. The two mechanisms always present in amenorrheic women are psychologic stress and recent weight loss,[31] which also correlate highly with the female athlete triad. In addition, approximately 25–30% of women who are vegetarian athletes have menstrual irregularities, compared to 3–5% of women in the omnivorous population.[31] Many of these "health-conscious" females, and numerous others with atypical eating habits, are athletes. Irregular eating habits, combined with intense physical activity, may lead to weight loss. Peer and societal pressures to be thin and to accommodate a particular physique may cause some athletes to go to extreme measures. These adverse relationships advance the cycle of the female athlete triad and may contribute to its prevalence.

The duration of amenorrhea has also been found to be a powerful predictor of BMD.[4] It has been estimated that 40–60% of normal BMD develops during adolescence when sex hormones become active.[7] When a young athlete does not menstruate for an extended period of time, her bones may not accumulate sufficient mineral calcium to develop optimal strength and hardness and to achieve peak bone mass. Young amenorrheic female athletes in their early 20s who have consumed poor diets and produced inadequate amounts of estrogen, may have thin, fragile bones resembling women in their 70s.[7]

The female athlete triad represents the combination of disordered eating, amenorrhea, and osteopenia or osteoporosis. Although the typical group at risk tends to be high school and intercollegiate athletes and others in highly competitive settings, a large number of physically active girls and women are also at risk for developing the health problems associated with the triad. Good nutritional habits, in particular, are important for maintaining a high level of performance for all athletes. Low food intake of energy and inadequate consumption of many critical nutrients are of concern. Therefore, nutrition education of female athletes needs to receive greater emphasis in preventing the rising occurrence of sports-related injuries and other consequences of the female athlete triad. Alone, or in combination, these disorders may impair normal health and stamina and ultimately lead to fatigue, injury, future complications (including difficulties with childbearing), and fractures. All three components are integrally related and they should be treated as such.

REFERENCES

1. Wallace C. Female athletes at risk for the female athlete triad. Children's Hospital Medical Center of Akron News Source, 1996;12;1.
2. Nickols-Richardson SM, Lewis RD, O'Connor PJ, Boyd AM. Body composition, energy intake and expenditure, and body weight dissatisfaction in female child gymnasts and controls. J Am Diet Assoc 1997;9:A-14.
3. American College of Sports Medicine. The female athlete triad position stand. Med Sci Sport Exerc 1997;29:i.
4. Krucoff C. Female athletes at risk. Washington Post Health News Source 1997;8:16.
5. Ward A, Brown N, Treasure J. Persistent osteopenia after recovery from anorexia nervosa. Int J Eat Disord 1997;22:73.
6. Neumark-Sztainer D, Story M, Resnick MD, Blum RW. Adolescent vegetarians. A behavioral profile of a school-based population in Minnesota. Arch Pediatr Adolesc Med 1997;151:823.
7. Williamson DA, Netemeyer RG, Jackman LP, Anderson DA, Funsch CL, Rabalais JY. Structural equation modeling of risk factors for the development of eating disorder symptoms in female athletes. Int J Eat Disord 1995;17:387.
8. Strober M, Freeman R, Morrell W. The long-term course of severe anorexia nervosa in adolescents: survival analysis of recovery, relapse, and outcome predictors over 10–15 years in a prospective study. Int J Eat Disord 1997;22:339.
9. Broso R, Subrizi R. Gynecologic problems in female athletes. Minerva Ginecologica 1996;48:99.
10. Arena B, Maffulli F, Morleo MA. Reproductive hormones and menstrual changes with exercise in female athletes. Sports Med 1995;19:278.
11. Stone J, Milord N, Durkin C. Coaches, female athletes, and menstrual irregularities. Olympic Coach Magazine, 1994;2.
12. Barber-Murphy L. Missed "period" (amenorrhea). Healthy Devil Online-Duke University Women's Health 1994;1.
13. Benson JE, Engelbert-Fenton KA, Eisenman PA. Nutritional aspects of amenorrhea in the female athlete triad. Int J Sport Nutr 1996;6:134.
14. Anderson JJB, Stender M, Rondano P, Bishop L, Duckett A. Nutrition and bone in physical activity and sport. Nutrition in Exercise and Sports 3rd ed. Boca Raton, FL: CRC Press; 1998, p. 219.
15. Farrell PA, Gustafson AB, Gaarthwaite TL, Kalthoff RK, Cowley AW, Morgan WP. Influence of endogenous opioids on the response of selected hormones to exercise in humans. J Appl Physiol 1986;61:1051.
16. Loucks AB, Mortola JF, Girton L, Yen SSC. Alterations in the hypothalamic-pituitary-ovarian and hypothalamic-pituitary-adrenal axes in athletic women. J Endocrinol Metab 1989;68:402.
17. Haberland CA, Seddick D, Marcus R, Bachrach LK. A physician survey of therapy for exercise-associated amenorrhea: a brief report. Clin J Sport Med 1995;5:246.
18. Anderson JJB. Introduction. In: Nutritional concerns of women. Boca Raton, FL: CRC Press; 1996, p. 36.
19. Sallis RE, Jones K. Stress fractures in athletes. Postgraduate Medicine, 1997; 1:89.
20. Brukner P, Bennell K. Stress fractures in female athletes. Sports Med 1997;24:419.
21. Bennell KA, Malcolm SA, Thomas SA, Reid SJ, Brukner PD, Ebeling PR, Wark JD. Risk factors for stress fractures in track and field athletes. A twelve-month prospective study. Am J Sport Med 1996;24:810.
22. Robinson TL. Bone mineral and menstrual cycle status in competitive female athletes: a longitudinal study. International Institution for Sports & Human Professionals 1996;1:230.
23. Robinson TL, Snow-Harter C, Taaffe DR, Gillis D, Shaw J, Marcus R. Gymnasts exhibit higher bone mass than runners despite similar prevalence of amenorrhea and oligomenorrhea. J Bone Miner Res 1995;10:26.
24. Keen AD, Drinkwater BL. Irreversible bone loss in former amenorrheic athletes. Osteoporosis International 1997;7:311.
25. Kirchner EM, Lewis RD, O'Connor PJ. Bone mineral density and dietary intake of female college gymnasts. Med Sci Sport Exerc 1995;27:543.
26. Kirchner EM, Lewis RD, O'Connor, PJ. Effect of past gymnasts participation on adult bone mass. J Appl Physiol 1996;80:226.
27. Fosgate H. Women athletes build body and bone. Resource Communication at the University of Georgia, 1998.
28. Ogawa A, Andrews AFB, Armstrong DW, Drake AJ. Weight bearing exercise predicts total bone mineral content in female midshipmen. J Am Diet Assoc 1997;9:A-19.
29. Dook JE, Henderson NK, James C, Price RI. Exercise and bone mineral density in mature female athletes. Med Sci Sports Exerc 1997;29:291.
30. Resch M. The female athletes' triad: eating disorders, amenorrhea, osteoporosis. Orvosi Hetilap 1997;138:1393.
31. Talbott S. The female triad. Strength and Conditioning, 1996;4:128.
32. Alfredson H, Nordstrom P, Lorentzon R. Bone mass in female volleyball players: a comparison of total and regional bone mass in female volleyball players and non-active females. Calcif Tissue Int 1997;60(4):338–342.
33. Kirchner EM, Lewis RD, O'Connor PJ. Bone mineral density and dietary intake of female college gymnasts. Med Sci Sport Exerc 1995;27(4):543–549.
34. Young N, Formica C, Szmukler G, Seeman E. Bone density at weight-bearing and nonweight-bearing sites in ballet dancers: the effects of exercise, hypogonadism and body weight. J Clin Endocrinol Metab 1994;78:449.
35. Haenggi W, Casez JP, Birkhaeuser MH, Lippuner K, Jaeger P. Bone and mineral density in young women with long-standing amenorrhea: limited effect of hormone re-

placement therapy with ethinylestradiol and desogre-strel. Osteoporos Int 1994;4:99.

36. Rutherford OM. Spine and total body bone mineral density in amenorrheic endurance athletes. J Appl Physiol 1993;74:2904.

37. Myerson M, Gutin B, Warren MP, Wang J, Lichtman S, Pierson RN. Total bone density in amenorrheic runners. Obstetrica Gynecologica 1992;79:973.

38. Wolman RL, Clark P, McNally E, Harries MG, Reeve J. Dietary calcium as a statistical determinant of spinal trabecular bone density in amenorrheic and estrogen-replete athletes. Bone and Mineral 1992;17:415.

39. Snead DB, Stubbs CC, Weltman JY, Evans WS, Vwldhuis JD, Rogol AD, Teates CD, Weltman A. Dietary patterns, eating behaviors, and bone mineral density in women runners. Am J Clin Nutr 1992;56:705.

Lee E. Thrash, a BS graduate in public health nutrition from the University of North Carolina at Chapel Hill, is currently a dual-degree graduate student in nutrition and public health at the University of Tennessee-Knoxville.

John J.B. Anderson, PhD, is Professor of Nutrition in the Schools of Public Health and Medicine at the University of North Carolina at Chapel Hill and President of the American College of Nutrition. His research focuses on calcium an bone metabolism as they are influenced by dietary intake.

The authors thank Sanford C. Garner, PhD, for critiquing the manuscript. The critical reading of the manuscript by Agna Boass, PhD, is also appreciated.

From *Nutrition Today*, September/October 2000, pp. 168-174. © 2000 by Nutrition Today. Reprinted by permission from Lippincott Williams & Wilkins.

UNIT 4
Obesity and Weight Control

Unit Selections

Key Points to Consider

- As the incidence of obesity increases, how can it best be prevented?

- What sort of health risks can be affected by some of the more popular weight-loss methods?

- What are some of the causes behind a person's becoming obese?

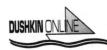 **Links: www.dushkin.com/online/**
These sites are annotated in the World Wide Web pages.

American Anorexia Bulimia Association/National Eating Disorders Association (AABA)
    http://www.nationaleatingdisorders.org/
American Society of Exercise Physiologists (ASEP)
    http://www.asep.org/
Calorie Control Council
    http://www.caloriecontrol.org
Eating Disorders: Body Image Betrayal
    http://www.bibri.com/home/index.htm
Shape Up America!
    http://www.shapeup.org

Being overweight and obesity have become epidemic in the United States during the last century and are rising at a dangerous rate worldwide. Approximately 5 million adults are overweight or obese according to the new standards set by the U.S. Government, which use a body mass index (BMI) of 30 to 39.9. Reports suggest that by the year 2050, half of the U.S. population will be considered obese. This problem is prevalent in both genders and all ages, races, and ethnic groups. Twenty-five percent of U.S. children and adolescents are overweight or at risk, which emphasizes the need for prevention, as obese children become obese adults. The catastrophic health consequences of obesity are heart disease, diabetes, gallbladder disease, osteoarthritis, and some cancers. The cost for treating this degenerative disease in the United States is approximately $100 billion per year.

Even though professionals have tried hard to prevent and combat obesity with behavior modification, a healthy diet, and exercise, it seems that these traditional ways have not proven effective. In a society where fast-food eateries are the mainstay meals, where "big," including food servings, is better, where there is a universal reliance on automobiles, and where the food industry is more interested in profit than in the health of the population, we should not be surprised that obesity has become an epidemic. Barbara Rolls discusses in depth how large portions and readily available energy-dense foods contribute to "adult onset" of diabetes and high blood pressure even among youth. Incorporating nutrition education as part of health education in schools, limiting the sale of soft drinks and snack foods in schools, learning to read labels, offering incentives to the food industry may improve nutrition and reduce portion sizes.

Thus, there is also a great need for a multifaceted public health approach that would include health officials, researchers, educators, legislators, transportation experts, urban planners, and businesses, which would cooperate in formulating ways to combat obesity. A sound public health policy would require that weight-loss therapies have long-term maintenance and relapse-prevention measures built into them. Healthy People 2010 is the U.S. government's prevention agenda designed to ensure high quality of life and reduce health risks. One of the 28 areas it focuses on, is overweight and obesity. Its main objectives are to reduce the proportion of overweight and obesity of children, teens, and adults to 15% and increase the proportion of adults who are at a healthy weight. Twice as many teens from poor households are overweight in comparison to those from middle-high-income. Women with less education and lower incomes have high rates of obesity, and the rates of obesity are higher among African-American women than Caucasian. Gender differences in the incidence of obesity have been observed in Hispanic and African Americans, with the rates of obesity 80% greater women than men.

Irresponsible, biased science reporting is adding to the distorted information about the role nutrients play in regulating body weight thus confusing the public even more. The sorry state of science journalism can be seen in the case of Gary Taubes who reported on the Atkins diet, trying to debunk research that has been conducted on the relationship of dietary fat and protein and degenerative disease by respected scientists. He chose to selectively report what supported his case, which is especially frightening not only for the public but for the science community as a whole. More evidence against increasing fat consumption as in the Atkins diet, comes from the International Agency for Research on Cancer. Studies have concluded that obesity predisposes humans to uterine, kidney, breast, colon, and esophageal cancers.

The long-term effect of low-carbohydrate high-protein diets on human health is currently being studied. Margo Denke discusses the detrimental long-term effects of the above diets on humans and why these diets should be avoided by the general public. Science News discusses the dietary transition of the U.S. population in replacing fat with high processed sugars and starches and the resultant obesity epidemic.

In the article "Losing Weight, More Than Counting Calories," Linda Bren describes a series of successful weight losers—setting realistic goals, changing eating habits, learning how to read food labels and use them when shopping, and increasing physical activity are some of the secrets of successful "losers."

For people who are frustrated trying to lose weight but are too busy or too embarrassed to be with a group of people, help is on the way. Virtual weight-loss centers are here and people find the structure and moral support helpful in achieving their goals. Nutritionists from Tufts University have thoroughly researched some weight-loss websites to help consumers in their decisions.

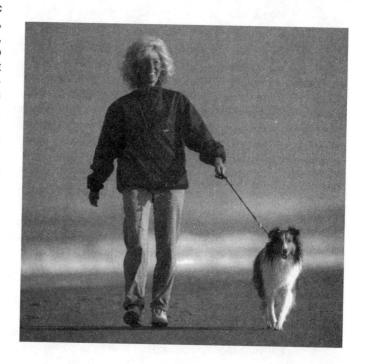

Healthy People 2010: Overweight and Obesity

Healthy People 2010 is the US prevention agenda for the next decade, designed to reduce health risks and increase the quality and years of healthy life. Ten Leading Health Indicators are selected as priority areas from the 28 sections. One of these is overweight and obesity, which is major part of the nutrition section.

What Is Healthy People 2010?

Healthy People 2010 is the document that sets the prevention agenda for the United States for the next 10 years. It is designed to identify the most significant preventable threats to health and establish national goals to reduce these threats.

The two overarching goals of Healthy People 2010 are (1) to increase the quality and years of healthy life for everyone—to add years to our lives and life to our years—and (2) to eliminate health disparities so that all people have access to better health care and opportunities.

The report includes 28 focus areas with 467 objectives in a large two-volume format. To make this more manageable, 10 Leading Health Indicators are selected as priority areas. These will provide a quick measure of progress—a snapshot of the health of the nation.

Healthy People 2010 was developed by leading federal agencies with input from more than 350 national membership organizations and 250 state health, mental health, substance abuse, and environmental agencies. Additionally, through a series of regional and national meetings and an interactive website, more than 11,000 public comments on the draft objectives were received.

Many of the objectives focus on interventions designed to reduce or eliminate illness, disability, and premature death among individuals and communities. Other focus on broader issues, such as improving access to quality health care, strengthening public health services, and improving the ability and dissemination of health-related information. Each objective has a target for specific improvements to be achieved by the year 2010. These targets will be the measure for assessing the progress of a wise array of federal and local programs.

Healthy People 2010 offers a simple but powerful idea: profile the objectives in a format that enables diverse groups to combine their efforts and work as a team. It is to be a road map to better health for all, used by many different people, communities, professional organizations, businesses, and state and federal programs who are encouraged to integrate it into current programs, special events, publications, and meetings to improve health for all. Most states are now working with community coalitions, developing their own versions tailored to their specific needs.

Healthy People 2010 is coordinated by and available from the Office of Disease Prevention and Health Promotion, US Department of Health and Human Services, Room 738G, 200 Independence Avenue SW, Washington, DC 20201 (202-205-8583). For more information, visit www.health.gov/healthpeople or call 1-800-336-4797.

The two main objectives for tracking progress in this priority area are

- Reduce the proportion of children and adolescents who are overweight or obese.

- Reduce the proportion of adults who are obese.

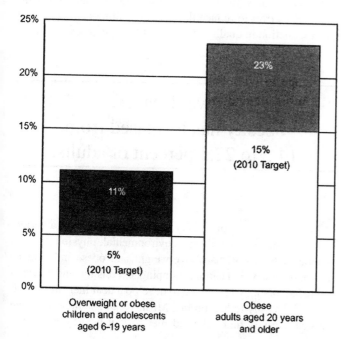

Figure 1 Overweight and obesity, US, 1988–1994.

Baseline data (Figure 1) show that 11 percent of youth age 6 to 19 are overweight or obese using the definition of measuring at or above 95th percentile (US Growth Charts, 2000). The target is to reduce this to 5 percent. Baseline data for adults age 20 and over show that 23 percent are obese using the definition of a body mass index (BMI) of 30 or more, including 20 percent of males and 25 percent of females. The target is 15 percent.

A third objective aims to

- Increase the proportion of adults who are at a healthy weight.

Only 42 percent of adults are considered at the healthy weight, defined as a BMI of 18.5 to less than 2.5 (Table 1). This includes 38 percent of males and 45 percent of females. The target is 60 percent.

Overweight (BMI of 25–29.9) and obesity (BMI of 30 or more) affect a large percent of the US population: 55 percent of adults. In two decades, obesity has increased from 14.5 to 22.5 percent of adults (Table 2). There is much concern about the increasing prevalence of obesity in children, that it may persist into adulthood and increase the risk of some chronic diseases later in life. Almost twice as many adolescents from poor households are overweight as from middle- and high-income households.

An estimated 107 million adults in the United States are overweight or obese, and rates are especially high among women with lower incomes and less education, according to this report. Obesity is more common among African-American and Hispanic women than among Caucasian women. Among African Americans, the number of women who are obese is 80 percent higher than for men. This gender difference is also seen among Hispanic women and men, but the percentage of Caucasian women and men who are obese is about the same.

Table 1. Healthy weight. Adults age 20 years and older, 1988–1994. Age adjusted to the year 2000 standard population. Categories without data are omitted from this chart. Objective 19–1.

	Healthy Weight, %		
	Total	Female	Male
Total	42	45	38
Race and ethnicity			
Black or African American	34	29	40
Caucasian	42	47	37
Hispanic or Latino			
Mexican American	30	31	30
Not Hispanic or Latino			
Black or African American	34	29	40
Caucasian	43	49	38
Age			
20–39 years	51	55	48
40–59 years	36	40	31
60 years and older	36	37	33
Family income level			
Lower income (≤130 percent of poverty threshold)	38	33	44
Higher income (> 130 percent of poverty threshold)	43	48	37
Disability status			
Persons with disabilities	32	34	30
Persons without disabilities	41	45	36
Select populations			
Persons with arthritis	36	37	34
Persons without arthritis	43	47	40

Although BMI alone is used to screen for overweight and obesity, it is not entirely satisfactory, the report acknowledges. A truly health-oriented definition would be based on the amount of excess body fat at which health risks begin to increase; however, no such definitions currently exist.

Table 2. Prevalence of obesity. Adults age 20 years and older, 1988–1994. Age adjusted to the year 2000 standard population. Categories without data are omitted from this chart. Objective 19–2.

	Obesity, %		
	Total	*Female*	*Male*
Total	23	25	20
Race and ethnicity			
Black or African American	30	38	21
Caucasian	22	24	20
Hispanic or Latino			
Mexican American	29	35	24
Not Hispanic or Latino			
Black or African American	30	38	21
Caucasian	21	23	20
Age (not age adjusted)			
20–39 years	18	21	15
40–59 years	28	30	25
60 years and older	24	26	21
Family income level			
Lower income (≤130 percent of poverty threshold)	29	35	21
Higher income (> 130 percent of poverty threshold)	21	23	20
Disability status			
Persons with disabilities	30	38	21
Persons without disabilities	23	25	22
Select populations			
Persons with arthritis	30	33	27
Persons without arthritis	21	23	19

Overweight and obesity are associated with increased risk of illness from high blood pressure, high cholesterol, type 2 diabetes, heart disease, stroke, gallbladder disease, arthritis, sleep disturbances and problems breathing, and endometrial, breast, prostate, and colon cancers. Obese individuals may also suffer from social stigmatization, discrimination, and lowered self-esteem. Thus, maintenance of a health weight is a major goal in the effort to reduce the burden of illness and its consequent reduction in quality of life and life expectancy.

In two decades, obesity has increased from 14.5 to 22.5 percent of adults.

The development of obesity is a complex result of a variety of social, behavioral, cultural, environmental, physiologic, and genetic factors. For many overweight and obese individuals, substantial change in eating, shopping, exercising, and even social behaviors may be needed to develop a healthier lifestyle. It is noted that any reduction in BMI in youth should emphasize physical activity and balanced diet so that healthy growth is maintained.

Note

Tables and figures in this article taken from Healthy People 2010 (Conference Edition). Washington, DC: January 2000, *www.health.gov/healthypeople*.

From *Healthy Weight Journal*, January/February 2001, Vol. 15, No. 1, pp. 4-5. © 2001 by Healthy Weight Journal. Reprinted by permission.

The Supersizing of America

Portion Size and the Obesity Epidemic

Although we are just beginning to understand how environmental factors such as portion size affect eating behavior, the available data suggest that large portions of energy-dense foods are contributing to the obesity epidemic. Serveral possible strategies for adjusting portions to bring intake back in line with energy requirements are discussed. The continuing rise in the rates of obesity calls for urgent action.

Barbara J. Rolls, PhD

In the United States, an obesity epidemic is rapidly becoming the most challenging public health problem that we have faced as a nation. Despite the known health consequences, the prevalence of both overweight and obesity has continued to increase. The National Health and Nutrition Examination Surveys show that the percentage of adults who were overweight or obese increased from 55.9% in 1988 through 1994 to 64.5% in 1999 through 2000.[1] During this same period, the percentage of overweight teenagers increased from 10.5% to 15.5%.[2] It is unlikely that our biology has changed during this short time, so other explanations for this surge in obesity rates must be found.

Both food supply data (which give an estimate of energy availability per person) and large-scale dietary surveys indicate that US adults are eating more calories per day than they were in the late 1970s. [3,4] One possible reason for this increase is that the environment in Western societies has changed, so that overconsumption of calories has become easier. At the same time, opportunities for physical activity have declined. Thus, it is increasingly difficult for individuals to match energy intake to energy output to maintain a healthy body weight. Although energy expenditure plays an important role in the obesity epidemic, this article focuses only on energy intake. Some of the changes in the eating environment that encourage overeating are the increasing availability of inexpensive high-calorie foods, the variety of palatable foods, the increasing frequency of meals consumed outside of the home, and the rise in portion sizes. Although all of these changes may stimulate excess intake, this article presents data that suggest that increasing portion sizes are contributing to the obesity epidemic. We will also suggest strategies to deal with the overconsumption associated with "megaportions."

Overconsumption is part of the obesity problem.

Supersizing: The Expanding Size of Portions

An obvious place to start in addressing the relationship between portion size and obesity is to ask whether increases in portion size have indeed occurred, and, if so, whether they coincide with the rise in obesity rates. It is critical, however, when considering such associations to remember that they do not prove causality. Young and Nestle (4) compared current portions of restaurant foods, grocery products, and recipes in cookbooks with comparable older data. They found a rise in portion size in all food categories except bread. The expansion of portions started in the 1970s, increased sharply in the 1980s, and has continued to rise. As portions have grown, they have become more dissociated from recommended serving sizes such as those in the Food Guide Pyramid and on food labels.

We are now surrounded by "huge food"; muffins can weigh half a pound, and pasta bowls in restaurants hold more than 2 pounds. A plate of steak or fish that weighs more than a pound is no longer unusual restaurant fare. In a movie house, a "medium" popcorn is 16 cups (with up to 1,000 calories), and the soft drink that accompanies it may contain 500 calories. Two recent analyses of nationally representative survey data find that the reported portion sizes consumed of several foods have increased between 1977 and 1998.[5,6] Of particular interest was the finding that portion sizes increased both outside and inside the home, with the largest increase being at fast-food establishments.[5] This demonstration that *portion sizes and obesity rates have increased in parallel*, although not proving causality, supports the hypothesis that portion size could play a role in increasing body weights.

Studies Showing That Portion Size Affects Intake

In addition to the data showing that there is an association between increasing portions and the prevalence of overweight and obesity, *recent controlled studies show directly that portion size affects energy intake*. When we tested how adults responded to 4 different portions of macaroni and cheese served on different days, we found that the bigger the portion, the more participants ate[7]. The participants consumed 30% more energy (162 kcal) when offered the largest portion (1000 g) compared to the smallest portion (500 g). Particularly interesting is that participants reported similar ratings of hunger and fullness after eating despite the intake differences. The results were not affected by subject characteristics including gender, body mass index, or concern about food intake or body weight. After the study, fewer than half (45%) of the subjects reported noticing that there were differences in the portions served. It is surprising that in a controlled laboratory setting where the main focus was food and eating, many participants in the study were unaware of the changes in the amount of food offered and the subsequent effect on their intake, hunger, and satiety. It is likely that in situations where there are more distractions, such as when eating out, consumers would be even less aware of portion size.

People eat in units, and larger units mean they eat more.

It could be argued that the effects of portion size on intake are specific to foods such as macaroni and cheese that are amorphous in shape. It is particularly difficult to judge the portion size of such foods, especially when the portions are large.[8] We conducted further studies to test whether intake is also influenced by the portion size of other types of foods, such as those with clearly defined shapes or units.

People eat in units. That is, if they are offered a food that comes in a preportioned unit, such as a cookie, most people will eat the whole cookie.[9] One of the most common unit foods is the sandwich. In most fast-food establishments, there is a choice of sandwich sizes; often the larger sandwiches are purchased because they are perceived as being a better value because they offer more food per dollar.[10] The key question is: if consumers

choose a larger sandwich, are they likely to eat more either at that meal or throughout the entire day? To test this, on 4 different days we offered men and women submarine sandwiches that varied in size: 6, 8, 10, and 12 inches.[11] We found a systematic and significant effect of portion size on intake for both men and women. When served the 12-inch sandwich compared to the 6-inch sandwich, women consumed 31% more energy (159 kcal) and men consumed 56% more energy (355 kcal). Hunger and fullness ratings after lunch did not differ significantly when subjects were served the 8-, 10-, and 12-inch sandwiches, despite the increase in energy intake. When served bigger portions, consumers override or adjust their level of satiety to accommodate greater energy intakes.

The amount of food in a package or container may also influence how much is eaten. Certainly, some prepackaged foods come in several sizes. For example, bags of potato chips range from 1-ounce (28 g) single-serving bags to 20-ounce (560 g) family-size bags. To test how the size of the bag affects intake, on 5 different occasions we served men and women an afternoon snack that consisted of 28, 42, 85, 128, or 170 g of potato chips in a plain unlabeled foil bag.[12] Participants ate directly from the bag so that they had few visual cues to guide consumption. The results showed that portion size had a significant effect on snack intake for both the men and the women. Many individuals ate all of the chips in the two smaller bags, but most did not consume all of the chips in the 85-g package. However, when they were served the 170-g package, women ate 18% more and men ate 37% more than when served the 85-g package. When dinner was served several hours later, participants did not adjust their intakes to compensate for the differences in snack intake. Thus, bigger portions of a prepackaged snack increased energy intake in the short-term. It is not clear that all prepackaged foods have a similar effect. It is possible that the effect will be greatest for highly palatable foods, such as potato chips, that people find difficult to stop eating. It is also possible that the effect will be different in other situations, such as when the snack is poured into a bowl so that the consumer can more readily assess the amount.

Additional studies conducted in various situations confirm that the package or container size of several foods can affect how much food is prepared and eaten.[13] When women were given a 2-pound box of spaghetti and asked to take out enough to make a dinner for two, they removed an average of 302 strands. But when given a one-pound box, they removed only 234 strands. When frying chicken, women poured 4.3 ounces of cooking oil from a 32-ounce bottle, but only 3.5 ounces from a 16-ounce bottle. When people were asked how many M&Ms they would eat when watching a movie by themselves, participants poured 63 from a small package that contained 114 candies, 103 from a package double in size, and 122 from a package triple in size. That is, they poured about twice as much from a jumbo bag, a difference of approximately 250 calories.[13] In a movie theater, consumers were given either a medium (120 g) or large (240 g) bucket of popcorn. Subjects rated the taste of the popcorn and were divided into two groups depending upon whether they perceived the taste as favorable or unfavorable. The results showed a large effect of the portion size of popcorn on intake in both groups. The larger package led to 49% more intake by those who rated the popcorn favorably (94 versus 63 g) and 61% more by those who rated the popcorn as relatively unfavorable (92 versus 57 g).[14] Thus, it is not just the sensory attributes or the perceived pleasantness of foods that is driving intake when large portions are available.

Several controlled studies show that in both the laboratory and more naturalistic situations, the portion size and package size of numerous foods can affect energy intake in adults in the short-term. A key question is whether after a bout of overeating stimulated by large portions, compensatory mechanisms limit subsequent intake. We tested this in a study in which the portion size of all foods served during a 2-day period was increased.[15] The results showed a highly significant effect of portion size on energy intake throughout the 2 days, with no indication that the effect decreased over time. When portions were 50% larger than the baseline portions, mean daily intake increased by 16% (328 kcal in women and 522 kcal in men); when portions were 100% larger, mean intakes increased by 26% (531 kcal for women and 806 kcal for men). Thus, these results show that the effects of portion size can persist for several days and are associated with highly significant increases in daily intakes.[15]

Portion Size and Intake in Children

Although it has been shown that adults respond to increasing portions by eating more, they probably did not start life responding in this way. A recent analysis of food survey data during a 20-year period showed that despite changes in the eating environment, there has been remarkable stability in the average portion size of foods consumed by children in the second year of life.[16] A controlled laboratory-based study that we conducted confirms *that in young children, intake is relatively unaffected by environmental cues such as portion size.* When we fed 3-year-old children 3 different portions of macaroni and cheese at 3 separate lunches, they ate the same amount at each meal. Their intake was therefore unaffected by portion size. In contrast, 5-year-old children were similar to adults because they responded to increasing portions by eating significantly more.[17]

We hypothesize that environmental influences, such as rewarding children for cleaning their plates, may undermine the ability to respond appropriately to physiologic cues related to hunger. This suggestion is supported by a study in 4-year-old children, which indicated that children's ability to self-regulate food intake was disrupted by focusing their attention on environmental cues, such as food rewards and the amount of food remaining on their plates.[18] When two experimental groups were compared, it was found that children who were taught to focus on the fullness in their stomachs adjusted their intake better to the energy content of food than did children who were rewarded for cleaning their plates. It will be interesting to test whether teaching older children, and even adults, to be more sensitive to cues related to hunger and satiety will help them to eat appropriate amounts when faced with large portions.

Eating Out and Portion Size

Although there is some evidence that portions consumed at home are increasing,[4,5] the large portions served in restaurants may be a bigger problem for weight management. The increase in the prevalence of obesity since the 1970s coincides with an increase in the number of meals eaten outside the home) Studies show that in both adolescents and adults, the frequency of eating out is associated with an increase in energy and fat intake[19] and with a higher body mass index.[20] In particular, eating in fast-food restaurants is associated with increased energy intake[21,22] and body fatness.[23] When eating out, portion size is one of numerous variables that could affect consumption. Several palatable foods, a convivial atmosphere with friends, and alcohol consumption may also increase energy intake. In particular, the tendency to choose foods high in energy density (calories per gram) is likely to increase calorie intake,[24] and these foods become particularly problematic when served in large portions.

Let us consider how the size of the portions offered in restaurants is determined. Although few published data are available, in one small study in Scotland of how caterers decide on portion sizes, the factors rated as most important were cost of the food, personal experience, and nutritional content. When caterers were asked what portions they would serve of several foods, the responses varied widely. For example, portions of rice varied from 80 to 380 g and French fries from 70 to 260 g.[25] Clearly, customers should not rely on the restaurant to serve a portion that is related to their energy needs. Indeed, it is hard to imagine how this can be accomplished. Information is needed about the customer's body mass index, when he or she last ate, his or her activity level and metabolic rate, and how hungry he or she is. Because such "personalized portions" are unlikely to become a reality, we must consider other ways to manage portion size.

Food cues, such as portion size and ready availability, override physiologic satiety cues.

Value Meals

Restaurants have found that customers appreciate good value, and this translates into large portions at a low price. Because food is only a small percentage of the cost of a restaurant meal, giving customers more food is an excellent economic strategy if it increases total sales. Thus the practice of "supersizing," (giving customers a lot more food and calories for only a small additional cost) is widespread, particularly in fast-food establishments. For example, when ordering a cheeseburger, spending $1.57 more can buy 600 extra calories; for French fries, 64 cents can buy 330 more calories; and for some soft drinks, 37 cents can buy 450 more calories.[10]

Restaurants may be giving consumers what they want in terms of value, but the crucial issue is whether people can adjust their energy intake to their energy needs when tempted with huge portions of energy-dense palatable foods. Faced with a lack of data in the scientific literature, the American Institute for Cancer Research[26,27] commissioned several surveys examining consumers' perceptions of the portions they are served. The surveys found that 78% of the respondents believed that the type of food they eat is more important for weight management than the amount of food. Furthermore, 62% were unaware that portions served in restaurants have increased in size during the past 10 years. Regardless of the amount served, 67% said they finish their entrees most of the time or always. *Many consumers are eating what is served, whether or not it is appropriate for their energy needs.*

We recently tested how increasing the portion size of a popular dish, while keeping the price the same, would affect intake in a restaurant setting.[28] An entree, baked ziti, was offered 10 times throughout 5 months, and 180 adult customers purchased the dish during that period. On different days, the portion was varied between a standard portion (248 g, 422 kcal) and a large portion (377 g, 633 kcal). Results showed that portion size significantly affected intake such that mean intake of the standard portion was 235 g and of the larger portion was 340 g. Thus, when customers were served 52% more food, they ate 45% more, equivalent to 172 kcal. A survey completed by the customers showed no difference in ratings of the appropriateness of the two portions. Thus, in restaurants as well as in the laboratory, portion size has a significant effect on energy intake, and it is likely that the consumers are unaware of this effect.

Large portions and high energy density are culprits—even small decreases in energy density can help.

The restaurant industry knows that there is an obesity epidemic and that some of the blame is being placed on their shoulders. In their rebuttal, the National Restaurant Association shifts the blame for excessive consumption to the consumer.[29] The association states:

> All of this finger pointing assumes that Americans have no self-control over what (or how much food) they put into their mouths. Is it true then that people today cannot control the foods they eat? Is it the responsibility of restaurants to compensate for this loss of control by limiting food choices for their customers by banning large portions? In the restaurant industry, we believe the answer is a resounding "No" to both questions. Customers clearly vote with their pocketbooks every day.

I Ate It Because It Was There!

Clearly, consumers are responsible for what and how much they choose to eat. But several different studies show that people find it difficult to resist large portions and the ready availability of food. An interest in the way that portion size affects intake can be found as far back as 1957 when Siegel[9] published a short article titled The Completion Compulsion in Human Eating. He showed that young

men eat foods in units. Thus, when a range of foods was preportioned into arbitrary units or servings, the men ate whole units rather than intermediate amounts. We observed this tendency in our study of varying sizes of submarine sandwiches, particularly when the men were eating the smaller sandwiches.[11]

Perhaps related to this observation is the not-surprising finding that in some individuals there is a tendency to eat all the food put in front of them, or to "clean the plate."[30] This was demonstrated in a study conducted in the late 1970s. Researchers served people soup from normal bowls to determine each person's customary intake.[31] On the fourth day, without telling anyone, the researchers substituted a "trick bowl" that slowly refilled itself from a hidden reservoir under the table so that it was never empty. Regardless of whether the participants were obese or lean, the continual presence of food in the bowl stimulated them to eat more than their usual portion. After one day, the subjects were told about the trick, and their intake was then measured during the next 6 days. The normal-weight individuals adjusted their intake to baseline levels, whereas the participants who were obese continued to overeat, apparently unable to resist the food in the bowl. These data suggest that some individuals, when given information about the foods they are eating and appropriate portions, may adjust their intake and resist overeating in the face of the continual availability of food.

Other studies confirm that simply making food more readily available increases consumption. For example, in a large hospital cafeteria, when the lid was kept on an ice-cream cooler, only 3% of participants who were obese and 5% of normal-weight participants selected ice cream. But when the lid was taken off the cooler, allowing people to see the ice cream and reach it more easily, the percentages rose: 17% of the participants who were obese and 16% of the participants who were lean chose ice cream.[32] In another recent study, the visibility and accessibility of chocolate candy was varied in workers' offices throughout 3 weeks. Both variables significantly affected the amount eaten: an average of 9 candies per person were consumed when the chocolate was visible on the desk, 6 were consumed when the candies were in a drawer of the desk, and only 3 were consumed when they were out of sight 2 m from the desk.[33]

Fortunately, the principle of easy availability also works with foods low in energy density, such as soup and fruits. Simply stockpiling soup in the house can increase the frequency of soup consumption. Even the position of fruit in the house affects intake. In one study, people were asked to put fruit in the refrigerator, in a bowl in the kitchen, or in a bowl in the dining room.[34] The participants ate the most fruit when it was in a bowl in the kitchen and the least when it was in the refrigerator.

Collectively, these studies show that we are responsive to environmental food cues. Whether or not we need food, when it is put in front of us, we eat. Many of us eat all of it. *Physiologic satiety cues are readily overridden by food cues, such as large portions and the ready availability of food.* The studies also suggest that it may be possible to decrease energy intake by structuring the environment so that large portions of foods low in energy density are readily available, while limiting the portion size and availability of foods higher in energy density.

re Big Portions Making Us Obese?

the 1970s, researchers believed that individuals who were
ese were more responsive to food cues than individuals who
ere lean. Now we know that there is an enormous variability
such responsiveness, and many individuals who are lean are
st as responsive as those who are overweight.[35] There is also
nsiderable variability in the size of the portions consumed by
dividuals within body weight categories. There are data from
od diaries that indicate, however, that women who are obese
ke larger portions of foods with a high energy density than do
omen who are not obese. Furthermore, women who are obese
ke smaller portions of foods low in energy density than do
omen who are not obese.[36]

Standard portions and actual portions are quite different.

Data showing that adults who are obese eat bigger portions
energy-dense foods do not prove that portion size plays a role
the etiology of obesity. Indeed, at this time we know of no
ta showing such a causal relationship. One recent analysis
es indicate, however, that a relationship between portion size
d body mass index (BMI) is evident at an early age?[37] An
aluation of reported intakes and body mass indices in children
ged 2 to 5 years in the Continuing Survey of Food Intake by
dividuals (1994-1996) indicated that children with a higher
MI consumed portions of many foods that were as much as
0% larger than those consumed by children with a lower
MI. Thus, these data suggest that an association between body
eight and portion size starts at an early age.

Eat Less" Is Not Always the Best Advice

ften the advice for dealing with large portions is simply to eat
ss. This advice is of little practical value because *it is not just
ortion size that increases energy intake, but rather, large por-
ons of calorie-laden energy-dense foods.* Indeed, large por-
ons of foods low in energy density, such as vegetables, fruits,
d broth-based soups, can aid weight management by pro-
iding satisfying portions with few calories.[38]

Recent research indicates that the energy density of foods is
major determinant of caloric intake.[24] The main components
f food that influence energy density are the fat content, which
creases energy density, and the water content, which lowers
. The influence of energy density on energy intake was dem-
nstrated in a study in which participants could eat as much as
ey wanted of foods provided in our laboratory throughout 2
ays. In 3 experimental conditions, all of the foods offered
aried in energy density from low- to medium- to high-energy
ensity. The energy density of mixed dishes, such as casseroles
d salads, was lowered by increasing the proportion of water-
ch vegetables. Of particular interest was the finding that al-
ough the foods in the low-energy-density condition had one-
ird fewer calories than those in the high-energy-density con-
ition, the participants liked them just as much. Participants did

not notice that the foods differed in calories, and they ate similar
portions during the 2 days in all 3 conditions. Thus, they ate
one-third fewer calories during the 2 days when they had the
low-energy-density foods than when they had the high-energy-
density foods. Despite the reduced calorie intake, participants
rated themselves equally full and satisfied.[39,40] Other studies
show that *even small reductions in energy density can lead to
significant reductions in energy intake.*[41]

These studies suggest one possible strategy for reducing the
effects of large portions on energy intake. Even modest reductions in the energy density of popular foods, such as burgers, submarine sandwiches, and pizza, could have a significant effect on
energy intake. With unit foods such as these, consumers will
order and consume their usual portion size. Therefore, when
eating their customary amount of food, they will be consuming
fewer calories but are likely to feel just as full and satisfied. If the
reduction in energy density does not compromise palatability or
increase the cost, it is unlikely to affect acceptability.

Portion Control and Weight Management

Another approach to handling the influence of portion size on
food intake is to consume portion-controlled meals. This approach has been used successfully in the dietary treatment of
obesity. Providing patients with preportioned liquid meal replacements is associated with better compliance and greater
weight loss compared with self-selected diets for periods as
long as 4 years.[42] Provision of preportioned solid meals has also
aided weight loss efforts.[43]

Estimating Portion Sizes

Another way to deal with the effect of portion size on intake is
to help consumers to become more aware of appropriate portion
sizes. Part of the problem is that there is a dissociation between
recommended serving sizes and the portions that are offered to
consumers. A study that illustrates how confused we are about
portion sizes was conducted among undergraduate nutrition students. The students were asked to bring in a "medium" portion
of a bagel, muffin, cookie, or baked potato. The amounts that
were brought varied widely; most were twice the US Department of Agriculture's (USDA's) recommended serving size or
more. For example, a "medium" bagel averaged 4 ounces or 4
servings. The average muffin was 5.2 ounces—more than 3
muffin servings. Cookies averaged 1 ounce, which is 2 cookie
servings. The baked potatoes averaged 6.7 ounces, nearly
double the USDA's 3.9 ounce definition of a medium baked potato.[44]

For several years, nutrition educators and dietitians studied
various methods to improve the estimation of portion size. The
research emphasized training subjects to use numerous reference tools that can be used for estimation. These tools included
standard household measures (cups) or objects (decks of cards,
baseballs), rubber models of foods, drawings and photographs
of foods, and the hand or fist. It is not clear how these reference
tools compare in terms of accuracy and ease of use, and it is

Some steps:

- Education and consumer awareness
- Food labels with portion size
- More point-of-purchase nutrition information
- Incentives and rewards for food industry to improve nutrition guidance and reduce portion sizes.

Meal replacements and structured meals may help to reduce the influence of environmental food cues and the number of decisions that have to be made about the type and amount of food to eat. Past researchers believed that meal replacements, although useful, did not teach people how to deal with the complexities of eating in the real world. This may be true, but replacing just one meal a day with a preportioned food helped with weight management.[42] These studies underline the importance of developing strategies to deal with an eating environment that is constantly compelling people to eat more than they need. One such strategy is to limit the frequency of uncontrolled eating opportunities.

likely that there will be variations that depend upon the type of food being assessed and who is doing the assessment. In a review of the many studies on this topic, Young and Nestle[45] conclude that indeed there are differences in estimation that depend upon subject characteristics, such as gender, age, body weight, and level of training, and that the error in estimation becomes greater as portions increase. However, the bottom line is that virtually everyone has difficulty estimating portion sizes accurately, and there is little research to suggest which methods would be the most successful for teaching individuals about appropriate portions.

Young and Nestle[45] outline several research priorities to improve the estimation of portion size. These priorities include identifying the best methods for determining portion sizes and for effectively educating the public about the relationship of portion size to caloric intake. The authors also recommend that there should be a reassessment of how the public is guided toward appropriate portions. Currently, confusion surrounds the discrepancy between recommended servings and actual portion sizes. Young and Nestle suggest that "Standards should provide cues to the public about appropriate portion sizes. Standards that more closely reflect actual intake levels might well help the public to understand better the relationship between food intake, caloric intake, and health."[45(p155)]

Public Policy and Portion Size

Young and Nestle[45] made their recommendations in 1995. Since then, little has been done to improve the situation. However, with the increasing girth of the nation, some policy makers have cited portion size as a dietary factor that requires special attention. For example, part of *The Surgeon General's Call to Action to Prevent and Decrease Overweight and Obesity*[46] includes promoting "healthier food choices, including at least five servings of fruits and vegetables each day, and reasonable portion sizes at home, in schools, at worksites, and in communities." In schools, the report specifically recommends "reducing access to foods high in fat, calories, and added sugars and to excessive portion sizes." The Dietary Guidelines[47] also emphasize the importance of choosing sensible portion sizes (Figure 1).

- If you're eating out, order small portions, share an entree with a friend, or take some of the food home (if you can chill it immediately).
- Check product labels to see how much food is considered a serving. Many items sold as single portions actually provide 2 servings or more—such as a 20-ounce soft drink, a 12-ounce steak, a 3-ounce bag of chips, or a large bagel.
- Be especially careful to limit the portion size of foods high in calories, such as cookies, cakes, other sweets, French fries, fats, oils, and spreads.

Figure 1. These recommendations on portion size in the Dietary Guidelines [47] are a good start, but we need to give consumers more immediate information about portions when they are deciding how much to eat.

The Future: What Can Be Done About Megaportions?

Restaurants are giving customers what they want—value for their money in portions and calories. Now that consumers are accustomed to big portions, getting portions back in synchrony with energy needs will be difficult. Successful strategies to achieve this goal require cooperation between researchers, the food and restaurant industries, and policy makers. *Ultimately, solutions depend upon consumers understanding and accepting the value to their health of eating reasonable portions.* Here are some possible approaches to dealing with megaportions:

Education and consumer awareness campaigns. The public is confused about the role of food in weight management. Many individuals believe that the kinds of foods and macronutrients that they eat are more important than the amount of food, and many are unaware of appropriate portions and the calorie content of foods. Targeted and appealing clear messages that educate the public on these issues are needed. In a recent article in *Nutrition Today*, Tillotson[48] points out that the food and restaurant industries use state-of-the-art marketing strategies to convince consumers that their products meet their desires and lifestyles. This is perfectly acceptable and expected in a free-market economy. However, if consumers are to understand the long-term health effects of eating huge portions of energy-dense foods, either food providers must moderate their promotion of these foods or public policy makers must mobilize to provide a well-funded counter-strategy, using marketing and psychologic techniques as sophisticated as those being used by industry.[48]

Food labels that give clear information about portion size. Recommended serving sizes are often unrelated to actual portions that are available. Consumers need clearer information about how the calories in the foods they buy relate to their daily energy needs. Although this information is available on the Nutrition Facts label, innovative ways to make it more prominent and easily understood by the public should be developed.

More point-of-purchase nutrition information. When eating out, nutritional information is often difficult to obtain. Sometimes it is available upon request, or the customers may be referred to a Web site. In its recent report, the National Alliance for Nutrition and Activity[10] calls for point-of-purchase nutrition information, including portion size information. A barrier to demanding that policy makers require the restaurant industry to provide such information is that the effects on consumer behavior are not well understood. For example, the effects that nutrition labels have on food choices are influenced by the consumer's attitudes toward healthy options when eating out and the type of food offered.[49] Clearly, we need a better understanding of how to best convey information about portion sizes and the energy content of foods to consumers.

Incentives and rewards for the food industry to improve nutritional quality and reduce portion sizes. Although there have been suggestions that penalties such as "sin taxes" should be levied against some types of foods, including high-fat snacks and soda, these have not been embraced. Deciding which foods should be taxed is just one of many issues that makes this proposal a political "hot potato." Often rewards work better than punishments when attempting to motivate change. It is worth considering whether rewarding companies that provide foods in reasonable portions could be implemented. Part of this strategy could be to encourage the availability of a greater range of portion sizes and initiatives to make smaller portions more appealing.

Develop an understanding of the interaction of biologic and environmental influences on children's eating behaviors. Studies indicate that until approximately 3 years of age, children eat in response to energy requirements. However, during this period, they are rapidly learning about different foods, developing preferences, and responding to the eating environment. By age 5 years, they show an adult response to portion size, eating more as the portions increase. Several studies suggest strategies to modify the influence of portion size in children. In one study, teaching children to attend to cues related to hunger and fullness rather than cleaning their plates was associated with better intake regulation.[18] In another study, children consumed 25% less of an entree when allowed to serve themselves than when served a large portion by someone else.[50] With the recent surge in obesity rates in children, it is critical to understand influences on their eating behavior so that healthy habits can be established early. Once established, eating habits are difficult to change. Parents and other caretakers need clear guidelines on appropriate portions for children of various ages and on how to maintain eating behaviors that match energy needs.

Consider how foods can be modified to give consumers satisfying portions, good value and taste, and fewer calories.

Should scientists and consumers be angry about the food on offer? Should we be militant and adopt a "tobacco model," involving litigation to force change? Are the recent cases brought against some fast-food chains, in which they are blamed for clients' obesity, frivolous or the opening of the floodgates? There is unlikely to be agreement on the answers to these questions. However, it is not clear that putting the food industry on the defensive will provide an incentive for change. A more positive approach is for scientists and the food industry to work together to develop foods appropriate for weight management that are acceptable to the consumer and profitable for the retailer.

Food modifications that involve little change in consumer behavior show promise. For example, a study in New Zealand suggests that if vendors were taught how to vary the method of cooking French fries so that less fat was absorbed, a significant reduction in per-capita fat consumption would result, with no change in the portions consumed.[51] Reductions in fat are one approach to reducing the calorie content without changing portion size, but a better approach is likely to be a reduction in the energy density. While reducing fat decreases the energy density of foods, the component of foods that has the greatest influence on energy density is the water content.[24] The combination of a reduction in fat content with the addition of water-rich vegetables would significantly reduce the energy density of popular foods, such as burgers and sandwiches (Figure 5). Consumers could eat their usual portions, but with fewer calories.

Food providers should focus on how to make such changes without affecting acceptability and perceived value. Another consideration is whether such changes should be made "silently" or accompanied by an advertising campaign. At issue is that some consumers will perceive any move toward calorie or fat reduction as being associated with a loss of palatability. This will be just one of the many challenges the food industry will face when attempting to maintain its profits while reducing the energy density of foods and keeping them tasty and reasonably priced.

Urgent Action Needed

Although we are just beginning to understand how environmental factors, such as portion size, affect eating behavior, there are enough data to suggest that large portions of energy-dense foods are contributing to the obesity epidemic. Although it is not yet clear which will be the most effective strategies for bringing intake back in line with energy requirements, *the continuing rise in the rates of obesity calls for urgent action.* Interventions must be initiated and their efficacy monitored in several settings. The complexity of the issues involved—economic, political, psychologic, educational—demands cooperation among scientists and the public and the private sectors. Clearly, individuals bear the ultimate responsibility for how much they eat, but innovative initiatives to help them to resist our abundant environment could help to slow the obesity epidemic. Above all, when considering the influence of portion size, remember that it is not portion size that is the problem, but rather big portions of energy-dense foods that encourage excess energy intake. Large portions of foods low in energy density, such as fruits and vegetables, not only are acceptable but also should be encouraged.

ACKNOWLEDGMENTS

The author thanks the Department of Nutritional Sciences, The Pennsylvania State University, University Park.

Barbara J. Rolls, PhD, holds the Helen A. Guthrie Chair in Nutrition in the Department of Nutritional Sciences at The Pennsylvania State University. Her studies examine influences on human ingestive behavior and body weight regulation. She is particularly interested in how properties of foods influence hunger and satiety. The practical implications of this work for weight management have been published in *The Volumetrics Weight-Control Plan*, HarperTorch, 2003.

This work was supported by NIH grants DK39177 and DK59853.

Corresponding author: Barbara J. Rolls, PhD, Department of Nutritional Sciences, 226 Henderson Building, The Pennsylvania State University, University Park, PA 16802-6501 (e-mail: bjr4@psu.edu).

REFERENCES

40. Flegal KM, Carroll MD, Ogden CL, Johnson CL. Prevalence and trends in obesity among US adults, 1999-2000. JAMA. 2002;288:1723-1727.

41. Ogden CL, Flegal KM, Carroll MD, Johnson CL. Prevalence and trends in overweight among US children and adolescents, 1999-2000. JAMA. 2002;288:1728-1732.

42. Harnack J, Jeffery RW, Boutelle KN. Temporal trends in energy intake in the United States: an ecologic perspective. *Am J Clin Nutr*. 2000;71:1478-1484.

43. Young LR, Nestle M. The contribution of expanding portion sizes to the US obesity epidemic. *Am J Public Health*. 2002;92:246-249.

44. Nielsen SJ, Popkin BM. Patterns and trends in food portion sizes, 1977-1998. JAMA. 2003;289:450-453.

45. Smiciklas-Wright H, Mitchell DC, Mickle SJ, Goldman JD, Cook A. Foods commonly eaten in the United States, 1989-1991 and 1994-1996: are portion sizes changing? *J Am Diet Assoc*. 2003;103:41-47.

46. Rolls BJ, Morris EL, Roe LS. Portion size of food affects energy intake in normal-weight and overweight men and women. *Am J Clin Nutr* 2002;76:1207-1213.

47. Slawson DL, Eck LH. Intense practice enhances accuracy of portion size estimation of amorphous foods. *J Am Diet Assoc*. 1997;97:295-297.

48. Siegel PS. The completion compulsion in human eating. *Psychol Rep*. 1957;3:15-16.

49. The National Alliance for Nutrition and Activity (NANA). *From Wallet to Waistline: The Hidden Costs of Super Sizing*. Washington, DC: NANA; 2002.

50. Ello-Martin JA, Roe LS, Meengs JS, Wall DE, Rolls BJ. Increasing the portion size of a unit food increases energy intake. *Appetite*. 2002;39:74.

51. Kral TVE, Roe LS, Meengs JS, Wall DE, Rolls BJ. Increasing the portion size of a packaged snack increases energy intake. *Appetite*. 2002;39:86.

52. Wansink B. Can package size accelerate usage volume? *J Marketing*. 1996;60:1-14.

53. Wansink B, Park SB. At the movies: how external cues and perceived taste impact consumption volume. *J Database Marketing*. 2000;7:308-320.

54. Kral TVE, Meengs JS, Wall DE, Roe LS, Rolls BJ. Effect on food intake of increasing the portion size of all foods over two consecutive days. *FASEB J*. In press.

55. McConahy KL, Smiciklas-Wright H, Birch LL, Mitchell DC, Picciano MF. Food portions are positively related to energy intake and body weight in early childhood. *J Pediatr*. 2002;140:340-347.

56. Rolls BJ, Engell D, Birch LL. Serving portion size influences 5-year-old but not 3-year old children's food intakes. *J Am Diet Assoc*. 2000;100:232-234.

57. Birch LL, McPhee L, Shoba BC, Steinberg L, Krehbiel R. Clean up your plate: effects of child feeding practices on the conditioning of meal size. *Learn Motiv*. 1987;18:301-317.

58. Clemens LHE, Slawson DL, Klesges RC. The effect of eating out on quality of diet in premenopausal women. *J Am Diet Assoc*. 1999;99:442-444.

59. Binkley JK, Eales J, Jekanowski M. The relation between dietary change and rising US obesity *Int J Obes*. 2000;24:1032-1039.

60. French SA, Harnack L, Jeffrey RW. Fast food restaurant use among women in the Pound of Prevention study: dietary, behavioral and demographic correlates. *Int J Obes*. 2000;24:1353-1359.

61. French SA, Story M, Neumark-Sztainer D, Fulkerson JA, Hannah P. Fast food restaurant use among adolescents: associations with nutrient intake, food choices and behavioral and psychosocial variables. Int J Obes. 2001;25:1823-1833.

62. McCrory MA, Fuss PJ, Hays NP, Vinken AG, Greenberg AS, Roberts SB. Overeating in America: association between restaurant food consumption and body fatness in healthy adult men and women ages 19-80. *Obes Res*. 1999;7:564-571.

63. Rolls BJ, Bell EA. Dietary approaches to the treatment of obesity. In: Jensen MD, ed. *Medical Clinics of North America*. Volume 84. Philadelphia: W.B. Saunders; 2000:401-418.

64. Kinghorn Y, Wise A, Blwyddin G. How do caterers decide on portion sizes? *P Nutr Soc*. 1995;54:198A.

65. American Institute for Cancer Research. New survey shows Americans ignore importance of portion size in managing weight. American Institute for Cancer Research home page. Available at: http://www.aicr.org/r032400.htm. Accessed November 8, 2001.

66. American Institute for Cancer Research. As restaurant portions grow, vast majority of Americans still belong to "clean plate club," new survey finds. American Institute of Cancer Research home page. Available at: http://www.aicr.org/r011501.htm. Accessed November 8, 2001.

67. Diliberti N, Bordi PL, Conklin MT, Rolls BR. Increasing the portion size of a restaurant entree results in increased food intake. *FASEB J*. In press.

68. Cohn SR, Grover SF Doing battle with the "fat" police. *Restaurant Hospitality*. 2000;84:62-64.

69. Krassner HA, Brownell KD, Stunkard AJ. Cleaning the plate: food left over by overweight and normal weight persons. *Behav Res Ther*. 1979;17:155-156.

70. Pudel VE, Oetting M. Eating in the laboratory: behavioral aspects of the positive energy balance. *Int J Obes*. 1977;1:369-386.

71. Meyers AW, Stunkard AJ, Coll M. Food accessibility and food choice. *Arch Gen Psychiatry*. 1980;37:1133-1135.

72. Painter JE, Wansink B, Hieggelke JB. How visibility and convenience influence candy consumption. *Appetite*. 2002;38:237-238.

73. Chandon P, Wansink B. When are stockpiled products consumed faster? A convenience-salience framework of post-purchase consumption incidence and quantity. *J Marketing*. 2002;39:321-335.

74. Bell EA, Rolls B. Regulation of energy intake: factors contributing to obesity. In: Bowman B, Russell R, ed. *Present Knowledge in Nutrition*. 8th ed. Washington, DC: ILSI Press; 2001:31-40.

75. Westerterp-Plantenga MS, Pasman WJ, Yedema MJW, Wijckmans-Duijsens NEG. Energy intake adaptation of food intake to extreme energy densities of food by obese and non-obese women. *Eur J Clin Nutr*. 1996;50:401-407.

76. McConahy KL, Picciano MF Smiciklas-Wright H, Mitchell DC. Portion size, energy intake, and weight status are positively as-

sociated among low-income children aged 4- to 5-years but not 2- to 3-years [abstract]. *FASEB J*. 2001;15:A738.

77. Rolls B, Barnett RA. *The Volumetrics Weight-Control Plan: Feel Full on Fewer Calories*. New York: Avon, HarperCollins Publishers; 2003.

78. Bell EA, Castellanos VH, Pelkman CL, Thorwart ML, Rolls BJ. Energy density of foods affects energy intake in normal-weight women. *Am J Clin Nutr*. 1998;67:412-420.

79. Bell EA, Rolls BJ. Energy density of foods affects energy intake across multiple levels of fat content in lean and obese women. *Am J Clin Nutr*. 2001;73:1010-1018.

80. Rolls BJ, Bell EA, Castellanos VH, Chow M, Pelkman CL, Thorwart ML. Energy density but not fat content of foods affected energy intake in lean and obese women. *Am J Clin Nutr*. 1999;69:863-871.

81. Ditschuneit HH, Flechtner-Mors M. Value of structured meals for weight management: risk factors and long-term weight maintenance. *Obes Res*. 2001;9:284S-289S.

82. Wing RR, Jeffery RW. Food provision as a strategy to promote weight loss. *Obes Res*. 2001;9:271S-275S.

83. Young LR, Nestle M. Variation in perceptions of a "medium" food portion: implications for dietary guidance. *J Am Diet Assoc*. 1998;98:458-459.

84. Young LR, Nestle M. Portion sizes in dietary assessment: Issues and policy implications. *Nutr Rev*. 1995;53:149-158.

85. US Department of Health and Human Services. The Surgeon General's Call to Action to Prevent and Decrease Overweight and Obesity. Rockville, Md: US Department of Health and Human Services, Public Health Service, Office of the Surgeon General, 2001. Available at: http://www.surgeongeneral.gov/topics/obesity/. Accessed September 4, 2002.

86. USDA Center for Nutrition Policy and Promotion. *Nutrition and Your Health: Dietary Guidelines for Americans*. 5th ed. Washington, DC: U.S. Department of Agriculture, 2000. Available at: http://www.usda.gov/cnpp. Accessed August 9, 2002.

87. Tillotson JE. We're fat and getting fatter! What is the food industry's role? *Nutr Today*. 2002;37:136-138.

88. Stubenitsky K, Aaron JI, Catt SL, Mela DJ. The influence of recipe modification and nutritional information on restaurant food acceptance and macronutrient intakes. *Public Health Nutr*. 2000;3:201-209.

89. Fisher JO, Rolls BJ, Birch LL. Large portions increase children's bite size and intake relative to age-appropriate and self-selected portions. *Am J Clin Nutr*. In press.

90. Morley-John J, Swinburn BA, Metcalf PA, Raza F. Fat content of chips, quality of frying fat and deep-frying practices in New Zealand fast food outlets. *Aust NZ J Public Health*. 2002;26:101-106.

Big Fat Fake

The Atkins diet controversy and the sorry state of science journalism

Michael Fumento

IT WAS EXACTLY what millions of obese Americans wanted to hear: Diet guru Robert Atkins has been right all along; conversely, the "medical establishment" that has routinely criticized him has been entirely wrong. Unlimited-calorie, high-fat meals are the key to low-fat bodies. So claimed award-winning science writer Gary Taubes in an 8,000-word *New York Times Magazine* blockbuster that appeared last July, "What If It's All Been a Big Fat Lie?"

The magazine's cover was even juicier than the title: It featured a slab of steak topped with butter and asked, "What If Fat Doesn't Make You Fat?" In fact, Taubes declared in his article, the consumption of *too little* fat could explain the explosion in obesity.

Atkins quickly wrote an editorial for his Web site claiming the article "validated" his work. Gushingly favorable follow-up stories appeared on NBC's *Dateline*, CBS' *48 Hours*, and ABC's *20/20*. *Dr Atkins' New Diet Revolution*, with 11 million copies already in print, shot up from No. 5 to the top spot on the *New York Times* paperback bestseller list for "Advice, How-To, and Miscellaneous" books. It went from No. 178 to No. 5 in Amazon's rankings. Taubes himself landed a book contract from publisher Alfred A. Knopf for a big fat $700,000.

Dr. Atkins claims that by simply minimizing your carbohydrate intake you can quickly lose massive amounts of weight, even while pigging out daily on fatback, pork rinds, and lard.

But there were serious problems with this revolutionary argument about one of our nation's most serious health problems. For example, Taubes omitted any reference to hundreds of refereed scientific studies published during the last three decades that contradicted his position. Researchers from whom he could not pull even a single useful quote supportive of his thesis were banished from the piece, while many of those whom Taubes did end up quoting now complain that he twisted their words.

"I was greatly offended by how Gary Taubes tricked us all into coming across as supporters of the Atkins diet,"
says one such source, Stanford University cardiologist John Farquhar. "I think he's a dangerous man. I'm sorry I ever talked to him."

Upon closer examination, Taubes' "What If It's All Been a Big Fat Lie?" turns into a big fat mess. The misguided hoopla over the *New York Times Magazine* article and the Atkins Diet is a short study in the sorry state of scientific and medical reporting, not to mention a diet industry that routinely panders to people's worst impulses.

The Fat Shall Set Ye Free?

In *Dr. Atkins' New Diet Revolution*, Robert Atkins claims that by simply minimizing your carbohydrate intake you can quickly lose massive amounts of weight, even while pigging out daily on fatback, pork rinds, and lard. He also claims his diet will relieve "fatigue, irritability, depression, trouble concentrating, headaches, insomnia, dizziness, joint and muscle aches, heartburn, colitis, premenstrual syndrome, and water retention and bloating."

Claims like those should make anyone suspicious, even those who have barely scraped through high school biology. Gary Taubes has gone well beyond that level. He's a contributing correspondent to America's preeminent scientific journal, *Science*. He has won the National Association of Science Writers' Science in Society Journalism Award three times—the maximum allowed. Only one other writer has ever achieved that status.

Nonetheless, at the very outset of his piece (viewable in its entirely at www.atkinsdiet.com) Taubes set forth the proposition that Atkins was crucified by the "American medical establishment," which claimed his diet was ineffective and possibly dangerous and in so doing encouraged the "rampaging epidemic of obesity in America."

There is a nugget of truth in Taubes' criticisms of establishment dietary fat advice. Well-meaning but misguided health officials and health reporters, joined by opportunistic anti-fat diet book gurus, have convinced much of the public that the major culprit—perhaps the *only* culprit—in obesity is dietary fat. Avoid fat, we were told, and you won't get fat. Given license to eat as many calories as we wanted from the other nutrient groups, many of us have done exactly that. This goes far to explain why almost one-third of us are obese and two-thirds of us are overweight. But even here Taubes is no pioneer; the damage caused by fat-free fanaticism was pointed out long before. (See, for example, my own 1997 book, *The Fat of the Land*.)

Moreover, the Atkins-Taubes thesis of "fat won't make you fat" encourage obesity in a similar way: It offers carte blanche for consuming limitless calories, only this time swapping carbohydrates for fat. Taubes made that swap while presenting a far less scientific case than is presented in an Atkins infomercial.

Ask Stanford endocrinologist Gerald Reaven. He's best known for calling attention to "Syndrome X," a cluster of conditions that may indicate a predisposition to diabetes, hypertension, and heart disease. Among Reaven's recommendations for lowering the risk of that syndrome is to reduce consumption of highly refined carbohydrates such as those present in soft drinks and table sugar. But that's where the overlap with Atkins ends.

"I thought [Taubes'] article was outrageous," Reaven says. "I saw my name in it and all that was quoted to me was not wrong. But in the context it looked like I was buying the rest of that crap." He adds, "I tried to be helpful and a good citizen, and I ended up being embarrassed as hell. He sort of set me up." When I first contacted Reaven, he was so angry he wouldn't even let me interview him.

But his position on Atkins was all over the Internet in interviews posted long before Taubes talked to him. Do "low-carb diets like *The Zone* [by Barry Sears] and Atkins work?" one asked. Answer: "One can lose weight on a low-calorie diet if it is primarily composed of fat calories or carbohydrate calories or protein calories. It makes no difference!"

The very person with whom Taubes chose to end his article, Stanford's John Farquhar, was as livid as Reaven. Taubes said that Farquhar had sent Taubes "an e-mail message asking the not-entirely-rhetorical question, 'Can we get the low-fat proponents to apologize?'" On this powerful note, the article ended.

But it's Taubes whom Farquhar wants to apologize. "I was greatly offended by how Gary Taubes tricked us all into coming across as supporters of the Atkins diet," he wrote in an e-mail he broadcast to reporters and to colleagues who were stunned that Farquhar might actually hold the beliefs Taubes attributed to him. "We are against the Atkins Diet," he wrote, speaking for himself and Reaven. "It told him [Taubes] there is the minor degree of merit" to the idea that "people are getting fatter because too much emphasis is being placed on just cutting fats," Farquhar told me. But "once I give him that opening—bingo—he was off and running, even though I said about six times that this is *not* the cause of the obesity epidemic."

Diets and Data

Taubes proved as adept at clipping data as at clipping quotes. Thus he claimed that one of the "reasons to suggest that the low-fat-is-good-health hypothesis has now effectively failed the test of time" is "that the *percentage* of fat in the American diet has been decreasing for two decades." (Emphasis added.)

That's true, but irrelevant. The *amount* of fat consumed has been steadily climbing, as has consumption of all calories. Individual caloric consumption jumped from 3,300 calories per day in 1970–79 to 3,900 in 1997, an 18 percent increase. Per-person consumption of fat grams increased from 149 to 156, a 4.5 percent increase. "We're eating just too darned much of everything," says Farquhar.

Taubes also shoved aside decades of published, controlled, randomized clinical trials comparing nutrient intake and weight loss. His apparent justification in the article was that the "research literature [is] so vast that it's possible to find at least some published research to support virtually any theory." But that's sheer nihilism. Good science is cautious and skeptical, not permanently open-ended. That's why terms like *weight of the evidence* are used. And the evidence against Atkins-like low-carbohydrate diets is crushing.

In April 2002, for example, the *Journal of the American Dietetic Association (JADA)* published a review of "all studies identified" that looked at diet nutrient composition and weight loss. It found over 200, with "no studies of the health and nutrition effects of popular diets in the published literature" excluded. In some, subjects were put on "ad libitum" diets, meaning they were allowed to eat as much as they wanted as long as they consumed fat, protein, and carbohydrates in the directed proportions. In others, subjects were put on controlled-calorie diets that also had directed nutrient proportions. The conclusion: Those who *ate* the least fat *carried* the least fat.

An alternative method of comparing diets is a meta-analysis, which means not looking at the sum of the whole but actually combining the data. One such meta-analysis, covering 16 ad libitum studies and almost 2,000 people, appeared in the *International Journal of Obesity and Related Metabolic Disorders* in December 2000. The conclusion: Those on low-fat diets had "a greater reduction in energy intake" and a "greater weight loss than control groups."

Well-meaning but misguided health officials and health reporters, joined by opportunistic anti-fat diet book gurus, have convinced much of the public that the major culprit—perhaps the only culprit—in obesity is dietary fat.

"Aren't all these studies highly relevant to the issue of whether an Atkins-like diet works, and don't they indicate that it does not?" I ask Dr. Louis Aronne, director of the Comprehensive Weight Control Program at New York's Weill Cornell Medical Center. "I agree completely," he says. "You're absolutely right."

This wasn't the first time Taubes had published a lengthy article on fat while leaving out this vital information. He also did so in one of his award-winning pieces, a precursor to the "Big Fat Lie" article called "The Soft Science of Dietary Fat" that appeared in *Science* in March 2001. In a subsequent letter to the journal, three obesity research co-authors, including James Hill, director of the University of Colorado Center for Human Nutrition in Denver, noted, "What Taubes does not mention are the meta-analyses of intervention studies comparing ad libitum intakes of higher fat diets with low-fat diets that clearly show reduced caloric intake and weight loss on the low-fat diet." Taubes responded to the letter but again refused to address these studies.

Why? "They're not worth mentioning," he told me in a telephone interview. They weren't done correctly. None of them? None. The one meta-analysis Taubes thinks was properly conducted appeared in 2002 in *The Cochrane Library*. Yet it, too, found no advantage to low-carbohydrate diets, merely that "fat-restricted diets are no better than calorie restricted" ones.

Where, I ask Taubes, did all these researchers go wrong? The problem is inherent to an intervention study, he says. "When you counsel people you change their behavior." But doesn't that apply to all the groups in a study? Yes, he grants. "But the idea is to make the intervention effect equal for everyone, whichever diet they happen to be on," he says. "If the interventions aren't the same, then you just don't know how to interpret the results." That may be true, but it's also irrelevant. There's no reason to think persons on either low-fat or high-fat diets got more or less intervention in these myriad studies. Indeed, in some of them virtually all the intervention emphasis was on *exercise*, with little nutrition counseling one way or the other.

Finally, the comprehensive *JADA* review published last April also looked at persons who weren't in intervention studies at all but rather were part of the U.S. Department of Agriculture's Continuing Survey of Food Intake by Individuals. An updated report on the survey appeared last June in the *Journal of the American College of Nutrition*. Both survey reports came to the same conclusion as the intervention studies.

Dr. Aronne is quick to point out that this wealth of data supporting lower-fat diets "is not an endorsement for eating unlimited amounts of nonfat muffins and soda simply because they're fat-free." All carbohydrate sources are not equal. For example, fiber appears to play a powerful role in weight control, but there is no more fiber in a soda than there is in a steak. That said, a high-fat diet does carry an inherent metabolic disadvantage in that fat has nine calories per gram, while carbohydrates and protein each have four.

Abstract Weight Loss

Having circumvented this mass of peer-reviewed literature readily open to public scrutiny in libraries and often online, Taubes instead tried to make his case with a mere *five* studies. All five were (and are) available only in abstract form. That is, they are summaries of about 300 words each that have been presented at various obesity conferences. "The results of all five of these studies are remarkably consistent," Taubes averred. "Subjects on some form of the Atkins diet… lost twice the weight as the subjects on the low-fat, low-calorie diets."

One of the five studies, conducted at the Durham Veterans Administration Medical Center in North Carolina, was funded by the Atkins Center. Those researchers repeatedly have publicized their interpretation of their findings and unsurprisingly have conferred their full blessings on the diet. They did so most recently in late November, garnering tremendous favorable media attention. (See "Hold the Lard" at www.reason.com/hod/mf120502.shtml.) The authors of the other four studies, however, have been reticent about releasing their data, in part because pre-publicity in the lay press makes it more difficult to get published in medical journals. But when I interviewed researchers for two of the other studies, they all insisted Taubes grossly mischaracterized their findings.

"The Atkins diet produces weight loss, as does the grapefruit diet, the rotation diet, and every other fad diet out there," says one of the researchers, Colorado's James Hill. "I haven't seen any data anywhere saying Atkins is better than these other diets for weight loss. Taubes is trying to fly in the face of the scientific evidence." Referring to the book deal, he says, "Taubes sold out."

Hill's co-researcher, Gary Foster of the University of Pennsylvania, says "the probable explanation for the greater weight loss in the groups on the Atkins regimen" is that it "gives people a framework to eat fewer calories, since most of the choices in this culture are carbohydrate driven…. You're left eating a lot of fat, and you get tired of that. Over time people eat fewer calories." That would make the Atkins plan nothing more than a low-calorie diet in disguise.

Another of the abstracts came from the University of Cincinnati. The Atkins-like group "did have twice as much weight loss, and to completely lose that point would be unfair," says one of the co-authors, Randy Seeley of the university's Obesity Research Center. But his explanation is similar to Foster's, if more colorful. "If you're only allowed to shop in two aisles of the grocery store, does it matter which two they are?" he asks.

All the researchers I interviewed also insisted the studies weren't long enough to be conclusive, with none lasting more than a year. And the kicker is that all five were *intervention studies*, conducted using the same methodology that Taubes cites to dismiss the mountain of published material that undercuts his position.

Seeley and co-researcher David D'Alessio were also upset that Taubes made use of their material at all and not just because it hurt their chances of publication. "One of the things I object to most in the Taubes article is the idea that we're going to carry out this scientific debate in the lay press with data that's unavailable for scientists to review," says Seeley. "I believe in the peer-review process." Indeed, one "danger of trying to conduct this out in the lay press," he says, is that "you have a guy like Taubes going through it and just picking up the pieces that support his opinion."

3,000 MIAs

Taubes also ignored the approximately 3,000 members of a database called the National Weight Control Registry. For 10 years, the registry has tracked people who have lost at least 30 pounds and kept it off for at least a year. The average member has maintained a loss of about 60 pounds for about five years.

Co-administered by Hill in Denver and Rena Wing of the University of Pittsburgh, the registry is aimed at finding out what works and what doesn't. According to its members, what *doesn't* work is a high-fat diet. On average, they consume only 23 percent of calories from fat. "Almost nobody's on a low-carbohydrate diet," Hill says. Another important lesson that may be drawn from the registry is that the importance of *any* type of diet in weight control may be overemphasized. Ninety-one percent of the subjects said they regularly exercised.

While relying on self-interpretation of unpublished abstracts is valid methodology to Taubes, he insists the registry is so unscientific as to be worthless. One problem, he told me, is that it represents only a tiny fraction of all those who have succeeded at weight loss. Further, the sample is entirely self-selected rather than randomized. "Its method of recruiting could bias the selection toward those who use low-fat diets," he says.

Yet the registry data have been considered valid and important enough to have been written up in such peer-reviewed medical publications as the *American Journal of Clinical Nutrition*, the *Journal of the American Dietetic Association*, the *International Journal of Obesity*, *Health Psychology*, and *Obesity Research*.

"You can't get around" the problem of self-selection, says Suzanne Phelan, a co-investigator of the registry at Brown University Medical School. "But why would non-Atkins people select in and Atkins ones stay out?" Atkins dieters, she notes, "seem to be very dedicated." (Other researchers have described them as having an almost religious fervor.) Originally, recruits were selected "based on a random-digit dialing procedure," she says. But that proved onerous, and "as media such as *USA Today* and *CNN* began talking about the registry, we just let them take over" the recruiting process. "There's no reason to think that people who see those media are more likely to have a certain diet," Phelan says.

The amount of fat Americans consume has been steadily climbing, as has consumption of all calories. Individual caloric consumption jumped from 3,300 calories per day in 1970–79 to 3,900 in 1997, an 18 percent increase.

Oh, and there's another place where joining the registry has been promoted: the Atkins Web site. So we're left wondering why successful low-fat eaters would be especially likely to select into the registry or why the purchasers of over 11 million Atkins diet books consistently opt out.

Feeling Full

For all its 8,000 words, there were few actual data in the Taubes piece. It was rather like reading a treatise explaining how the Chicago Cubs may well be the best team in baseball history without being informed they haven't won a pennant since 1945. Instead readers were regaled with explanations of physiological mechanisms—the basis for which, Taubes wrote, is "endocrinology 101"—that might explain how dieters shed pounds and inches. *Endocrinology 101* is a term popularized by Dr. David Ludwig, who runs the pediatric obesity clinic at Children's Hospital Boston.

According to Taubes, Endocrinology 101 "requires an understanding of how carbohydrates affect insulin and blood sugar and in turn fat metabolism and appetite." In brief, it says there are aspects of a high- or low-carbohydrate diet that affect both how much we want to eat (referred to as "satiety") and how efficiently the body converts the various nutrients into body fat. And the theory says an Atkins-like diet is both more satiating and less efficient in converting calories to fat.

Yet the published literature that Taubes ignored says otherwise. The aforementioned review of over 200 studies in the *Journal of the American Dietetic Association* expressly nixed the idea that any type of food converts less efficiently to body fat. "None of the popular diet research we reviewed suggests a metabolic advantage with respect to weight loss," it declared.

Nor can Taubes fall back on his five studies, according to Seeley. "Ultimately our data do not support *any* of the mechanisms" for why a low-carbohydrate diet might be especially effective in inducing weight loss "that Atkins and proponents of the diet have [suggested]," he told me. Indeed, each explanation that Taubes presents for how an Atkins diet *might* cause weight loss collapses under the weight of the published research he ignores.

Consider the matter of satiety. How, Taubes wondered, could a low-calorie regimen "suppress hunger, which Atkins insisted was the signature characteristic of the diet." One possibility, he said, was, yes, "Endocrinology 101: that fat and protein make you sated and, lacking carbohydrates and the ensuing swings of blood sugar and insulin, you stay sated."

But is there any empirical support for this? No, according to an April 2002 review of studies in the *Journal of the American College of Nutrition* that summarized "high and low fat treatments when subjects were allowed to eat ad libitum." It found "energy intake on the low-fat diets ranged from 16 percent to 24 percent less than those on high fat diets."

"We've done masses of studies on fat and satiety," says Barbara Rolls, professor of nutrition at Pennsylvania State University, where she has authored four books and written about 60 medical journal articles on human food intake. She's widely considered the nation's top authority on satiety. Some of her experiments involved ingestion; in others, "We directly infused pure fat and pure carbohydrates both directly into [human] veins and directly into stomachs." Says Rolls, "We found very little difference between fats and carbohydrates."

Rolls does say there is some evidence that high-protein diets may be more satiating, but Atkins isn't really high protein; it's just high fat. According to an analysis in the journal *Circulation*, Atkins starts off at 36 percent protein from calories and declines to 24 percent in the "maintenance" stage.

What really counts when it comes to satisfying hunger, Rolls says, is "foods that give big portions without a lot of calories. We call these low-energy-density foods." She adds, "The Atkins diet would not be a good way to reduce energy density at all, especially with the restrictions on fruits and vegetables that are really the keys to a low-energy diet." Further, because fat contains more than twice the energy per ounce as either carbohydrates or protein, "high-fat foods are so energy-dense that it's really easy to eat excessive portions."

Rolls says she sent a big pile of her material on satiety to Taubes, but he "just brushed it aside." She says he also interviewed her for over six hours, but every last sentence disappeared into a black hole. Likewise for the interviews Taubes conducted with James Hill and at least five other top obesity researchers from whom he apparently couldn't extract even a single useful line: Dr. F. Xavier Pi-Sunyer of St. Luke's-Roosevelt Hospital in New York; Marion Nestle, chairwoman of the Department of Nutrition and Food Studies at New York University; Dr. Arne Astrup of Denmark; and Dr. Jules Hirsch, whom Taubes interviewed in his office at Rockefeller University in New York. "I just kept telling him, it doesn't matter what kind of calories you eat," says Hirsch.

Taubes is "very selective in what he chooses to include because he's trying to sell a specific line," Rolls says. "He is a good writer; that's the thing that scares me. This is such a good example of how you can pick and choose your facts to present the story you want. But that's not how science should be done. You can't interview everybody and simply ignore the people you don't want to hear." She means that rhetorically, of course.

Gorging on Theory

Stacking theory atop theory, Taubes roared on. Something called "hyperinsulinemia" could also favor the Atkins dieter, he insisted. When carbohydrates are ingested they are broken down in the intestine into glucose and other sugars. Glucose then stimulates cells in the pancreas to secrete insulin to remove that glucose and take it into tissues to be used as fuel or stored. Protein and fat consumption don't have nearly the same impact on insulin production because the whole point of insulin is to maintain the stability of the sugar level.

The Atkins hyperinsulinemia theory, explained Taubes, is that carbohydrates can "cause a spike of blood sugar and a surge of insulin within minutes. The resulting rush of insulin stores the blood sugar away and a few hours later, your blood sugar is lower than it was before you ate." The brain receives a signal that the body needs more food, and the vicious circle repeats itself. Carbohydrates at the top of what's called the "hypoglycemic index" are the most evil of the evil, since they cause blood sugar to rise the fastest. The index ranks potatoes as slightly worse than jelly beans.

For support, Taubes once again fell back on "Endocrinology 101." David Ludwig "notes that when diabetics get too much insulin, their blood sugar drops and they get ravenously hungry," wrote Taubes. "They gain weight because they eat more, and the insulin promotes fat deposition." But according to Seeley, this applies to diabetics injecting massive amounts of insulin into the bloodstream, not to carbohydrate consumers.

"Yes," Seeley says, "if you give people a big wallop of insulin they do eat a lot, but do people under normal circumstances ever get close to that by *eating*? No. Is it possible that *some* people are that reactive? Yes. Is it likely that lots of people fall into that category? No."

Taubes presented University of Washington endocrinologist Michael Schwartz, whom he had interviewed, as a proponent of the idea that blood insulin levels as altered by carbohydrates could be a significant contributor to weight gain. But a commentary in the same magazine Taubes writes for, *Science,* sharply contradicted that position. "Although the concept that insulin triggers weight gain has little scientific merit, it remains a key selling point for advocates of diets that are low in carbohydrate and high in protein and fat," it read. "If hyperinsulinemia has adverse consequences, obesity does not appear to be among them," it concluded. Who wrote that? Michael Schwartz.

Indeed, Schwartz was also the primary author of a study concluding that obese people whose systems secrete insulin at high levels may be *protected* against further weight gain. "Relatively reduced insulin secretion," he concluded, "is a significant and independent predictor of the tendency to gain weight and adiposity in Pima Indians."

The American Medical Association explained why the diet didn't work, mocking Atkins' basic thesis that fat and protein cannot cause weight gain in the absence of carbohydrate consumption as a "thermodynamic miracle."

The Pima in Arizona have been the focus of a tremendous amount of research because even by American standards they are incredibly obese and suffer horrific rates of diabetes and heart disease. Comparisons of the Arizona Pima with genetically similar Pima in Mexico find that the Arizonans eat about twice as much fat (although the Mexicans also do far more manual labor) and are almost 60 pounds heavier on average. A National Institutes of Health evaluation of the traditional Pima diet (that is, back when they were thin and healthy) found that it was extremely high in carbohydrates, from 70 percent to 80 percent.

Schwartz says it's not that he believes insulin *can't* play a role in promoting weight gain, but he rejects "Endocrinology 101" based on what he calls "Scientific Methodology 101." "Before you draw conclusions you need data," he says. "There is no compelling evidence that in normal individuals day-to-day fluctuations of the blood glucose level are an important determinant of how much food is consumed."

The Diet Revolution That Isn't

Two distinct controversies have always swirled around the Atkins diet. First, is it effective for long-term weight loss? Second, could those using it be harming themselves by raising their blood lipids (cholesterol and triglycerides)? The five unpublished abstracts do seem to indicate that for people who manage to stick to a high-fat Atkins diet, it may not be as harmful as was once generally believed. But this finding is quite preliminary and in any case certainly must depend greatly on which types of fat are consumed.

This is a distinction Taubes decided to lose.

Thus he quoted or invoked the name of the chairman of the Department of Nutrition at the Harvard School of Public Health, Walter Willett, seven times during his piece. Willett protests, however, that "I told Taubes several times that red meat is associated with higher risk of colon and possibly prostate cancer, but he left that out." And don't forget the illustration on the cover of *The New York Times Magazine;* that wasn't a flounder with heart-healthy flaxseed oil sitting on top of it.

Taubes also told readers that a metabolic process called ketosis, often invoked to show the Atkins diet could be dangerous, was quite harmless, providing reassuring words from National Institutes of Health researcher Richard Veech that "ketosis is a normal physiologic state." Veech told me by e-mail that the quote was correct, but that Taubes "omitted to say that I strongly urged people to not use the Atkins diet without the supervision of a physician because of the likely elevation of blood cholesterol and lipid on a high fat diet." But you don't have an impact if you insist that a fad diet be supervised by a doctor.

There's nothing "revolutionary" about the Atkins diet. A similar diet appeared in an 1863 booklet by a British undertaker named William Banting, who got the idea from a surgeon. It has popped up in various guises ever since, including a 1946 book extolling the virtues of eating whale blubber, and a 1958 book, *Eat Fat and Grow Slim,* written by a psychiatrist.

Likewise, there has long been convincing evidence that the diet fails to live up to its claims. Taubes wrote that "when the American Medical Association (AMA) released its scathing critique of Atkins' diet in March 1973, it acknowledged that the diet probably worked but expressed little interest in why."

The heavily endnoted document, which appeared in the June 4, 1973, issue of *The Journal of the American Medical Association* but unfortunately is not available on the Internet even in abstract form, was indeed scathing. But the rest of Taubes' description is false.

"The notion that sedentary persons, without malabsorption or hyperthyroidism, can lose weight on a diet containing 5,000 calories a day is incredible," the article says. Statements such as "No scientific evidence exists to suggest that the low-carbohydrate ketogenic diet has a metabolic advantage over more conventional diets for weight reduction," and "there is no reason to associate a diet rich in carbohydrate with obesity" hardly seem to acknowledge "that the diet probably worked." Other terms the AMA used to described Atkins' theories included "naïve," "biochemically incorrect," "inaccurate," and "without scientific merit."

It also explained *why* the diet didn't work, mocking Atkins' basic thesis that fat and protein cannot cause weight gain in the absence of carbohydrate consumption as a "thermodynamic miracle."

Three additional decades of research have merely played "pile on" with the AMA's findings. The explanation for weight loss on Atkins given by Foster and Seeley was right there. "When obese patients reduce their carbohydrate intake drastically, they are apparently unable to make up the ensuing deficit by means of an appreciable increase in protein and diet," said the AMA.

Girth of a Nation

What *has* changed drastically in the last three decades is the girth of a nation. American obesity is increasing at a terrifying rate.

Since the publication of Taubes' article, numerous doctors, scientists, and health writers have picked apart various pieces of his argument. A fatlash has formed against Taubes, *The New York Times Magazine,* and Knopf. Originally riding an adulatory wave, Taubes complained bitterly to the weekly *New York Observer* in November that he was "being attacked by sleazebags."

The New York Times Magazine has printed no clarification or retraction of any kind. Yet not only should the magazine's editors have known there were serious problems with the piece, but Farquhar says he told them so outright, based on what he had gleaned from two fact checkers. He says he told those checkers that if Taubes "tries to make it look like I'm saying that I was supporting the idea that the obesity epidemic was from overloading on carbohydrates that this was so far off the mark that I would have to vomit."

At Knopf, Taubes' acquisitions editor, Scott Segal, has wrapped himself in the flag, telling the *Observer,* "It's a free country: First Amendment," as if he believes the Constitution requires publishers to hand out $700,000 checks to all authors. Equally bizarre is his effort to distance the book acquisition from the article. They "chose to put a certain picture on the cover and to use a certain approach to the subject in 5,000 [*sic*] words, but that's not the book," he said. Critics "are reacting to a magazine piece I had nothing to do with." Yet Taubes told me that his article had barely hit the stands when Knopf's offer dropped in his lap, as did an even larger offer from another publisher that he says he rejected because it's the publisher of Atkins' book and it might hurt his credibility.

But obesity and the millions of individual tragedies it has produced are ultimately far more important than this skirmish over a single story. Louis Aronne says, "I think people are getting increasingly confused about what to do. I'm afraid they'll just give up." Randy Seeley says journalism like Taubes' "just makes people confused and frustrated."

Taubes "gave his readers what they wanted to hear," says James Hill. "But what people want to hear is killing them."

Michael Fumento is a senior fellow at the Hudson Institute and author of The Fat of the Land: The American Obesity Epidemic and How Overweight Americans Can Help Themselves *(Viking, 1997). His next book, on biotechnology, will be published in the spring by Encounter Books.*

Losing Weight:
MORE THAN
COUNTING CALORIES

By Linda Bren

Americans are eating less fat, but getting fatter. We're putting on the pounds at an alarmingly rapid rate. And we're sacrificing our health for the sake of supersize portions, biggie drinks, and two-for-one value meals, obesity researchers say.

More than 60 percent of U.S. adults are either overweight or obese, according to the Centers for Disease Control and Prevention (CDC). While the number of overweight people has been slowly climbing since the 1980s, the number of obese people has nearly doubled since then.

No Laughing Matter

Excess weight and physical inactivity account for more than 300,000 premature deaths each year in the United States, second only to deaths related to smoking, says the CDC. People who are overweight or obese are more likely to develop heart disease, stroke, high blood pressure, diabetes, gallbladder disease and joint pain caused by excess uric acid (gout). Excess weight can also cause interrupted breathing during sleep (sleep apnea) and wearing away of the joints (osteoarthritis).

Carrying extra weight means carrying an extra risk for cancer. "[Our] researchers have concluded that obesity increases the risk for many of the most common cancers worldwide, and perhaps cancer in general," says Melanie Polk, R.D., director of nutrition education at the American Institute for Cancer Research (AICR), a nonprofit research and education organization in Washington, D.C.

In their review of more than 100 studies and international reports on obesity and cancer risk, completed in October 2001, researchers at the AICR concluded that obesity is consistently linked to post-menopausal breast cancer, colon cancer, endometrial cancer, prostate cancer, and kidney cancer.

The public health epidemic of being overweight or obese in the United States has become so serious that Surgeon General David Satcher has prepared a national action plan to address the issue.

Are You Overweight?

Overweight refers to an excess of body weight, but not necessarily body fat. Obesity means an excessively high proportion of body fat. Health professionals use a measurement called body mass index (BMI) to classify an adult's weight as healthy, overweight, or obese. (See the BMI chart, "Are You at a Healthy Weight?") BMI describes body weight relative to height and is strongly correlated with total body fat content in most adults.

BMI is determined by dividing a person's weight in kilograms by height in meters squared. To get your approximate BMI using pounds and inches, multiply your weight in pounds by 700, then divide the result by your height in inches, and divide that result by your height in inches a second time. (Or you can use the interactive BMI calculator at *www.nhlbisupport.com/bmi/bmicalc.htm.*)

A BMI of 18.5 to 24.9 is considered healthy, from 25 to 29.9 is overweight, and 30 or higher is obese. Generally, the higher a person's BMI, the greater the risk for health problems, according to the National Heart, Lung and Blood Institute (NHLBI). However, there are some exceptions. For example, very muscular people, like body builders, may have a BMI greater than 25 or even 30, but

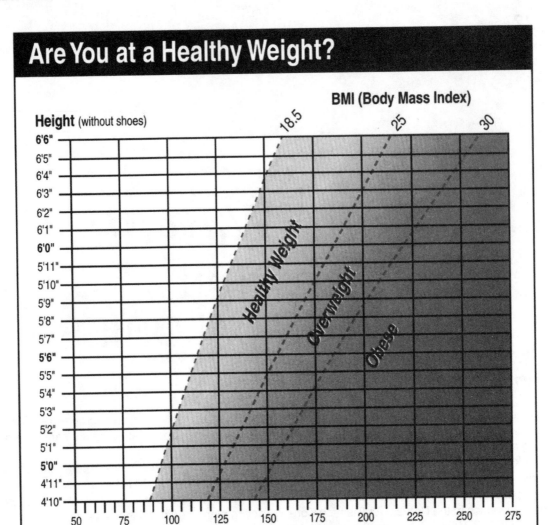

Are You at a Healthy Weight?

BMI (Body Mass Index)

Height (without shoes)

Healthy Weight

Overweight

Obese

Pounds (without clothes)

The BMI ranges shown above are for adults. They are not exact ranges of healthy and unhealthy weights. However, they show that health risk increases at higher levels of overweight and obesity. Even within the healthy BMI range, weight gains can carry health risks for adults.

Directions: Find your weight on the bottom of the graph. Go straight up from that point until you come to the line that matches your height. Then look to find your weight group.

- **Healthy Weight:** BMI from 18.5 up to 25 refers to healthy weight.
- **Overweight:** BMI from 25 up to 30 refers to overweight.
- **Obese:** BMI 30 or higher refers to obesity. Obese persons are also overweight.

Source: *Report of the Dietary Guidelines Advisory Committee on the Dietary Guidelines for Americans*, 2000.

this reflects increased muscle rather than fat. "It is excess body fat that leads to the health problems such as type 2 diabetes, high blood pressure, and high cholesterol," says Eric Colman, M.D., of the Food and Drug Administration's division of metabolic and endocrine drug products.

In addition to a high BMI, having excess abdominal body fat is a health risk. Men with a waist of more than 40 inches around and women with a waist of 35 inches or more are at risk for health problems.

Obesity, once thought by many to be a moral failing, is now classified as a disease. The NHLBI calls it a complex chronic disease involving social, behavioral, cultural, physiological, metabolic, and genetic factors. Although experts may have different theories on how and why people become overweight, they generally agree that the key to losing weight is a simple message: Eat less and move more. Your body needs to burn more calories than you take in.

Successful 'Losers'

A popular weight-loss myth is that everyone who loses weight eventually gains it back, says Rena Wing, Ph.D., a professor of psychiatry at Brown Medical School. Wing, the co-developer of a research study known as the National Weight Control Registry, has worked to deflate this myth.

Tucked away in the registry's database is information about the weight-control behaviors of more than 3,000 American adults who have lost an average of 60 pounds and have kept it off for an average of six years.

How do they do it?

These successful losers report four common behaviors, says Wing. They eat a low-fat, high-carbohydrate diet, they monitor themselves by weighing in frequently, they are very physically active, and they eat breakfast. Eating breakfast every day is contrary to the typical pattern for the average overweight person who is trying to diet, says Wing. "They get up in the morning and say 'I'm going to start my diet today,' and they eat little or no breakfast and a light lunch. Then they get hungry and consume most of their calories late in the day. Successful weight losers have managed to change this pattern."

Six years after their weight loss, most of the registry's successful losers still report eating a low-calorie, low-fat diet, with about 24 percent of calories from fat. (The Dietary Guidelines for Americans recommend no more than 30 percent of daily calories from fat.) They also exercise for about an hour or more a day, expending about 2,800 calories per week on a variety of activities. This is equivalent to walking 28 miles a week, or four miles a day, says Wing.

Wing also reports that more than 70 percent of the registry's weight losers became overweight before age 18.

Although Barbara Croft of Columbus, Ohio, was not an overweight child, she gained weight once she left home and started cooking for herself. Replacing the plain and simple meals she had as a child with pizza, sodas, and meat and vegetables laden with sauces, the 5-foot-5-inch Croft worked her way up to 350 pounds. "I always ate from all the food groups—I just ate huge portions and I ate in between meals," says Croft.

When she was diagnosed with type 2 diabetes in February 1999, Croft got scared. "I worried about the health consequences—about going blind. I already have a little numbness in my feet."

Croft went on a diet and lost 200 pounds in 19 months. She has kept it off for a year and a half. "This is the third time I've lost over 100 pounds," says the 52-year-old, 150-pound Croft, "but this is the longest I've been able to keep

the weight off." In her two previous weight losses, Croft ate nutritious meals, but didn't exercise. This time, she started walking for exercise, but could only walk about a block at first. "My husband went with me because he was afraid I wouldn't make it," she says. Now, Croft walks on a treadmill for 50 minutes a day—25 minutes each morning and night.

She still eats balanced meals, but restricts her portions. And she always eats breakfast. "I have Egg Beaters, two pieces of low-calorie bread, fruit, decaf coffee, and 8 ounces of water." Croft dines out almost every night, typically eating half her dinner of grilled chicken or salmon and a vegetable or salad. She sends the other half back, so she isn't tempted to overeat.

"Losing the weight was easy—maintaining it is much harder," says Croft.

Croft had tried commercial weight-loss programs in the past, but this last time she did it on her own. "You have to find out what works for you," she says. "If I eat butter or cheese, that seems to do me in. Beef is also a problem."

"It's hard to accept that I'm never going to be able to eat what I want," says Croft. But she knows the tradeoff is her health. Her diabetes is under control now without medication. And Croft says her knees don't hurt anymore, she can buy clothes in a regular store, and she started traveling again now that she can fit into an airplane seat.

Setting a Goal

The first step to weight loss is setting a realistic goal. By using the BMI chart above and consulting with your health-care provider, you can determine what is a healthy weight for you.

Studies show that you can improve your health with just a small amount of weight loss. "We know that physical activity in combination with reduced calorie consumption can lead to the 5 to 10 percent weight loss necessary to achieve remission of the obesity-associated complications," says William Dietz, M.D., Ph.D., director of the division of nutrition and physical activity at the CDC. "Even these moderate weight losses can improve blood pressure and help control diabetes and high cholesterol in obese or overweight adults."

To reach your goal safely, plan to lose weight gradually. The NHLBI recommends a weight loss of 1 to 2 pounds per week by decreasing the calories eaten or increasing the calories used by 500 to 1,000 calories per day. (Some people with serious health problems due to obesity may lose weight more rapidly under a doctor's supervision.) If you plan to lose more than 15 to 20 pounds, have any health problems, or take medication on a regular basis, a doctor should evaluate you before you begin a weight-loss program.

Food Guide Pyramid

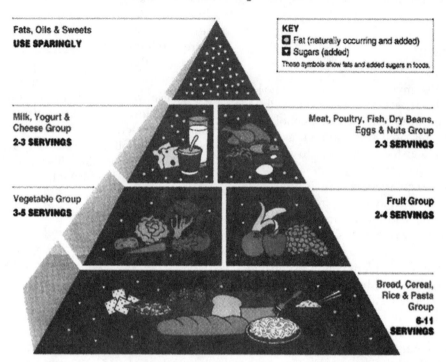

Fats, Oils & Sweets
USE SPARINGLY

KEY
◻ Fat (naturally occurring and added)
▾ Sugars (added)
These symbols show fats and added sugars in foods.

**Milk, Yogurt &
Cheese Group**
2-3 SERVINGS

**Meat, Poultry, Fish, Dry Beans,
Eggs & Nuts Group**
2-3 SERVINGS

Vegetable Group
3-5 SERVINGS

Fruit Group
2-4 SERVINGS

**Bread, Cereal,
Rice & Pasta
Group**
**6-11
SERVINGS**

Changing Eating Habits

Dieting may conjure up visions of eating little but lettuce and sprouts—but you can enjoy all foods as part of a healthy diet as long as you don't overdo it on fat (especially saturated fat), sugars, salt and alcohol. To be successful at losing weight, you need to change your lifestyle—not just go on a diet, experts say.

Limit portion sizes, especially of foods high in calories, such as cookies, cakes, other sweets, french fries, and fats, oils, and spreads. Reducing dietary fat alone—without reducing calories—will not produce weight loss, according to the NHLBI's guidelines on treating overweight and obesity in adults.

Use the Food Guide Pyramid, developed jointly by the U.S. Department of Agriculture (USDA) and the Department of Health and Human Services, to help you choose a healthful assortment of foods that include vegetables, fruits, grains (especially whole grains), skim milk and fish, lean meat, poultry, or beans. Choose foods naturally high in fiber, such as fruits, vegetables, legumes (such as beans and lentils), and whole grains. The high fiber content of many of these foods may help you to feel full with fewer calories.

All calories are not created equal. Carbohydrate and protein have about 4 calories per gram, but fat has more than twice that amount (9 calories per gram). Just as for the general population, weight-conscious consumers should aim for a daily fat intake of no more than 30 percent of total calories.

Keep your intake of saturated fat at less than 10 percent of calories. Saturated fats increase the risk for heart disease by raising blood cholesterol. Foods high in saturated fats include high-fat dairy products (like cheese, whole milk, cream, butter, and regular ice cream), fatty fresh and processed meats, the skin and fat of poultry, lard, palm oil, and coconut oil.

If you drink alcoholic beverages, do so in moderation. Alcoholic beverages supply calories but few nutrients. A 12-ounce regular beer contains about 150 calories, a 5-ounce glass of wine about 100 calories, and 1.5 ounces of 80-proof distilled spirits about 100 calories.

Limit your use of beverages and foods that are high in added sugars—those added to foods in processing or preparation, not the naturally occurring sugars in foods such as fruit or milk. Foods containing added sugars provide calories, but may have few vitamins and minerals. In the United States, the major sources of added sugars include non-diet soft drinks, sweets and candies, cakes and cookies, and fruit drinks and fruitades.

Using the Food Label

Under regulations from the FDA and the USDA, the food label, found on almost all processed foods, offers more complete, useful and accurate nutrition information than ever before. Even when restricting calories and portions, you can use the part of the food label called the Nutrition Facts panel to make sure you get all the essential nutrients

How to Use the Nutrition Facts Label

Macaroni & Cheese

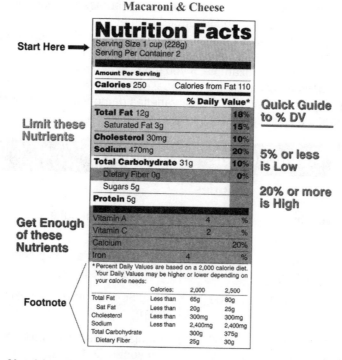

Use the **Nutrition Facts** Label not only to **limit** those nutrients you want to cut back on, but also to **increase** the ones you want to consume in greater amounts.

Look at the % Daily Value (%DV) column to see whether a food is high or low in nutrients. If you want to **limit** a nutrient (such as fat, saturated fat, cholesterol, sodium), choose foods with a lower %DV. To consume **more** of a nutrient (such as calcium, fiber, vitamins or minerals), choose foods with a higher %DV.

As a **quick guide**, foods with 5% DV or less contribute a small amount of that nutrient to your diet, while those with 20% DV or more contribute a large amount.

Remember, serving sizes are not recommended amounts, but are close to amounts people actually eat. They can help you compare similar foods.

for good health (see "How to Use the Nutrition Facts Label").

You'll find the serving size and the number of servings per package listed at the top of the Nutrition Facts panel. The serving size affects all the nutrient amounts listed on the panel. For example, if there is one cup in a serving and the package contains two servings, you need to double the calories and other nutrient numbers if you eat the whole package. Many items sold as single portions—like a 20-ounce soft drink, a 3-ounce bag of chips, and a large bagel—actually provide two or more servings.

"If you zero in on the 'amount per serving' section of the Nutrition Facts panel, you can tell at a glance how many calories a serving has and whether a food is high in total fat, saturated fat, cholesterol, and sodium," says

Naomi Kulakow, coordinator of food labeling education in the FDA's Center for Food Safety and Applied Nutrition. "These are items you should think about limiting in your diet."

The Nutrition Facts panel also shows how much dietary fiber, vitamin A, vitamin C, calcium, and iron are contained in a serving. These are nutrients you need for good health.

Also listed on the Nutrition Facts panel are the amounts of carbohydrates, protein, and sugars contained in a serving. Use the panel to compare the amount of total sugars among similar products, and try to choose ones lower in sugars.

In addition to listing some nutrients by weight, the panel also gives this information as a percentage of Daily Value (%DV). The percentage of Daily Value shows how

Fat-Free vs. Regular Calorie Comparison

You can lose weight by eating fewer calories and by increasing your physical activity. Reducing the amount of total fat and saturated fat that you eat is one way to limit your overall calorie intake. However, eating fat-free or reduced-fat foods isn't always the answer to weight loss. This is especially true when you eat more of the reduced fat food than you would of the regular item. For example, if you eat twice as many fat-free cookies as you would regular cookies you actually have increased your overall calorie intake. The following list of foods and their reduced-fat varieties demonstrates that just because a product is fat-free, it doesn't mean that it is "calorie-free."

Fat-Free or Reduced-Fat	Calories	Regular	Calories
Reduced-fat peanut butter, 2 T	187	Regular peanut butter, 2 T	191
Reduced-fat chocolate chip cookies, 3 cookies (30 g)	118	Regular chocolate chip cookies, 3 cookies (30 g)	142
Fat-free fig cookies, 2 cookies (30 g)	102	Regular fig cookies, 2 cookies (30 g)	111
Nonfat vanilla frozen yogurt (< 1% fat), ½ cup	100	Regular whole milk vanilla frozen yogurt (3-4 % fat), ½ cup	104
Light vanilla ice cream (7 % fat), ½ cup	111	Regular vanilla ice cream (11% fat), ½ cup	133
Fat-free caramel topping, 2 T	103	Caramel topping, homemade with butter, 2 T 103	103
Low-fat granola cereal, approx. 1/2 cup (55 g)	213	Regular granola cereal, approx. ½ cup (55 g)	257
Low-fat blueberry muffin, 1 small (2 ½ inch)	131	Regular blueberry muffin, 1 small (2 ½ inch)	138
Baked tortilla chips, 1 oz.	113	Regular tortilla chips, 1 oz.	143
Low-fat cereal bar, 1 bar (1.3 oz.)	130	Regular cereal bar, 1 bar (1.3 oz.)	140

Infographic By Renée Gordon

Source: National Heart, Lung and Blood Institute.
Nutrient data taken from Nutrient Data System for Research, Nutrition Coordinating Center, University of Minnesota.

a serving of a food fits in with recommendations for a healthful diet and allows consumers to make comparisons between similar products.

For example, shoppers can use the %DV figures to find out which frozen dinner is lower in saturated fat—particularly when it involves a comparative nutritional claim, such as reduced-fat. "You don't need to know the precise definition of 'low' or 'reduced,'" says Kulakow. "Just look at the percentage of Daily Value and see which is higher or lower in the nutrient you are interested in." Foods with 5 percent or less of the Daily Value are considered low in a nutrient, while those with 20 percent or more are high in the nutrient.

The percentages of Daily Value are based on a 2,000-calorie daily diet. But even if you eat less than 2,000 calories, the percentage of Daily Value can be used to determine whether a food is high or low in a particular nutrient.

"People use the food label too often to just restrict calories and fat—not to get enough nutrients," says Kulakow. While restricting calories is important for weight loss, "most people have no idea how many calories they consume every day—especially if they eat out." The percentage of Daily Value gives you a frame of reference and can be used to make dietary trade-offs, says Kulakow. "For example, if you eat a favorite food that's high in fat

Avoid 'Fad' Diets

The cabbage soup diet, the low-carbohydrate and high-protein diet, and other so-called "fad" diets are fundamentally different from federal nutrition dietary guidelines and are not recommended for losing weight.

Fad diets usually overemphasize one particular food or type of food, contradicting the guidelines for good nutrition, which recommend eating a variety of foods. These diets may work at first because they cut calories, but they rarely have a permanent effect. A high-protein diet is one fad diet that has remained popular over the years. "High-protein items may also be high in fat," says Robert Eckel, M.D., professor of medicine at the University of Colorado Health Sciences Center in Denver. High-fat diets can raise blood cholesterol levels, which increases a person's risk for heart disease and certain cancers.

High-protein diets force the kidneys to try to get rid of the excess waste products of protein and fat, called ketones. A buildup of ketones in the blood (called ketosis) can cause the body to produce high levels of uric acid, which is a risk factor for gout (a painful swelling of the joints) and kidney stones. Ketosis can be especially risky for people with diabetes because it can speed the progression of diabetic renal disease, says Eckel.

"It's important for the public to understand that no scientific evidence supports the claim that high-protein diets enable people to maintain their initial weight loss," says Eckel. "In general, quick weight-loss diets don't work for most people."

—L.B.

at one meal, balance it with low-fat foods at other times of the day."

Kulakow advises caution when choosing foods that are labeled "fat-free" and "low-fat." Fat-free doesn't mean calorie-free. To make a food tastier, sometimes extra sugars are added, which adds calories (see "Fat-Free vs. Regular Calorie Comparison"). So dieters should always check the Nutrition Facts panel to get complete information, says Kulakow.

For further guidance on using the Nutrition Facts panel, see *www.cfsan.fda.gov/~dms/foodlab.html*.

Increasing Physical Activity

Most health experts recommend a combination of a reduced-calorie diet and increased physical activity for weight loss. All adults should get at least 30 minutes of moderate physical activity on most, and preferably all, days of the week. But only 1 in 5 U.S. adults get the rec-

ommended amount of physical activity, according to a 1996 Surgeon General's report.

In addition to helping to control weight, physical activity decreases the risk of dying from coronary heart disease and reduces the risk of developing diabetes, hypertension, and colon cancer. Researchers also have found that daily physical activity may help a person lose weight by partially lessening the slow-down in metabolism that occurs during weight loss.

Exercise does not have to be strenuous. Moving any part of your body, regardless of how fast or slow, is considered physical activity. And studies show that short sessions of exercise several times a day are just as effective at burning calories and improving health as one long session.

To lose weight and to maintain a healthy weight after weight loss, many adults will likely need to do more than 30 minutes of moderate physical activity daily.

Prescription Weight-Loss Drugs

For obese people who have difficulty losing weight through diet and exercise alone, there are a number of FDA-approved prescription drugs that may help. "On average, individuals who use weight-loss drugs lose about 5 percent to 10 percent of their original weight, though some will lose less and some more," says the FDA's Colman.

Tips for Eating Out

- Choose foods that are steamed, garden fresh, broiled, baked, roasted, poached or stir-fried.
- Share food, such as a main dish or dessert, with your dining partner.
- Take part of the food home with you, and refrigerate immediately. You may want to ask for a take-home container when the meal arrives. Spoon half the meal into it, so you're more likely to eat only what's left on your plate.
- Request your meal to be served without gravy, sauces, butter or margarine.
- Ask for salad dressing on the side, and use only small amounts of full-fat dressings.

—L.B.

All of the prescription weight-loss drugs work by suppressing the appetite except for Xenical (orlistat). Approved by the FDA in 1999, Xenical is the first in a new class of anti-obesity drugs known as lipase inhibitors. Lipase is the enzyme that breaks down dietary fat for use by the body. Xenical interferes with lipase function, decreasing dietary fat absorption by 30 percent. Since undigested fats are not absorbed, there is less calorie intake, which may help in controlling weight. The main side effects of

For More Information

Weight-control Information Network (WIN)
National Institute of Diabetes and Digestive and
Kidney Diseases
1-877-946-4627
www.niddk.nih.gov/health/nutrit/win.htm

American Dietetic Association
1-800-877-1600, or 800-366-1655
for recorded food/nutrition messages
www.eatright.org

American Obesity Association
1-800-98-OBESE (1-800-986-2373)
www.obesity.org

National Weight Control Registry
1-800-606-NWCR (1-800-606-6927)
www.nwcr.ws
This study gathers information from people who have successfully lost weight and kept it off. The registry would like to hear from anyone 18 or older who has lost at least 30 pounds and maintained that weight loss for at least a year.

Xenical are cramping, diarrhea, flatulence, intestinal discomfort, and leakage of oily stool.

Meridia (sibutramine), approved by the FDA in 1997, increases the levels of certain brain chemicals that help reduce appetite. Because it may increase blood pressure and heart rate, Meridia should not be used by people with uncontrolled high blood pressure, a history of heart disease, congestive heart failure, irregular heartbeat, or stroke. Other common side effects of Meridia include headache, dry mouth, constipation and insomnia.

Other anti-obesity prescription drugs that were approved by the FDA many years ago based on short-term, limited data include: Bontril (phendimetrazine tartrate), Desoxyn (methamphetamine) and Ionamin and Adipex-P (phentermine). These drugs are only to be taken for a few weeks.

"There is no magic pill for obesity," says David Orloff, M.D., director of the FDA's division of metabolic and endocrine drug products. "The best effect you're going to get is with a concerted long-term regimen of diet and exercise. If you choose to take a drug along with this effort, it may provide additional help."

Until September 1997, two other drugs, fenfluramine (Pondimin and others) and dexfenfluramine (Redux), were available for treating obesity. But at the FDA's request, the manufacturers of these drugs voluntarily withdrew them from the market after newer findings suggested that they were the likely cause of heart valve problems. The FDA recommended that people taking the drugs stop and that they contact their doctor to discuss

their treatment. (For the latest information on this topic, visit *www.fda.gov/cder/news/feninfo.htm*.)

Prescription weight-loss drugs are approved only for those with a BMI of 30 and above, or 27 and above if they have other risk factors, such as high blood pressure or diabetes.

Beware of Unproven Claims

Some dietary supplement makers claim their products work for weight loss. These products are not reviewed by the FDA before they are marketed. "Under our existing laws, manufacturers have the responsibility for ensuring that their dietary supplement products are safe and effective," says Christine Lewis Taylor, Ph.D., R.D., director of the FDA's office of nutritional products, labeling, and dietary supplements.

Many weight-loss products claim to be "natural" or "herbal," but this does not necessarily mean that they're safe. These ingredients may interact with drugs or may be dangerous for people with certain medical conditions. If you are unsure about a product's claims or the safety of any weight-loss product, check with your doctor before using it.

Over-the-Counter Drugs

Over-the-counter (OTC) weight-control drugs contain the active ingredient phenylpropanolamine, which is also used as a nasal decongestant. The FDA recently asked drug manufacturers to discontinue marketing products containing phenylpropanolamine, based on evidence linking the substance to an increased risk of hemorrhagic stroke (bleeding in the brain). In addition, the FDA issued a public health advisory in November 2000, warning consumers to stop using products containing this ingredient.

The FDA is proposing to classify phenylpropanolamine as "not generally recognized as safe," and is proceeding with regulatory actions that will likely remove this ingredient from the market.

Worth the Effort

"Losing weight requires major lifestyle changes, including diet and nutrition, exercise, behavior modification, and—when appropriate—intervention with drug therapy," says Judith S. Stern, Sc.D., professor of nutrition and internal medicine at the University of California, Davis, and vice president of the American Obesity Association. "But it is always worth making the effort to improve your health."

From *FDA Consumer*, January/February 2002, pp. 18-25. © 2002 by FDA Consumer.

Metabolic Effects of High-Protein, Low-Carbohydrate Diets

Margo A. Denke, MD

Weight-losing diets appeal to the growing population of overweight Americans. Fad diets promise rapid weight loss, easy weight loss, limited restrictions on portion sizes of favorite foods, and above all an enhanced sense of well being. The popularity of fad diets points out the honest promises of traditional weight loss diets. Traditional weight loss diets promise slow weight loss of 0.45 to 0.9 kg/week. The weight loss is nothing but easy, because portion sizes of nearly all foods except low-calorie "free foods" must be continuously evaluated and tracked. Claiming an enhanced sense of well being is hardly appropriate for a traditional diet— most patients report dissatisfaction from the constant vigilance over dietary intake. Through discipline and perseverance, traditional weight loss programs try to teach a patient a new lifestyle of healthy eating. Unfortunately, 70% of successful weight losers return to their old habits and within 2 years regain at least half of the weight lost. These patients typically have little insight into the reasons why the weight was regained, and consider themselves "failures" to traditional diet programs. They become prime targets for diets promising rapid and easy weight loss.

Prototypes of the High-Protein, Low-Carbohydrate Diets

High-protein, low-carbohydrate diets have a long history of cyclic popularity. Greek Olympians ate high meat, low vegetable diets >2,000 years ago to improve athletic performance. Dr. William Harvey recommended a diet prohibiting sweet and starchy foods and permitting ad lib consumption of meats for patients who needed diuresis. As the basic understanding of nutrition and essential vitamins developed, these diets fell out of favor. They regained popularity in the late 1960s and early 1970s with the publication of the Atkins' Diet, Stillman's Diet, The Drinking Man's Diet, the Scarsdale Diet, and the Air Force Diet. The American Medical Association strongly criticized these diets,[1] leading to their submergence on the popular diet trend.

Resurgence of low-carbohydrate diets has been fueled by rising obesity and insulin resistance in the general population. Although the Atkins' Diet is the prototype of the low-carbohy-drate diet, The Sugar Busters Diet, Carbohydrate Addicts Diet, Protein Power Diet, and the Zone Diet are all variations on this common theme.

Several diets promise that, as long as you restrict carbohydrates, you will lose weight and you can eat as much food as you want. There may be a kernel of truth to this claim. For some patients, high-protein intake suppresses appetite.[2] For other patients, ketosis from carbohydrate restriction suppresses appetite. Restricting carbohydrate eliminates some popular foods that are often consumed in excess such as bread, cereal, soft drinks, french fries, and pizza. By simply excluding carbohydrate foods, patients following the Atkins diet typically consume 500 fewer calories a day.[3]

How Low-Carbohydrate Diets Produce Initially Greater Weight Loss

Reducing caloric intake by 500 kcal/day should result in a 0.45- to 0.9-kg weight loss each week. However, low-carbohydrate, high-protein diets typically produce a 2- to 3-kg weight loss in the first week. This added weight loss is not due to the miracle of "switching the body's metabolism over to burning fat stores." It is due to a diet-induced diuresis. When carbohydrate intake is restricted, 2 metabolic processes occur, both of which simultaneously reduce total body water content. The first process is mobilization of glycogen stores in liver and muscle. Each gram of glycogen is mobilized with approximately 2 g of water. The liver stores approximately 100 g of glycogen and muscle has 400 g of glycogen. Mobilization glycogen stores result in a weight loss of approximately 1 kg. Patients notice this change as a reduction in symptoms of "bloating" and are very pleased with the effect. The second process is generation of ketone bodies from catabolism of dietary and endogenous fat. Ketone bodies are filtered by the kidney as nonreabsorbable anions.[4] Their presence in renal lumenal fluids increases distal sodium delivery to the lumen, and therefore increases renal sodium and water loss.

In a study comparing an 800-calorie mixed diet with an 800-calorie low-carbohydrate, high fat diet,[5] 10-day weight loss was 4.6 kg on the ketogenic diet and 2.8 kg on the mixed diet. Energy-nitrogen balanced studies documented that the difference in weight lost was all accounted for by losses in total body water.

Long-term Weight Loss Is Influenced by Caloric Restriction, Not Carbohydrate Restriction

The diuretic effect of low-carbohydrate intake is limited to the first week of the diet. The remaining weight loss is a function of the laws of energy balance. Calories from any source determine the success of additional weight loss.

In the only published study of Atkins' diet, patients following the diet reduced caloric intake by 500 kcal/day. The average weight loss was 7.7 kg at 8 weeks, which is no greater than that expected from caloric restriction alone.[6] The ability of low carbohydrate intake to generate ketones has been touted as a relative advantage for losing weight. However, this advantage was not confirmed in a 1-month study comparing ketogenic with nonketogenic hypocaloric diets.[7] Most comparison studies have evaluated the relative advantages of either a low-carbohydrate or low fat hypocaloric diets; some studies found a slight 1- to 3-kg greater weight loss on a low-carbohydrate diet,[8,9,10,11] others a slight advantage with a high-carbohydrate diet,[12] but most studies have observed no statistical advantage of a low-carbohydrate diet.[13-18] The preponderance of evidence suggests that as long as caloric intake remains constant,[19] there is no intrinsic advantage to cutting carbohydrate intake.[20]

Untoward Metabolic Effects

Complications from Ketosis

Eucaloric ketogenic diets have been prescribed as part of an antiepileptic regimen in children with refractory seizure disorders. Children following these ketogenic diets have higher rates of dehydration, constipation, and kidney stones. Other reported adverse effects include hyperlipidemia, impaired neutrophil function, optic neuropathy, osteoporosis, and protein deficiency.[21]

Because ketogenic diets affect the central nervous system, it has been suspected that ketogenic diets may alter cognitive function. In a randomized weight loss study comparing a ketogenic with a nonketogenic hypocaloric diet, subjects consuming the ketogenic diet had impairments in higher order mental processing and flexibility than those following the nonketogenic diet.[7]

Complications from High Saturated Fat Intake

Despite the beneficial effects of weight loss, diets that promote liberal intake of high fat meats and dairy products raise cholesterol levels. In a study 24 subjects following the Atkins'-type 4-week induction diet, then 4 weeks maintenance diet,[6] low-density lipoprotein cholesterol levels increased significantly from

127 to 151 mg/dl. Similar increases in total cholesterol (13%) were reported in a study of patients following the Stillman diet.[22]

Complications from High Fat Intake

High fat diets increase free fatty acid flux and circulating free fatty acids. Fasting plasma free fatty acids may have a pro-arrhythmic effect in cardiac muscle. A number of mechanisms have been suggested including a possible detergent effect of circulating free fatty acids on cell membranes and direct effects of acylcarnitine on cellular ion channels and exchangers.

Complications from Exclusion of Fruits, Vegetables, and Grains

Because they exclude fruits, vegetables, and grains, low-carbohydrate, high-protein diets are deficient in micronutrients. Children consuming low-carbohydrate ketogenic diets have reduced intakes of calcium, magnesium, and iron.[21] Two sailors following a low-carbohydrate, high-protein hypocaloric diet during an extended voyage developed optic neuropathy from thiamine deficiency.[23] Although vitamin deficiencies can be circumvented by supplemental multivitamins, even supplemented low-carbohydrate diets will still be deficient in a growing number of important, biologically active phytochemicals present in fruits, vegetables, and grains.

Complications from High Protein Intake

Increasing the protein content of a diet significantly increases glomerular filtration rate.[24,25] Increases in glomerular filtration rate are likely explained by increased renal capillary permeability. Unfortunately, this compensatory response to the greater production of nitrogen is insufficient to clear protein by-products, and blood urea nitrogen levels increase. High protein diets significantly lower urinary pH by increasing titratable acid concentrations.[25,26] High protein intakes provide a greater uric acid load to the kidney. Despite increases in urinary uric acid excretion, increases in serum uric acid are observed.[6,26]

Untoward Long-term Effects

Development of Nephrolithiasis

Hypercalciuria is a risk factor for nephrolithiasis. High-protein diets induce hypercalciuria by several different mechanisms. High-protein diets increase glomerular filtration rate and decrease renal tubular reabsorption of calcium. The relation between dietary protein intake and calcium excretion (Table 1) is clearly linear.[27]

The stone-forming propensity of the hypercalciuria induced by high-protein diets is aggravated by other changes in urine composition. A high animal protein diet reduces gastrointestinal alkali absorption, leading to reduced urinary citrate.[28] Hyperuricemia and hyperuricosuria are also associated with excess

TABLE 1 Graded Effects of High-Protein Diets on Urinary Calcium Excretion

Diet Duration	% Calories from Protein*	No.	Creatinine Clearance (ml/min)			Urinary Calcium Excretion (mg/24 h)		
			Low	Medium	High	Low	Medium	High
15 d	1%/12%/25%	6	98	105	122	51	99	161
4 d	8%/12%/25%	16	85	95	107	108	129[†]	196[†]
15 d	8%/16%/24%	33				168	240[†]	301[†]
15 d	8%/16%/24%	9				217	303[†]	426[†]
15d	8%/16%/24%	9				168	240[†]	301[†]

*Percent calories calculated assuming 70-kg average subject weight, 2,400-calorie diet.

[†]Significantly different from low-protein diet.

intake of animal protein. Animal protein is a rich source of sulfur-containing amino acids; amino acids have a greater propensity to lower urinary pH.

Adding a carbohydrate restriction to a high-protein diet exacerbates many of these parameters. Low-carbohydrate intake further reduces urinary pH by inducing ketosis. Limiting the intake of vegetables and fruits further reduces urinary citrate by reducing dietary sources of alkali. Thus, high-protein, low-carbohydrate diets are associated with hypercalciuria, hyperuricosuria, and hypocitraturia, which can all contribute to renal calculi formation.

Development of Osteoporosis

High-protein, low-carbohydrate diets generate a high acid load, resulting in a subclinical chronic metabolic acidosis. Metabolic acidosis promotes calcium mobilization from bone.[29] Osteoclasts and osteoblasts respond to small changes in pH in cell culture; thus, a small decrease in pH results in a large burst of bone resorption.

The effects of varying dietary protein intakes on bone turnover has been carefully documented in young women consuming metabolic diets. High-protein diets increase renal calcium excretion, raise parathyroid hormone levels, and raise urinary N-telopeptide concentrations. Markers of bone formation (alkaline phosphatase and osteocalcin) remain steady, suggesting that high-protein diets increase bone resorption without affecting the rate of bone formation.[27] These effects may be exaggerated in older persons who tend to have decrements in renal clearance of acid and higher serum parathyroid hormone concentrations.[29]

Progression of Chronic Renal Insufficiency

In several small, randomized, controlled dietary trials, dietary protein restriction retarded the progression of diabetic nephropathy to end-stage renal disease.[30] High-protein, low-carbohydrate diets have a weak effect at reducing creatinine clearance over time, and could potentially hasten renal failure in patients with baseline renal insufficiency.

Patients are inherently attracted to the simple, permissive dietary instructions: eat as much as you want of foods containing fat and protein, but don't eat foods containing carbohydrate. As promised, almost everyone loses weight during the first week. Low-carbohydrate diets cause a greater initial weight loss from a physiologic diuresis accompanying the obligate loss of glycogen stores and renal clearance of ketone bodies. Once glycogen stores have been liberated, and a new steady state for total body sodium has been achieved, these diets hold no greater promise for weight loss than any other caloric restricted diet. High-fat, low-carbohydrate diets can be harmful. The diet plan is deficient in micronutrients. Consuming ad libitum fatty meats raises total and low-density lipoprotein cholesterol levels. High-protein, low-carbohydrate intakes create a subclinical metabolic acidosis, and increase blood urea nitrogen and uric acid levels. Resultant urine acidification, hyperuricosuria, and hypercalciuria increase urine lithogenicity. Trying to convince a devotee to stop the diet uncovers yet another deleterious effect; ketogenic diets impair higher order cognitive function. High-protein, low-carbohydrate diets have untoward clinical consequences for patients with coronary artery disease, including progression of diabetic nephropathy, exacerbation of gouty diathesis, increases in circulating free fatty acids, and increases in low-density lipoprotein cholesterol levels. High-protein, low-carbohydrate diets are not superior weight-losing diets and should not be recommended.

References

1. Anonymous. A critique of low-carbohydrate ketogenic weight reduction regimens. A review of Dr. Atkins' diet revolution. JAMA 1973;224:1415–1419.

2. Johnstone AM Effect of overfeeding macronutrients on day-to-day food intake in man. Eur J Clin Nutr 1996;50:418–430.

3. Yudkin J. The treatment of obesity by the high fat diet. Lancet 1960;2:939–941.

4. Kolanowski J. On the mechanisms of fasting natriuresis and of carbohydrate-induced sodium retention. Diabetes Metab 1977;3:131–143.

5. Yang MU, Van Itallie TB. Composition of weight lost during short-term weight reduction. Metabolic responses of obese subjects to starvation and low-calorie ketogenic and nonketogenic diets. J Clin Invest 1976; 58:722–730.

6. LaRosa JC, Fry AG, Muesing R, Rosing DR. Effects of high-protein, low-carbohydrate dieting on plasma lipoproteins and body weight. J Am Diet Assoc 1980;77:264–270.

7. Wing RR, Vazquez J, Ryan C. Cognitive effects of ketogenic weight reducing diets. *Int J Obes Relat Metab Disord* 1995;19:811–816.

8. Lewis SB, Wallin JD, Kane JP, Gerich JE. Effect of diet composition on metabolic adaptations to hypocaloric nutrition: comparison of high carbohydrate and high fat isocaloric diets. *Am J Clin Nutr* 1977;30:160–170.

9. Rabast U, Kasper H, Schonborn J. Obesity and low-carbohydrate diets comparative studies. *Nutr Metab* 1977;21(suppl 1):56–59.

10. Alford BB, Blankenship AC, Hagen RD. The effects of variations in carbohydrate, protein, and fat content of the diet upon weight loss, blood values and nutrient intake in adult obese women. *J Am Diet Assoc* 1990;90:534–540.

11. Baron JA, Schori A, Crow B, Carter R, Mann JI. A randomized controlled trial of low carbohydrate and low fat/high fiber diets for weight loss. *Am J Publ Health* 1986;76:1293–1296.

12. Rabast U, Vornberger KH, Ehl M. Loss of weight, sodium and water in obese persons consuming a high- or low-carbohydrate diet. *Ann Nutr Metab* 1981;25:341–349.

13. Davie M, Abraham RR, Godsland I, Moore P, Wynn V. Effect of high and low-carbohydrate diets on nitrogen balance during calorie restriction in obese subjects. *Int J Obes* 1982;6:457–462.

14. Piatti PM, Pontiroli AE. Insulin sensitivity and lipid levels in obese subjects after slimming diets with different complex and simple carbohydrate content. *Int J Obes* 1993;17:375–381.

15. Rumpler WV, Seale JL. Energy intake restriction and diet composition effects on energy expenditure in men. *Am J Clin Nutr* 1995;53:430–436.

16. Low CC, Grossman EB, Gumbiner B. Potentiation of effects of weight loss by monounsaturated fatty acids in obese NIDDM patients. *Diabetes* 1996;45:569–575.

17. Golay A, Allaz AF, Morel Y, de Tonnac N, Tankova S, Reaven G. Similar weight loss with low- or high-carbohydrate diets. *Am J Clin Nutr* 1996;63:174–178.

18. Golay A, Eigenheer C, Morel Y, Kujawski P, Lehmann T, de Tonnac N. Weight-loss with low or high carbohydrate diet? *Int J Obes Rel Metab Disord* 1996;20:1067–1072.

19. Skor AR, Toubro S, Ronn B, Holm L, Astrup A. Randomized trial on protein vs. carbohydrate in ad libitum fat reduced diet for the treatment of obesity. *Int J Obes* 1999;23:528–536.

20. Shah M, Garg A. High fat and high carbohydrate diets and energy balance. *Diabetes Care* 1996;19:1142–1152.

21. Tallian K, Nahata M, Tsao CT. Role of ketogenic diet in children with intractable seizures. *Ann Pharmacother* 1998;32:349–361.

22. Rickman F, Mitchell N. Changes in serum cholesterol during the Stillman diet. *JAMA* 1974;228:54–58.

23. Hoyt CS III, Billson FA. Low-carbohydrate diet optic neuropathy. *Med J Aust* 1977;1:65–66.

24. Kerstetter JE, O'Brien KO, Insogna KL. Dietary protein affects intestinal calcium absorption. *Am J Clin Nutr* 1998;68:859–865.

25. Schuette SA. Studies of the mechanism of protein induced hypercalciuria in older men and women. *J Nutr* 1980;110:305–315.

26. Fellstrom B, Danielson BG, Karlstrom B, Lithell H, Ljunghall S, Vessby B. The influence of a high dietary intake of purine-rich animal protein on urinary urate excretion and supersaturation in renal stone disease. *Clin Sci* 1983;64:399–405.

27. Kerstetter JE, Mitnick ME, Gundberg CM, Caseria DM, Ellison AF, Carpenter TO, Insogna KL. Changes in bone turnover in young women consuming different levels of dietary protein. *J Clin Endocrinol Metab* 1999;84:1052–1055.

28. Breslau NA, Brinkley L, Hill KD, Pak CY. Relationship of animal protein-rich diet to kidney stone formation and calcium metabolism. *J Clin Endocrinol Metab* 1988;66:140–146.

29. Barzel US, Massey LK. Excess dietary protein can adversely affect bone. *J Nutr* 1998;128:1051–1053.

30. Kasiske BL, Lakatua JD, Ma JZ, Louis TA. A meta-analysis of the effects of dietary protein restriction on the rate of decline in renal function. *Am J Kidney Dis* 1998;31:954–961

Dietary Dilemmas

Is the pendulum swinging away from low fat?

Damaris Christensen

This time of year, thoughts turn from overloaded holiday tables to overweight bodies, the beach, and diet programs. Losing weight is not just a matter of looking good in a swimsuit. Packing on the pounds increases a person's risk of heart disease, diabetes, high blood pressure, stroke, and some cancers. Recent surveys estimate that more than 50 percent of adults in the United States are overweight. As the U.S. public has gotten fatter, public health officials have been pushing diets low in fat. A variety of epidemiological data supports this advice, but it's now being challenged as other types of weight-loss diets have gained support.

"As a country, our fat intake has decreased, but our calorie intake has increased, and obesity rates are going up," says Bonnie J. Brehm of the University of Cincinnati. "Over the last 10 years, Americans have been so obsessed with low fat that people have forgotten that carbohydrates have calories, too. The pendulum may be swinging back a bit."

Some recent studies—and provocative articles in the popular press—have suggested that low-carbohydrate diets, such as the Atkins diet, could be more effective for weight loss than low-fat diets are. However, the low-carb diets tend to be high in fat and protein. So, there are concerns about their potential health effects. Although scientists caution that these diets haven't yet been studied over long periods, several new trials have shown them to have surprisingly positive short-term effects.

Low-Fat Lunches

The idea behind cutting fat out of weight-loss diets was that fatty foods represent the densest source of calories that a person eats, says Jennie Brand-Miller of the University of Sydney in Australia. Dieters have been told to replace high-fat items with fruits, vegetables, and grains.

Various studies have shown that such diets can help people achieve and maintain a healthy weight. In 2001, the U.S.-based Diabetes Prevention Program showed that low-fat, low-calorie diets combined with exercise produced a 5 to 7 percent weight loss over 6 years (*SN: 9/8/01, p. 150*.

Last November at the American Heart Association meeting in Chicago, researchers reported that among 74,000 women, those who increased their fruit and vegetable intake over the 12-year study period were 26 percent less likely to become obese than were women who decreased their consumption of such foods.

However, some scientists argue that low-fat diets aren't more effective than tracking calories. Early last year, an analysis of six studies that compared low-fat and fixed-calorie diets concluded that participants lost about the same amount of weight, 5 to 10 pounds. "The review suggests that fat-restricted diets are no better than calorie-restricted diets in achieving long-term weight loss in overweight or obese people," concludes Sandi Pirozzo of the University of Queensland in Australia. Furthermore, she notes, "the overall weight loss…in all studies was so small as to be clinically insignificant."

One reason that nutritionists had thought that people would lose more weight on a low-fat diet than on other calorie-restricted diets was that traditionally low-fat foods have been bulkier and higher in fiber than fattier foods. The nutritionists reasoned that people feel fuller after eating low-fat foods than after dining on other foods.

Over the past decade, the food industry's introduction of many low-fat choices has altered the relationship between fat, bulk, and fiber. Brand-Miller says, "New low-fat foods are not necessarily bulky. Nor are they low in calories because they often have added sugars." That means that it's become easier for people to eat low-fat meals and still add pounds.

Nevertheless, low-fat eating may have health benefits beyond any weight loss. Many epidemiological studies have shown that people who report eating diets low in fat and high in fruits and vegetables are less likely to develop heart disease and diabetes than people eating higher-fat diets are. The review of six studies concluded that participants in the low-fat group were slightly more likely to show a drop in cholesterol concentrations in their blood than were those in the fixed-calorie group.

In fact, one of the widely used low-fat diets was developed a decade ago to help people with heart disease reduce fatty buildup in their arteries. Dean Ornish, a professor of medicine at the University of California, San Francisco School of Medicine, developed a high-fiber diet in which less than 10 percent of the calories come from fat. That's about a third of the fat of a typical U.S. diet.

Most national health organizations have weighed in on behalf of low-fat diets. However, critics of these diets point out that the studies often encourage participants to not only change their diets but also increase exercise and learn stress-management strategies. Thus, in these tests, it's difficult to tease out the effects of any diet on weight loss.

Critics also note that high carbohydrate consumption can result in overproduction of insulin and eventually in people's becoming less sensitive to it (SN: 4/8/00, p. 236). This condition, called insulin resistance, may eventually lead to diabetes.

"What's becoming increasingly clear is that low-fat diets for people with certain biological predispositions may increase their risk of developing the insulin-resistance syndrome," says endocrinologist David S. Ludwig of Children's Hospital Boston. He speculates that replacing fats with processed sugars and starches played a role in the development of current epidemics of obesity and diabetes.

Protein Power?

One of the most popular low-carbohydrate diets today was devised and has been promoted by Robert C. Atkins, a cardiologist in New York City. The diet restricts carbohydrate consumption to less than 10 percent of total calories eaten, whereas people in the United States often get more than 50 percent of their calories from carbohydrates such as bread, processed foods, starch in vegetables, and sugar in fruits. People on the Atkins diet tend to eat at least 40 percent of their calories in fat, while the average U.S. diet contains about 30 percent fat calories.

The body's reaction to very low carbohydrate load is a condition called ketosis. According to Atkins' many books and magazine articles, people in ketosis preferentially burn stored body fat for energy—and burning fat takes more energy than burning carbohydrates does. Thus, he argues, dieters can lose weight while eating foods higher in calories than their previous choices.

Some researchers think there's another factor at play. They speculate that any benefits of a low-carb diet stem not from ketosis but from the diet's effects on blood sugar and insulin. A diet higher than average in protein and fat, which are digested more slowly than carbohydrates, might avoid carbohydrate-induced spikes of insulin in the blood that force blood sugar concentrations so low that the person feels hungry soon after eating, says Ludwig.

Critics of the Atkins diet say that it is likely to have dangerous side effects. Bone health is one concern about it and other low-carb diets.

"The huge load of animal protein ingested in such diets leaches calcium from the bones and sends it through the kidneys into the urine," says Neal Barnard, president of the Washington, D.C.-based Physicians Committee for Responsible Medicine. High protein intake increases the acidity of blood. In response, acid-neutralizing calcium

gets pulled from bones. Also, excess urea from the protein pulls extra water into the kidneys, so dissolved calcium is expelled. "Over the long run, that can spell osteoporosis," says Barnard.

A study in the August 2002 American Journal of Kidney Diseases showed that after 6 weeks on the Atkins diet, the 10 participants made urine containing 55 percent more calcium than it had at the start of the trial.

People on meat-heavy diets are also more prone to kidney stones, gout, colon cancer, and potentially cardiovascular problems, Barnard adds. A high-fat diet might also boost the cholesterol and triglycerides, or free fatty acids, in people's blood. High cholesterol and fatty acid concentrations are linked to heart disease.

"Low-carb diets remain a serious health risk," Barnard says. To investigate potential health effects, as well as the effectiveness of such a diet, Eric Westman of Duke University in Durham, N.C., undertook a study funded by the Robert C. Atkins Foundation. He tracked 60 overweight people following a diet with less than 30 percent of its calories from fat and 60 others following the Atkins diet. As part of the diet, the Atkins group took supplements of fish oil, borage oil, and flaxseed oil. Westman reports that participants were more likely to stick to the Atkins diet than to the low-fat regimen.

Over 6 months, the people in the Atkins group lost 31 pounds, compared with 20 pounds for the people in the low-fat group. The changes in blood characteristics associated with heart disease were more favorable in the Atkins group, Westman says. Low-density-lipoprotein-linked cholesterol (the bad cholesterol) didn't change in blood samples from either group, while high-density-lipoprotein-linked cholesterol (the good cholesterol) went up slightly in the Atkins group but not in the other group. Triglyceride concentrations dropped in the Atkins group members' blood by almost twice as much as in the low-fat group's members.

> ## "You can lose weight on any diet."
> —Gerald Reaven

"The findings were unexpected," Westman says, "but the results of several small studies seem to be consistent with ours."

With funding from the American Heart Association, Brehm also compared two diets. She randomly assigned 53 women to either a low-carbohydrate or a moderately low-fat regimen. On the low-carb diet, women were permitted to eat as much as they wanted as long as they kept carbohydrate calories to less than 10 percent of the diet. On the low-fat diet, the women were asked to eat between 1,200 and 1,500 calories per day.

At the end of 6 months, the low-carbohydrate dieters had lost about 18.7 pounds, including 10.6 pounds of body fat, while the low-fat dieters had lost 8.6 pounds, of which 4.4 pounds was body fat, Brehm and her colleagues reported at meetings late last year. "According to food records, both groups took in about the same amount of calories," Brehm says. Only the low-carb dieters showed signs of ketosis, she notes, so they burned more body fat for energy than the other group did.

Moreover, while blood concentrations of two markers of inflammation decreased in both sets of dieters, one marker decreased more in the low-carbohydrate group than in those on the low-fat diet. Inflammation has been linked with heart disease and diabetes (SN: 6/14/97, p. 374; SN: 8/31/02, p. 136.).

Blood pressure, cholesterol concentrations, and blood-sugar measurements weren't significantly different in the two groups and didn't change during the study. On the other hand, the amount of insulin in all the dieters' blood—measured before a meal—decreased in both groups during the 6-month study. That change typically indicates that a person is becoming more sensitive to insulin, a positive health sign.

A third major trial of an Atkins-style regimen enrolled 60 overweight men and women. Half followed a strict diet high in protein and low in carbohydrates, and the others adhered to a regimen lower in protein and higher in carbohydrates. Unlike the other trials, the researchers adjusted the volunteers' protein intakes to keep the percentage of fat the same in the two diets, says Peter M. Clifton of Australia's Commonwealth Scientific and Industrial Research Organisation in Adelaide. The two groups were matched for age and weight.

Over 16 weeks, the participants in both groups lost an average of about 18 pounds. Participants on the high-protein diet lost more fat and less muscle.

"There are subtle metabolic advantages for being on a high-protein diet, especially for women," says Clifton. The researchers measured no difference in blood-cholesterol concentrations between the two diet groups, but people on the high-protein diet had greater reductions of triglycerides in their blood. Also, over the course of the study, their sensitivity to insulin improved more than that of the other participants.

Several other small studies have shown similar results. All the researchers say they aren't prepared to recommend a low-carb diet ahead of other weight-loss plans, but they agree that the diet merits further investigation. The National Institutes of Health is funding a study that will track 360 participants at three universities for at least a year to compare the Atkins diet and a low-fat diet.

"We are trying to stay on top of the science here," says Robert Bonow, president of the Dallas-based American Heart Association. "People should not change their eating patterns based on very small, short-term studies. Bottom line, the American Heart Association says that people who want to lose weight and keep it off need to make lifestyle changes for the long term—this means reg-ular exercise and a balanced diet including lots of fruits and vegetables."

Weighing the Issues

There's certainly room for improvement in the typical Western diet, says Brand-Miller. "There are good and bad high-protein diets, and there are good and bad low-fat diets," she says.

Although proponents of the Atkins diet argue that low carbohydrate intake has specific metabolic effects, some researchers still hold that all dieting is basically a matter of eating less. "People will lose weight on any diet, like the Atkins diet, that cuts out major groups of food because people get bored of eating the same thing day after day. But, in my experience, people find these diets very difficult to stick to," says Brand-Miller.

Though difficult in execution, dieting is simple in concept, says endocrinologist Gerald Reaven of Stanford University. "If you do carefully controlled studies, a calorie is a calorie, and if you lower your calorie intake you lose weight. So, you can lose weight on any diet," he says.

The short-term dietary changes needed for weight loss are unlikely to have negative effects on health, he argues, especially given the benefits of weight loss.

However, he takes a different view of the diets that people use over the long term to maintain their lowered weight. For example, a low-fat diet may be bad for people who are resistant to the effects of insulin, he says. Likewise, he argues, a low-carb diet may be bad for people with high cholesterol.

STATS: $117 Billion
Cost of obesity in the United States

Reaven argues that the best long-term diet is one that contains moderate amounts of both fat and carbohydrates. Dietary recommendations released last year by the National Academy of Sciences suggest a diet of 10 to 35 percent protein, 45 to 65 percent carbohydrates, and 20 to 35 percent fat. Compared with previous guidelines, this new recommendation lowers the amounts of carbohydrates that people are told to eat and increases the permissible fat and protein, but it still rules out at least the initial phase of the Atkins diet, in which fruits or vegetables are strictly limited.

No matter how people do it, losing weight and keeping it off is a crucial public health issue. The federal government estimates that in 2000 the cost of obesity in the United States was more than $117 billion. Researchers agree that the rising numbers of overweight and obese people ensure that studies of diets and weight loss will be a burgeoning field for years to come.

A Guide to Rating the Weight-Loss Websites

MANY PEOPLE who are successful at weight loss go it alone. But research suggests that at least half use formal programs such as Weight Watchers or Jenny Craig. The structure and moral support offered by such programs help many reach their goals.

But what if you're caught in the middle? What if you're someone who's frustrated trying to lose weight solo but too embarrassed to attend meetings—or too busy for yet another activity? Enter virtual weight-loss centers.

That's right. An increasing number of ambitious weight losers are going online for help, signing on with one of a burgeoning number of websites created to bring dieters together with health professionals—and other dieters—who can guide and cheer them on. It's convenient and social, yet with privacy built in.

Does it work? Can virtual assistance lead to actual weight loss? Some preliminary research from Brown University suggests that joining a weight-loss website *can* be a practical alternative to in-person diet counseling. But how do you sort through the sites to find the right match?

By using the eight questions we've established to rate them. That's what we asked a Web-savvy dietitian from the Tufts community to do in assessing eight of the most popular weight-loss sites now operating.

None of the ones she looked at are all good or all bad. But different sites have different "personalities" that will appeal to some consumers and not others. For instance, a few, like **Cyberdiet** and **DietWatch**, provide strong online "communities" that offer a "we're in this together" camaraderie. Others, like **eFit**, are more

straightforward clearinghouses of information with less social interaction.

Some sites, like **eDiets** and **Shape Up and Drop 10**, charge a fee. It is not essential to pay for online weight-loss information—there are several good sites that provide free access to their dieting and fitness features. But a few of the sites that do charge money offer some pretty good personalized services that you can't get for free.

We do have some favorites among the sites we visited. Of the free sites, we'd choose the easy-to-use **Shape Up America** (the no-cost counterpart to Shape Up and Drop 10—both are operated by former Surgeon General C. Everett Koop, MD). For a fee, we'd opt for the great customer service offered by eDiets. But the sites profiled here are only a sampling of everything that's available online to potential dieters.

As you surf the choices out there, keep in mind that even an authoritative-looking home page doesn't guarantee that the author of a dieting site knows anything about dieting, healthful or otherwise. That's why it's particularly important to apply our set of questions—not just to see which site is the right "fit" for you but also to weed out those that aren't the right fit for *anybody*.

1. Who provides the diet plans and advice to members?

All the sites we visited except one, **Asimba**, provide diet plans that have been formulated by registered dietitians—health professionals trained in nutrition. Meal plans on Asimba are generated by a computer program that uses guidelines set by an exercise physiologist, and the lack of a dietitian's professional touch shows. One of the meal plans e-mailed to our dietitian reviewer included a lunch of cinnamon oatmeal,

a peach, 1/2 cup of grapes, and 3/4 cup of green beans—an odd combination of foods.

2. What claims are made by the site as to how much or how fast weight can be shed on its diet plan?

A reasonable rate of weight loss is about 1 to 2 pounds a week. Responsible websites should use a person's height, weight, age, and activity level (usually gathered at the outset) to suggest a calorie level that will allow for this moderate rate of weight loss. Ediets pushes the goal somewhat, promising new clients that they will lose 10 pounds within a month of joining.

Adults should not attempt to follow a diet that provides fewer than 1,200 calories daily. That's too little food to meet essential nutrient needs. None of the sites we reviewed, including eDiets, offered meal plans that were too low in calories.

3. What kind of meal plan does the site offer?

Some sites are able to customize meal plans more than others. Does the entry questionnaire ask about dietary restrictions, food preferences, and food allergies? Are vegetarian and/or vegan meal plans available? Ediets, for example, can adapt menus to accommodate low-sodium or low-cholesterol plans. The eDiets questionnaire also asks potential members to what extent they want convenience foods, like Healthy Choice frozen dinners, incorporated into their menus.

Several sites give dieters some do-it-yourself meal-planning options. Cyberdiet members, for example, can go one of three ways. Those whose dieting philosophy is "just tell me what to eat" can download 30 days' worth of menus. But those who want to make their own food choices can use one of two inventive meal planners.

	1. Who designs the diet plan?	2. Does the diet make reasonable weight-loss claims?	3. Does the meal plan consider dietary restrictions, food preferences?	4. Do members have access to staff professionals?	5. Is member-to-member support available?	6. Does the site include an exercise plan?	7. Cost/length of contract?	8. Does the site offer a weight maintenance plan?
Asimba (www. asimba.com)	Exercise physiologist	Yes	Vegetarian, non-dairy meal plans available	Option to sign up with a personal coach for a fee	Bulletin boards	Yes	Members pay for personal coach, other features free	No
Cyberdiet (www. cyberdiet. com)	Registered dietitian	Yes	No, but meal-planning options include meat-free, dairy-free food choices	Dietitian, chef, others host chats	Chat rooms, bulletin boards, e-newsletter	Yes	Free	Weight-mainte-nance bulletin board
Dietwatch (www. dietwatch. com)	No diet plan available	—	—	Dietitian hosts some chats	Chat rooms, bul-letin boards, e-newsletter	Yes	Free	No
eDiets (www. ediets.com)	Registered dietitian	Yes, but pushes the limit, saying you'll lose 10 pounds in the first month	Menus available for vegetarian, milk- or egg-free, low-sodium, low-cholesterol diets	Yes, by talking with a dietitian via e-mail or during moderated chat	Chat rooms, bul-letin boards, e-newsletter	Yes	$10/month	Members can receive weight-maintenance meal plans
eFit (www. efit.com)	Registered dietitian	Yes	Vegetarian, low-sodium menus available; meal plans can exlude fish, nuts, milk	No	E-newsletter	Yes	Free	Members can receive weight-maintenance meal plans
nutrio.com (www. nutrio.com)	Registered dietitian	Yes	Low-fat, low-cholesterol, low-sodium, vegetarian meal plans available	No	Bulletin boards, e-newsletter	Yes	Free	No
Shape Up America (www. shapeup.org)	Registered dietitian	Yes	No, but meal-planning options include meat-free, dairy-free food choices	No	Bulletin boards	Yes	Free	No
Shape Up and Drop 10 (www. shapeup.org)	Registered dietitian	Yes	Choose from regular, non-dairy, lacto-ovo, vegan meal plans	Members contact the dietitian through customer service	Bulletin boards	Yes	$10/week	Members can receive weight-maintenance meal plans.

One, the Express Menus feature, lets readers design their own meal plans from lists of food choices. Meals planned using this option really are express—dieters select items from lists that include fast foods like Mc-Donald's hamburgers, Taco Bell burritos, and frozen entrees from Stouffer's Lean Cuisine and Healthy Choice. The other, Cyberdiet's 1-2-3-Step program, provides even more flexibility—members can design meals around their own recipes. For instance, if you plug in your favorite meatloaf recipe, the program will tell you how big a slice you can have and still fit within your calorie level.

Dieters accessing Shape Up America enter the site's Cyberkitchen to plan their meals. Cyberkitchen is easy to use and includes lots of calorie-controlled meals to choose from. To come up with a meal, dieters click on a "breakfast," "lunch," or "dinner" icon to bring up a list of food choices. The available selection of items varies in calorie value, allowing dieters to make a higher-calorie choice for one meal and a lower one at the next. Try to go over the allotted calorie allowance for the day and the computer program says, "Oops, try again."

Shape Up and Drop 10 customers, who pay a fee, don't engage in their own menu planning. After filling out an assessment questionnaire they receive a meal plan with recipes. The recipes are nicely designed and also sized to serve a family rather than just one person—a practical consideration for dieters who cook for a crowd.

Nutrio.com and eFit provide calorie-controlled menus as well—a week's worth. They are standard meal plans that will look familiar to veteran dieters, but the menus are nutritionally balanced and include enough calories to allow for a reasonable rate of weight loss. Both sites also have features that let members make changes in their meal plans from a list of acceptable food substitutions. (EFit visitors should note, however, that an interactive feature that is supposed to make it easier for members to make substitutions was not working at the time of review.)

Asimba's meal-planning pages, as we said earlier, could use some retooling. The meal plans allow for a reasonable rate of weight loss but include some odd food combinations. Computer-generated menus make sense only if the computer is programmed to recognize acceptable food combinations that people consider "normal."

4. Do members have access to staff professionals?

When Brown University researchers looked into the effectiveness of computer-based weight-loss counseling, they found that people who had regular online interaction with a dietitian lost more weight than those who simply downloaded a weight-loss plan from their computers and followed it themselves.

But only the weight-loss sites that charge a fee really duplicate this personal touch. Ediets, in particular, tries hard to promote communication between staff and clients. Ediets clients can e-mail the site's support dietitian if they have any questions about their diet plan or some other aspect of the program. The questions we posed were answered the next business day. For general questions such as how to access the chat rooms, eDiets's customer service desk is reachable by e-mail or phone (toll-free) 7 days a week.

Shape Up and Drop 10 clients don't have direct access to a staff professional—questions are sent to the site manager to be forwarded to a registered dietitian—but our questions were still answered promptly the next business day.

While free sites do not usually give members one-on-one access to their professional staffs, some, like Cyberdiet and DietWatch, host dietitian-moderated chat sessions in which all members can receive nutrition advice—a nice touch for a site that does not charge a fee.

Free professional advice from Asimba is limited to a not very helpful "Ask the Expert" feature. Several questions that we posed went unanswered.

Those who want more personalized guidance from Asimba can hire an online diet or fitness coach for a fee. Clients choose their coaches from a list that includes registered dietitians and personal trainers and then contact them by e-mail. Fees for this service vary, as they are set by the coaches, not the site.

5. Can members share ideas and support?

DietWatch and eDiets members can sign up for a "diet buddy" to help them over the rough spots as they begin their weight-loss efforts. Communication is conducted via e-mail. But most of the member-to-member contact on diet sites is not one-on-one. Rather, it is conducted through chat rooms and bulletin boards.

A chat, if you're new to the cyberworld, is just what it sounds like: Members log on to a site at a preappointed time and communicate "live" with other members, and all chatters can read the conversation as it appears on the screen. Chat schedules are posted on the site so that members know when to log on. Some chat sessions on Cyberdiet, eDiets, and DietWatch are moderated by a health professional such as a dietitian, chef, or personal trainer and thereby give members a chance to ask questions on particular aspects of cooking, exercise, or weight control.

People new to chats might be confused by the relative chaos of online conversations. **Not everyone logs on to talk about dieting. During a recent DietWatch dietitian-moderated chat, we "listened" to a woman complain about a damaged planter in front of her house**. And a crowd participating in a dietitian-moderated chat on eDiets seemed to be more interested in chatting with each other than in speaking to the dietitian. In spite of the confusion, though, chats are a popular stop on most of the weight-loss sites we visited.

Bulletin boards are also just what they sound like—a place to post and receive messages. Members use them to pass on dieting tips, recipes, gripes, and encouragement. Cyberdiet, eDiets, and nutrio.com have very active bulletin boards. Both Shape Up America and Shape Up and Drop 10 have bulletin boards that let members exchange dieting tips and encouragement, but they do not appear to attract much traffic.

A word on chats and bulletin boards. They constitute the motivational backbone of most weight-loss sites, providing the much needed vir-

tual contact that is missing from an otherwise impersonal experience. Viewers should keep in mind, however, that while these interactive features are monitored for offensive material, there is no guarantee that the opinions posted are scientifically sound. A message we saw on one of the DietWatch bulletin boards, for instance, came from a member concerned about sudden hair loss. Of the seven readers who responded, only one suggested that the person seek medical help. The lesson here: While chat rooms and bulletin boards offer great opportunities for social dieting, they are not the best places to get health advice. Use them cautiously in that regard.

Note: eFit has no chat rooms or bulletin boards, only an e-mail newsletter. But its motivational ace is its "morphover" feature, which lets members submit a digitalized photo and receive a computer-altered image of themselves 15 pounds lighter.

6. Does the site focus only on diet, or are members encouraged to increase their physical activity?

Successful weight loss requires both diet *and* exercise, so consumers should look for a site that offers advice on how to work physical activity into their daily routines. Just like with choosing a diet plan, there is no one right exercise regimen that will fit everyone's needs, so potential members should visit several sites to find one that works for them.

EFit and Asimba are sports-oriented sites, with pages of advice on how to start and maintain a program of running, water sports, cycling, yoga, or walking. Both also provide members with individual activity plans. A nice feature on Asimba is its "very easy" walking program, a good place to start for novice exercisers. Members on this program start with a daily half-mile walk and work up to 2 miles a day within a month. EFit provides aerobic exercise routines that are explained in print as well as video clips (this feature requires users to download Real Media or Microsoft Media plug-in).

All of the exercise routines in the eDiets program are illustrated with animated graphics, using a virtual instructor who demonstrates how to do each activity. It's a really clever feature, kind of like the online version of an exercise video.

The "Health Club" pages of Cyberdiet are less high-tech, but they do provide easy-to-follow routines, explained via text and pictures, that focus either on strength training, aerobics, or increased flexibility. Nutrio.com features a similar type of exercise program, although its exercise pages do not include any pictures at all.

Shape Up America's fitness pages come with a big plus. They place a significant emphasis on "thinking around" barriers—like fatigue or a hectic work schedule—that can prevent some people from starting and maintaining a diet and exercise program. Too hot or too cold to exercise? Walk at the mall. Too busy? Break up a half-hour exercise routine into three 10-minute sessions. The site's

authors encourage dieters to keep a daily activity log in order to identify times of the day when a sedentary activity (like watching television or sitting at the computer) could be replaced with a more vigorous activity, like walking.

7. Does the site charge a fee? How long is the contract?

Sites that charge an access fee may offer a reduced rate to clients willing to sign up for several weeks or months at a time. Be wary, though, of getting locked into a long-term contract. While it may take several months to get comfortable with a particular weight-loss site, you might regret buying into a program that requests payment for 6 months or more up front. Neither of the two fee-for-use sites reviewed here requires a long-term commit-

ment. Shape Up and Drop 10 clients pay by the week, and eDiets clients pay in 3-month installments.

8. Does the site offer a weight-maintenance plan?

Unfortunately, there isn't much focus on weight maintenance on any of the sites we visited, although eFit, eDiets, and Shape Up America and Shape Up and Drop 10 offer weight-maintenance meal plans for interested members. Cyberdiet also acknowledges that the battle isn't over once the weight is lost and hosts a "weight maintenance" bulletin board to support those who have reached goal weight. Given how hard it is to hold onto hard-won weight goals, support for "maintainers" deserves more attention on all of these sites.

From *Tufts University Health & Nutrition Letter,* May 2001, pp. 1-4. © 2001 by Tufts University Health & Nutrition Letter, 50 Broadway, 15th Floor, New York, NY 10004.

UNIT 5
Health Claims

Unit Selections

Key Points to Consider

- How can consumers protect themselves from misinformation in the nutrition field?

- How do your interpret the different types of research studies so that you can get at the truth of health claims?

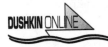 **Links: www.dushkin.com/online/**
These sites are annotated in the World Wide Web pages.

Federal Trade Commission (FTC): Diet, Health & Fitness
http://www.ftc.gov/bcp/menu-health.htm

Food and Drug Administration (FDA)
http://www.fda.gov/default.htm

National Council Against Health Fraud (NCAHF)
http://www.ncahf.org

QuackWatch
http://www.quackwatch.com

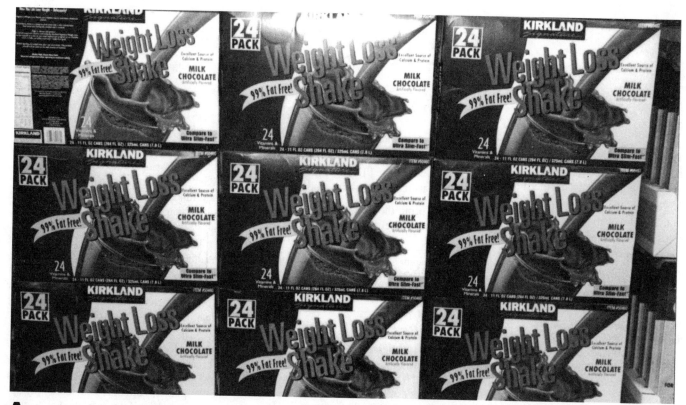

Americans spend approximately $25 billion per year on alternative treatments. According to an American Dietetic Association (ADA) Survey, 90% of consumers polled get their nutrition information from television, magazines, and newspapers.

It is very discouraging that Americans are confused and overwhelmed about the controversies surrounding food and health and that they have stopped paying attention to the contradictory claims reported by news media. Good science takes time to unfold. The media along with the public misinterpreting the results, simplify them, and take them out of context. Additionally the media are too eager to publish sensational information and not solid science. A new source of information is the Internet, which allows distribution and promotion of just about anything. About 29% of Americans turn to the Internet for information. We need to be vigilant as to the type of information we get from different websites.

The supplement industry is not regulated by the government. The consumer cannot trust what the label claims the supplement contains or how much, and does not guarantee that the supplement does not contain contaminants. Laboratory tests reveal that labels often overstate the amount of the active ingredient in a pill. The Food and Drug Administration (FDA) needs funding to enforce truth-in-labeling rules. Lists of approved "Health Claims" by the FDA and examples of food that carry deceptive claims is offered.

Functional foods are foods which may provide a health benefit beyond basic nutrition and are becoming one of the fastest growing segments of the food industry especially among affluent baby boomers. The U.S. government has no regulatory category of functional foods. Despite their popularity, their efficacy and safety is questionable due to lack of scientific evidence. So we are far from declaring them "magic bullets" to improve health and prevent disease. The consumer should be advised to eat a variety of foods in moderation and to view functional foods as part of an overall healthful diet.

Soy is one of the foods Americans are incorporating into their diet recently mostly due to evidence of soy's effects on the major degenerative diseases such as diabetes, CVD and cancer. The food industry is making advances in technology to meet the high consumer demand for new tasty and attractive soy products.

The food industry is also developing products that contain different types of pro-and prebiotics recognizing the importance of bacteria to human health. Foods such as Kefir, miso, tempeh that contain probiotics and oatmeal, flax, legumes etc that are good sources of prebiotics and their benefits to health are presented in one of the articles. Herbal supplements as other dietary supplements are also not regulated by the USDA.

Herbal supplements have become very popular in the U.S. but what the consumer does not know is that manufacturers have problems with quality control. Activity of the herbal product components depend on many factors and what the label describes is not usually what is in the bottle. Safety of herbal supplements and their interactions with other herbs and medications are generally unknown in our population and it is sad that we have to discover them through case-studies of people who experienced adverse health problems due to the above interactions.

Claims Crazy

Which can you believe?

Here's a quiz for the astute shopper: Which (one or more) of these claims can appear on a food or supplement label without approval from the Food and Drug Administration?

a. improves memory
b. relieves stress
c. suppresses appetite
d. helps reduce difficulty in falling asleep
e. supports the immune system

The answers: a, b, c, and e. They're called "structure/function claims," because they describe how a food or supplement affects the body's structure (say, the skeleton) or its function (for example, digestion). And manufacturers can slap one on virtually any food or supplement with or without evidence to back it up.

"The law says that structure/function claims can't be misleading, but the FDA has never said how much evidence a company needs to substantiate a claim," says Bruce Silverglade, director of legal affairs for the Center for Science in the Public Interest, publisher of *Nutrition Action Healthletter*.

Is one good study enough? What if that study is contradicted by a dozen others? "With no rules ensuring uniformity in structure/function claims, the resulting free-for-all could end up confusing consumers, and encouraging them to buy unhealthy foods," says Rep. Henry Waxman. The California Democrat is one of the strongest advocates of honest food labeling in Congress.

The FDA has no rules, in part because, until recently, structure/function claims only showed up on supplements.

No Approval Needed

In 1994, under strong industry pressure, Congress passed the Dietary Supplement Health and Education Act. The law gives supplement-makers free rein to make structure/function claims, as long as the companies:

- notify the FDA within 30 days after using a new claim, and
- print the following disclaimer on the label:

These statements have not been evaluated by the Food and Drug Administration. This product is not intended to diagnose, treat, cure or prevent any disease.

"Not evaluated" is right. "The FDA doesn't even look at the evidence behind structure/function claims," says Silverglade. "It just makes sure that the supplement doesn't make a disease claim—one that's approved only for drugs."

According to the law, a disease claim promises to "diagnose, cure, mitigate, treat, or prevent disease." If a supplement makes a disease claim, then legally it becomes a drug. "Drugs must be pre-approved for safety and effectiveness, so that would make the supplement illegal," explains Silverglade.

But the distinction between a structure/function claim and a disease claim can be subtle. For example, "helps restore sexual vigor, potency, and performance" is a disease claim, says the FDA. In contrast, "arouses sexual desire" is a structure/function claim.

Got that?

"Studies show that consumers can't distinguish between disease claims and structure/function claims," says Silverglade.

And if shoppers can't, why should food companies bother with health claims when they can say just about anything they want by using structure/function claims?

Textbook Talk

"For years, the law has allowed structure/function claims on foods," explains Silverglade. "But companies rarely made them, probably because they didn't have much appeal."

The classic example was a statement like "calcium builds strong bones." "Structure/function claims were supposed to be something you might read in a textbook," says Silverglade.

Instead, the industry was fired up about health claims—that a food could, "as part of an overall diet," help reduce the risk of heart disease, cancer, or osteoporosis. In 1990, Congress passed a law permitting health claims, but with clear limits.

"The FDA had to approve the claim, and the food couldn't be too high in harmful nutrients like saturated fat or sodium or too low in vitamins and minerals," says Silverglade. "And the FDA could only approve the claim if it was backed by 'significant scientific agreement.'" In other words, the claim had to be supported by strong and consistent evidence.

Since 1990, the FDA has approved 14 health claims (see "The 'A' List"). Apparently, that hasn't been enough for the food industry.

Tower of Babel

The Grocery Manufacturers of America, like other industry groups, has been hot under the collar over health claims for years.

The FDA approves claims "only where there is overwhelming science to support a diet/disease relationship, thus preventing the public from learning about new scientific developments until they have matured into hard science," a GMA spokesperson told Congress in May 2001. "As a result, the FDA has approved only a handful of disease/health claims…"

Not to worry, GMA. Last December, the FDA created a new kind of health claim. The agency announced that it would allow health claims for foods based on preliminary evidence as long as the label qualified it with a disclaimer like "this evidence is not conclusive."

These preliminary health claims haven't shown up on many foods yet. But even when they do, most companies will no doubt stick with anything-goes structure/function claims.

Why shouldn't they? Even preliminary health claims require approval and are prohibited on unhealthy or empty-calorie foods. What's more, structure/function claims have gotten jazzier. Goodbye, textbook. Hello, Madison Avenue.

"The supplement industry made a mint with structure/function claims," observes Silverglade. "Why should the food industry bother with health claims when they've got a free ride with structure/function claims? Food companies don't even have

to notify the FDA or print a disclaimer, like supplement companies do."

Structure/function claims are starting to hit the marketplace...and no one's watching. So far, many are showing up on decent foods, like fruit juice and fruit. But it's only a matter of time before they start to pop up in the cookie, chip, and soft-drink aisles.

Says Waxman: "The growth of structure/function claims for foods threatens to return us to the days when the Secretary of HHS called the food marketplace a 'Tower of Babel' for the consumer."

The Claim Game
Through the Lutein Glass

Even someone with lousy vision couldn't miss the "New! With Lutein for Healthy Eyes" sign on Prune Juice+. Sunsweet has added enough lutein to

supply 500 micrograms of the carotenoid per cup. Why?

"A growing body of scientific research links lutein consumption to a variety of eye health benefits, including a reduction in the incidence of macular degeneration, cataracts and retinal diseases," says the sign.

Sort of. In several studies, people who ate more lutein-rich foods had a lower risk of cataract surgery or degeneration of the retina's center (macula). And taking high doses of lutein (4,000 micrograms a day) raised the low levels of lutein in the retinas of patients with macular degeneration.

But no studies have tested whether lutein supplements reduce the risk of eye disease. That's why the National Eye Institute says that "claims made about an asso-

---

The "A" List

Approved Health Claims

Here are the 14 (slightly edited) health claims that the FDA has approved. Some are more popular than others. Words in [square brackets] vary according to the food bearing the claim.

- Diets rich in **whole grain foods** and other plant foods and low in total fat, saturated fat and cholesterol, may help reduce the risk of **heart disease** and certain **cancers**.
- Diets containing foods that are good sources of **potassium** and low in **sodium** may reduce the risk of **high blood pressure** and **stroke**.
- A diet low in **total fat** may reduce the risk of some **cancers**.
- Three grams of soluble fiber from [**oatmeal**] daily in a diet low in saturated fat and cholesterol may reduce the risk of **heart disease**. This [cereal] has [two] grams per serving.
- While many factors affect **heart disease**, diets low in **saturated fat** and **cholesterol** may reduce the risk of this disease.
- Diets low in **sodium** may reduce the risk of **high blood pressure**.
- Low fat diets rich in **fiber**-containing **grains**, **fruits**, and **vegetables** may reduce the risk of some types of **cancer**.
- Diets low in saturated fat and cholesterol that include 25 grams of **soy protein** per day may reduce the risk of **heart disease**. One serving of this product provides at least [6.25 g] of soy protein.
- Healthful diets with adequate **folate** may reduce a woman's risk of having a child with a **brain** or **spinal cord defect**.
- Two or three servings per day with meals, providing 3.4 grams of **plant stanol esters** daily, added to a diet low in saturated fat and cholesterol may reduce the risk of **heart disease**. [Benecol Spread] contains [1.7 g] stanol esters per serving.
- Diets low in saturated fat and cholesterol and rich in **fruits, vegetables,** and **grains** that contain some types of fiber, particularly **soluble fiber**, may reduce the risk of **heart disease**.
- Does not promote **tooth decay**.
- Low fat diets rich in **fruits** and **vegetables** containing **vitamin A, vitamin C,** and **fiber** may reduce the risk of some types of **cancer**.
- Regular exercise and a healthy diet with enough **calcium** helps teens and young adult white and Asian women maintain good bone health and may reduce their high risk of **osteoporosis** later in life.

NOTE: Each food that makes a health claim must meet specific criteria. For example, foods with the soy claim must contain at least 6.25 grams of soy protein per serving and be low in saturated fat and cholesterol. "Does not promote tooth decay" can only appear on sugar-free foods that contain maltitol, xylitol, or other sugar alcohols. Foods that make health claims must also meet general criteria. They can't be high in fat, saturated fat, cholesterol, or sodium and must have some naturally occurring nutrients.

ciation between lutein and eye health are speculative and should be viewed with caution."

Cautious or not, it won't hurt you to get extra lutein in your prune juice. Just remember that Sunsweet is jumping to conclusions when it says that "lutein acts as nature's defense system for the eyes."

The Antioxidant Rag

Strawberry Kiwi V8 Splash is 75 percent sugar and water and only 25 percent juice—carrot, apple, kiwi, and strawberry. To boost Splash's nutrition credentials, the label declares that the beverage is "Rich in Vitamins A, C, E." (The C and E are added.) Unfortunately, its claims are misleading:

- Vitamin A *"is essential for vision and healthy skin."* (People with severe vitamin A deficiency get skin lesions and go blind. But extra vitamin A won't do a thing for the average American's skin or sight.)

- Vitamin C *"is needed for healthy bones, gums and teeth."* (Yes, people with scurvy—severe vitamin C deficiency—have bleeding gums and weak bones. But there's no evidence that extra vitamin C can help yours.)

- Vitamin E helps "to protect cells from damage and promote a healthy immune system." (In theory, all antioxidants should protect cells, but studies that have tested vitamin E on people have found no drop in cancer or heart disease. And vitamin E may strengthen some immune functions, but no one has evidence that the vitamin prevents illness.)

You'll see A•C•E claims on many labels. Sounds good, but so far, no cigar.

So Proud

"Proud partners with the National Kidney Foundation," glows the label on Ocean Spray Cranberry Juice Cocktail. (You can choose your disease with Ocean Spray. Some bottles have the American Heart Association seal. Others

are "proud sponsors of the American Diabetes Association." It's a very proud company.)

"This delicious juice drink is good for you because it helps maintain urinary tract health," say labels that feature the Kidney Foundation. Maybe.

Of the five best trials testing cranberry juice's ability to prevent urinary tract infections (UTIs), only two found that it worked.

"The small number of poor quality trials gives no reliable evidence of the effectiveness of cranberry juice and other cranberry products," concludes the Cochrane Collaboration, an international organization that rigorously reviews medical treatments.

And that won't change no matter how much money Ocean Spray gives the National Kidney Foundation.

Raisin the Bar

"High in Antioxidants," boasts the banner on the Del Monte Raisins box. To prove its point, the box shows the "Fruit Antioxidant Score" of prunes, raisins, blueberries, strawberries, and oranges. Raisins wouldn't have come in second, but third (well behind prunes and blueberries and barely above strawberries and oranges) if Del Monte had compared one serving of each fruit instead of 100 grams—about 3 1/2 ounces—of each. (A serving is a small box of raisins, an orange, or half a cup of berries.)

It's not clear what those antioxidants can do for you anyway. People who eat more fruits and vegetables have a lower risk of heart disease, stroke, and some cancers. But so far, studies that have given people antioxidants—like vitamin E or beta-carotene—haven't found any lower risk.

Because raisins are low-fat, fiber-rich fruits, they qualify for the FDA-approved health claims on cancer and heart disease. But Del Monte implies that it's the antioxidant vitamins in raisins that lower the risk of those diseases...and "slow the effects of aging." Evidence? Who needs it?

Fruit Farce

Tropicana Twisters are only 10 to 15 percent juice. And despite names like

"Mango Tangerine Mambo," the few spoonfuls of juice in each cup are mostly orange, grape, or apple.

Maybe that's why Tropicana needed "now with FruitForce energy releasing B vitamins!" to help sell its sugared water. B-vitamins help cells convert food to energy, but taking B-vitamins doesn't make you feel more energetic.

Want more B-vitamins? Take a multivitamin, not a 140-calorie glass of sugar, water, and 10 percent of a day's worth of niacin and pantothenic acid thrown in.

Total Trick

"Lose More Weight with 100% Daily Value of Calcium," promises Total's box. "As part of a reduced calorie diet," says the smaller print. (That always helps.)

"Now a recent study from a major university suggests that increasing calcium intake while cutting calories may help you lose more weight than dieting alone," explains the package. In fact, the evidence is flimsier than a wet Total flake.

Susan Barr, a researcher at the University of British Columbia, examined 17 clinical trials on calcium supplements and weight loss. "Only one study found greater weight loss in the supplemented group," she wrote. "In the remaining studies, changes in body weight and/or body fat were strikingly similar between groups."

The bottom line: "A recent study" could be the only one the company could find to back its claim.

Lycopene Lore

Campbell's Tomato Juice, Hunt's Whole Tomatoes, V8 Vegetable Juice, and others are suddenly talking about the "long-term health benefits" of "diets rich in tomatoes," which may be explained by lycopene, a "natural antioxidant."

While men who eat more lycopene-rich foods have a lower risk of prostate cancer, it's not clear that lycopene makes the difference. There's no harm in eating tomato foods. Just choose carefully. Campbell's Tomato Juice has 750 mg of sodium in each cup—too much to bear a health claim (see "The 'A' List,"). But with structure/function claims like these, anything goes.

Q & A on Functional Foods

Q. What are "functional foods"?

"Functional foods" is simply a convenient way to describe foods or their components which may provide a health benefit beyond basic nutrition. In other words, functional foods do more than meet your minimum daily requirements of nutrients—they also can play a role in reducing risk of disease and promoting good health. While all foods are functional in that they provide nutrients, "functional foods" tend to be those with health-promoting ingredients or natural components that have been found to have potential benefit in the body. They can include whole foods as well as fortified, enriched or enhanced foods and dietary supplements that have a beneficial effect on health.

The concept of functional foods is not entirely new, although it has evolved considerably over the years. In the early 1900s, food manufacturers in the United States began adding iodine to salt in an effort to prevent goiter, representing one of the first attempts at creating a functional component through fortification. Today, researchers have identified hundreds of compounds with functional qualities, and they continue to make new discoveries surrounding the complex benefits of phytochemicals in foods.

Q. How does a food become "functional"?

Since many of these foods are just natural, whole foods with new information about their potential health qualities, they do not become "functional" except for the way we perceive them. On the other hand, functional foods can result from agricultural breeding or added nutrients/ingredients.

Many—if not most—fruits, vegetables, grains, fish, and dairy and meat products contain several natural components that deliver benefits beyond basic nutrition, such as lycopene in tomatoes, omega-3 fatty acids in salmon or saponins in soy. Even tea and chocolate have been noted in some studies as possessing functional attributes.

Agricultural scientists are able to boost the nutritional content of certain crops through the same breeding techniques that are used to bring out other beneficial traits in plants and animals—everything from beta-carotene-rich rice to vitamin-enhanced broccoli and soybeans, just to name a couple of examples. And research is under way to improve the nutritional quality of dozens of other crops.

Below is a sampling of a few functional foods, their components and their potential benefits for human health.

Functional Component	Source	Potential Health Benefit
Lutein	Green vegetables	Contributes to maintenance of healthy vision
Insoluble fiber	Wheat bran	May reduce risk of breast and/or colon cancer
Lactobacillus	Yogurt, other dairy	May improve gastrointestinal health
Soy protein	Soy-based foods	May reduce risk of cardiovascular disease
Omega-3 fatty acids	Salmon, tuna, fish/marine oils	May reduce risk of cardiovascular disease and improve mental, visual functions
Xylitol	Nutritional bars, beverages	Improves oral health; Does not promote tooth decay

Other foods may be specially formulated with nutrients or other ingredients. This is true of products such as orange juice fortified with calcium, cereals with added vitamins or minerals, or flour with added folic acid. In fact, more and more foods are being fortified with nutrients and other physiologically active components (such as plant stanols and sterols) as researchers uncover more evidence about their role in health and even disease risk reduction.

Q. What are some of the health benefits associated with functional foods?

The scientific community has only just begun to understand the complex interactions between nutritional components and the human body. However, there is already a large body of scientific evidence showing that eating foods with functional benefits on a regular basis as part of a varied diet can help reduce the risk of, or manage a number of health concerns, including cancer, heart and cardiovascular disease, gastrointestinal health, menopausal symptoms, osteoporosis and eye health, to name a few.

Q. How can I get more functional foods in my diet?

The most effective way to reap the health benefits from foods is to eat a balanced and varied diet, including fruits and vegetables as well as foods with added beneficial components. Watch labels and read articles for information about foods and health. Before you decide to make any major dietary changes, however, take the time to evaluate your personal health, or speak to your health care provider on ways to help reduce your risk of certain diseases. It is also important to remember that there is no single "magic bullet" food that can cure or prevent most health concerns, even when eaten in abundance. The best advice is to choose foods wisely from each level of the food guide pyramid in order to incorporate many potentially beneficial components into the diet.

Q. Where can I learn about scientific research related to the functional benefits of foods?

There are several universities and research institutions conducting scientific studies on various food components. You can find out more about current research by visiting the home page of the Functional Foods for Health program administered by the University of Illinois at Urbana-Champaign and Chicago. Information on functional foods research is also available from the U.S. Department of Agriculture's Agricultural Research Service, the Institute of Food Technologists, the American Dietetic Association, and the food science programs at Rutgers University and the University of California, Davis.

Q. Are functional foods regulated by the federal government?

Yes. "Functional foods" has no official meaning and do not constitute a distinctly separate category of foods. Most often they are simply natural whole foods we have been eating for thousands of years. Therefore, the Food and Drug Administration (FDA) regulates them in the same way they regulate all foods—safety of ingredients must be assured in advance, and all claims must be substantiated, truthful, and non-misleading.

A significant amount of credible scientific data is needed to confirm any "health claims"—messages pertaining to a relationship between dietary components and a disease or health condition, for example soy protein and heart disease. Foods also can bear another type of claim to convey their potential benefits, and those are called "structure/function claims." These statements describe or imply a relationship between the product itself, or its components, and normal bodily functions (for example, "may help support digestion"). All such claims must be adequately substantiated.

A 1994 law stipulates that dietary supplements-for example an herb, vitamin, mineral or other substance added to one's total diet—shall continue to be treated as foods for regulatory purposes, but with just a few differences in approach. Regardless of any differences in approach, like all other foods, supplements are regulated by FDA to assure safety and accuracy of label claims.

There has been some criticism of certain foods containing herbal ingredients—whether or not such ingredients are allowed in food and whether their label claims are substantiated. The FDA is looking into these allegations. While herb-containing foods may be considered "functional", it is important to keep in mind that they represent only a small number of the broad spectrum of foods that are thought of as "functional foods".

Consumers need to remember that functional foods represent an important breakthrough in understanding the connection between diet, health, and even disease risk reduction. With regard to all claims pertaining to diseases and health conditions, consumers may be reassured to know that they must be pre-approved by FDA and substantiated by a large body of credible scientific evidence. And, although structure/function claims do not require FDA pre-approval, they too must be adequately substantiated by the producers of the food.

Q. What health claims have been approved so far by FDA?

Since 1993, FDA has approved 14 health claims, eight of which are related to the functional benefits of food:

- Potassium and reduced risk of high blood pressure and stroke
- Plant sterol and plant stanol esters and coronary heart disease
- Soy protein and coronary heart disease
- Calcium and reduced risk of osteoporosis
- Fiber-containing grain products, fruits and vegetables and cancer

- Fruits, vegetables and grain products that contain fiber, particularly soluble fiber, and risk of coronary heart disease
- Fruits and vegetables and cancer
- Folate and neural tube birth defects
- Dietary soluble fiber, such as that found in whole oats and psyllium seed husk, and coronary heart disease
- Dietary sugar alcohol and dental caries (cavaties)

The remaining three are based on diets low in "negative" nutrients in food, such as sodium:

- Dietary fat and cancer
- Dietary saturated fat and cholesterol and risk of coronary heart disease
- Sodium and high blood pressure

Q. What is the relationship between biotechnology and functional foods?

While many of the nutritional compounds in functional foods are either naturally present or added during processing, some may be the result of agricultural breeding techniques, including conventional crossbreeding and biotechnology.

Crossbreeding a plant for a specific genetic trait, such as higher vitamin A content, can take as long as a decade or more. Modern biotechnology, however, makes it possible to select a specific genetic trait from any plant and move it into the genetic code of another plant in a much shorter time span, and with more precision than crossbreeding allows.

Researchers are working with farmers around the world to develop dozens of functional foods through the use of this promising technology.

From *International Food Information Council Foundation*, November 2002. © 2002 by International Food Information Council Foundation.

The Latest Scoop on Soy

Twenty-eight percent of Americans consume soyfoods or soy beverages once a week or more, according to the United Soybean Board's 2003–04 annual study, "Consumer Attitudes about Nutrition." According to the survey, soymilk, tofu, and soy veggie burgers are the top soy products regularly consumed (see table).

The USB study found that significantly more consumers are aware of soymilk, soy ice cream or cheese, miso, and tempeh compared to 2002. In addition to becoming more aware of soy products, consumers are also learning more about soy's health benefits. The study found that 74% of U.S. consumers perceive soy as healthy. Heart health is the main benefit that consumers associate with soy. Other areas of awareness include menopause relief, obesity prevention/ weight loss, cancer prevention, and protein source.

As awareness grows and as research accumulates, so do the soy ingredients that companies offer. Ingredients such as soy protein isolates, soy protein concentrates, soy isoflavones, soy flour, and soy nuggets have evolved through the years to become more functional for manufacturers' needs. Solubility and flavor of soy ingredients are two areas that have vastly improved.

Here's a brief update on some of the latest soy news related to health and ingredient offerings.

The Healthy Side of Soy

Soy is most commonly known for its cardiovascular benefits, particularly soy protein. This is evident in the Food and Drug Administration's approved soy protein health claim linking it to a reduced risk for heart disease. The health claim is based on clinical trials showing that consumption of soy protein can lower total and low-density-lipoprotein (LDL) cholesterol levels.

> Soy is most commonly known for its cardiovascular benefits [but] bone health, prostate cancer, and menopause are three main areas where consumers may soon be learning more about soy's benefits.

Additional research and clinical trials are pointing to other potential health benefits of soy protein and soy isoflavones. Bone health, prostate cancer, and menopause are three main areas where consumers may soon be learning more about soy's benefits.

Bone Health

"In my view, there is probably the most support for the skeletal benefits of soy protein and isoflavones," said Mark Messina, Adjunct Associate Professor at California's Loma Linda University and co-owner of Nutrition Matters Inc. "When soy protein is substituted for milk protein, several studies have found that urinary calcium excretion is decreased. The metabolism of the sulfur amino acids in protein leads to the production of acid, which requires buffering. The skeletal system is the largest source of buffering agent in the body. In response to acid, the bones are broken down, which leads to an increase in urinary calcium. Since soy protein contains lower amounts of sulfur amino acids than milk protein, it causes less calcium excretion."

In addition to soy protein, isoflavones may have possible skeletal benefits. Mes-sina discussed two studies that have drawn attention to this. "A recent one-year trial found that genistein, the main isoflavone in soybeans, was even more effective than conventional hormone replacement therapy (HRT) at reducing bone loss at the hip in postmenopausal women and was only slightly less effective than HRT at the spine," he said. "Another recently presented two-year trial found that isoflavone-rich soymilk reduced bone loss at the hip and spine in comparison to soymilk low in isoflavones."

He added that long-term studies are currently underway to firmly conclude that isoflavones have the same effect as HRT in reducing fracture risk. "Nevertheless, because soy protein is high quality, the current data justify recommending that isoflavone-rich soyfoods be part of an overall bone-healthy diet. When using soy in place of dairy products, calcium-fortified soy products should be used."

Breast and Prostate Cancer

"There is a large body of literature on the cancer prevention actions of a diet that includes soy. These data support a beneficial effect especially on breast cancer and prostate cancer risk," stated Debra Miller, Director, Nutrition Science Communications, The Solae Co., St. Louis, Mo.

For example, a recent Japanese study suggested that eating foods rich in isoflavones reduced the risk of breast cancer, especially in postmenopausal women. Frequent consumption of soy-rich miso soup was found to be particularly effective (Yamamoto et al., 2003).

Researchers from the National Cancer Center Research Institute in Japan evaluated the relationship between isoflavone consumption and breast cancer risk among women as part of the Ja-

What consumers say about soy foods, according to the United Soybean Board's 2003–04 annual study	
Soy products used regularly	**Soy products tried at least once during the year**
1. Soymilk (17%)	1. Tofu (48%)
2. Tofu (12%)	2. Soy veggie burgers (44%)
3. Soy veggie burgers (12%)	3. Soymilk (39%)
4. Soy protein bars (5%)	4. Soy nuts (26%)
5. Soy nuts (4%)	5. Soy protein bars (22%)

pan Public Health Center-based prospective study on cancer and cardiovascular diseases.

The JPHC study began in 1990, when nearly 22,000 Japanese female residents age 40–59 years from four public health center areas completed a questionnaire which included items about the frequency of soy consumption. Ten years later, 179 of these women had been diagnosed with breast cancer.

Researchers found that while soyfoods alone did not have a significant effect, both consumption of miso soup and overall isoflavone intake reduced the risk of breast cancer. In addition, the researchers reported that the association was found to be stronger in postmenopausal women.

Because of increasing evidence of the benefits of isoflavones, a European Union-funded project, called the Isoheart project, has recently been established to explore the physiological effects from eating foods with added soy-derived isoflavones. One of the project's aims is to establish the presumed health benefits of phytoestrogens in reducing the risk of heart disease in postmenopausal women, as well as to study the consumer acceptability of foods enriched with isoflavones.

In men, soy isoflavones are believed to help in preventing prostate cancer. "Personally, I am most excited about the role that soy may have in preventing and even treating prostate cancer," said Messina. "One key to preventing prostate cancer mortality is preventing the latent (small, clinically irrelevant) tumors from progressing to the larger tumors that can metastasize and which are life threatening," he said. "The International Prostate Health Council concluded that isoflavones stop this progression. Animal

studies are very supportive of this hypothesis, and a recent pilot study found that isoflavones were of benefit to prostate cancer patients resistant to conventional medical treatment. Still, all this remains speculative, although I strongly recommend that men consume soy."

Research presented at a recent American Urological Association meeting in Chicago showed that genistein reduced prostate-specific antigen (PSA) levels in men with untreated cancer, in some cases by almost two thirds.

PSA is a protein produced by the cells of the prostate gland. PSA levels tend to rise if the prostate gland is enlarged due to cancer. The researchers from the University of California Davis Cancer Center said their study suggested that genistein could help men at risk of developing prostate cancer.

The researchers studied 62 men known to have prostate cancer and elevated PSA levels. The men were given 5 g of a dietary supplement containing genistein every day for six months. Sixteen of the men had untreated prostate cancer—they were in the "watchful waiting" group, where the cancer is slow-growing and causing no symptoms. In this group, three had to stop the therapy because they suffered from diarrhea, but eight saw their PSA level fall between 3 and 61%. The remaining five (38%) saw their PSA levels rise, but the researchers say this is a far smaller proportion than in the remaining 46 men who had been treated for prostate cancer, 98% of whom saw a rise.

Ralph de Vere White, Director of the UC-Davis Cancer Center, said, "It must be interpreted cautiously because the numbers of men enrolled are small. He added, however, that "patients on watchful waiting may do better due to grade of

disease or distribution and concentration of genistein within the prostate."

Menopausal Symptoms

A number of studies have shown that consuming both soy protein and soy isoflavone extracts can help reduce the severity and frequency of hot flashes, said Miller. "It should be noted, however, that consuming soyfoods or supplements will not result in the powerful and quick results that HRT provides. However HRT has recently been associated with a number of long-term health risks such as heart attack, stroke, breast cancer, and Alzheimer's disease. In light of these risks, many women find consuming soyfoods a healthy option."

In an article in the *Journal of Medicinal Food*, Messina and Hughes (2003) reviewed the evidence to date on the impact of soyfoods and soy isoflavones on hot flush symptoms in women. They found a statistically significant relationship between initial hot flush frequency and treatment efficacy.

"Initial hot flush frequency explained about 46 percent of the treatment effects, and hot flush frequency decreased by about 5 percent (above placebo or control effects) for every additional initial hot flush per day in women whose initial hot flush frequency was five or more per day," the authors reported.

Soy has received attention as an alternative to HRT largely because it is a unique dietary source of isoflavones. However, there have been conflicting results from trials measuring the ability of isoflavones to reduce menopausal symptoms. In their review, Messina and Hughes eliminated trials on breast cancer patients. They also eliminated non-blinded trials.

Out of 11 studies on soyfoods, only one found that women showed a significant decrease in hot flush frequency. The researchers noted, however, that "the large placebo effect makes most of these trials underpowered to detect modest effects." In four out of six studies on isoflavone supplements, there was a positive link to reduced menopausal symptoms. But the baseline level of hot flush frequency was higher on average among participants in the supplement trials. This led the authors to the theory that efficacy increased with hot flush frequency, so that those women having around 10 hot flushes each day saw this frequency halved, while those experiencing only seven daily only saw a reduction of around three flushes, after taking isoflavones.

The researchers wrote that although conclusions based on the analysis should be considered tentative, "the available data justify the recommendation that patients with frequent hot flushes consider trying soyfoods or isoflavone supplements for the alleviation of their symptoms."

They added that future trials involving soyfoods and isoflavone supplements are warranted, "but should focus on women who have frequent hot flushes." The correlation between initial hot flush frequency and the extent of reduction of symptoms should also be studied, they said.

Weight Management/Diabetes Control

"Given the enormous problem with obesity and its secondary effects, such as type 2 diabetes in the Western world, many people are looking at alterations in diet. Many have opted for high protein/lower carbohydrate diets and found success with such diets," said Miller. "However, health professionals are concerned with long-term high animal protein consumption. Eating large amounts of meat, cheese, and eggs can cause calcium loss from bones and cause the kidneys to work harder than usual (a big risk factor for those who have type 2 diabetes already). Interestingly, soy protein, as a vegetable protein, does not cause calcium loss and is actually the protein recommended to many patients on dialysis to prevent protein malnutrition because

even patients with impaired renal function can tolerate soy protein."

Soy protein and its constituents have also been linked to enhancements in glucose tolerance and reductions in insulin resistance, added Miller. "This research is encouraging. Certainly adding soy protein to food in place of carbohydrates can help reduce the glycemic index of foods."

Soy proteins and isoflavones are becoming more versatile and functional for various products.

Cognitive Ability

"One of the most exciting areas of research regarding soy foods is the association with better recognition and recall ability in memory testing when people eat a diet high in soy compared to those on a low-soy diet," said Miller. Research is ongoing in this area.

Improvements in Soy Ingredients

"Who thought that soy protein would be used in cold cereal four or five years ago?" said Mian Riaz, Head of the Extrusion Technology Program and Research Scientist at the Food Protein Research and Development Center at Texas A&M University, College Station. "With improved ingredients, we will see more soy-cultured products with improved flavor and taste, real soy cheese and ice cream, which taste just like traditional cheese and ice cream products, soy water, soy tea, and soy candy."

He added that there is a lot of research going on to process a soy meat analog that is very close to real meat. "This meat texture will resemble fresh meat and have the same composition as real meat you buy from the butcher (with 70% moisture content)."

Novel soy products such as these would not have been possible if not for the continuous improvement of soy ingredients. From the following information from three soy suppliers, we can see that the ingredients are becoming more refined and tailored for specific food product applications. Both soy proteins and isofla-

vones are becoming more versatile and functional for various products.

New Soy Ingredient Developments

"What's happened overall with soy ingredients is that companies have figured out how to create better-tasting ingredients for different applications. That now has allowed us to put together food systems with better taste and texture," said Tony DeLio, Vice President, Marketing and External Affairs, Archer Daniels Midland Co., Natural Health and Nutrition Division, Decatur, Ill.

The company offers a range of soy products, from flours, to soy protein concentrates and isolates, to soy isoflavones. "It all depends on what your end product is. Our soy flours enable us to work in bread applications, for example. Utilizing our baking expertise, we can easily get 6.25 g of soy protein into two slices of sandwich bread without compromising texture and flavor," said DeLio.

A new addition to the company's *NutriSoy* line is *Wholebean Soy Powder*, an organic ingredient for soymilk and other dairy-like products. It offers the superior nutrition of whole soybeans—fiber and isoflavones—in a form that can be easily incorporated into virtually any dairy or dairy analog product, he said.

"We can also incorporate soy into chocolate coating systems and have worked with a number of companies to create soy rice crispies for nutrition bars," DeLio added. "On the meat analog side, we tend to use soy concentrates and isolates to get a higher level of protein. We are currently developing technology to simulate whole-muscle meat products. We hope to have this revolutionary new product on the market within the next six months."

Regarding isoflavones, approximately 125 different retail product labels carry the *NovaSoy* brand name. "Isoflavones have gone from being primarily in dietary supplements to functional foods such as beverages and snack bars," he said. "We provide all different concentration levels of isoflavones. We have recently licensed technology that allows the time release of isoflavones. For example, you could have a time-released steady stream of isoflavones in a product."

DeLio concluded that with the innovation in soy ingredients, there is no reason why the food industry can't have a line of branded soy products that cut across all food segments. This would be similar to the line of *Healthy Choice* products that cater to low salt and low fat demand. "The consumer interest is there and the time is right for somebody."

Concept Beverage with Soy Isoflavones.

A ready-to-drink raspberry tea that supports bone health was unveiled by Cargill Health & Food Technologies, Minneapolis, Minn., at the Institute of Food Technologists' Annual Meeting + Food Expo® last month. The prototype beverage, named *Bone Appetit*, contains Cargill's *AdvantaSoy*™ Clear isoflavones, *Oliggo-Fiber*™ inulin, and calcium. Proprietary processing technology results in beverages that retain their traditional flavor, color, and consistency. "*AdvantaSoy Clear* isoflavones allow us to meet the challenge of creating new functional beverages that promote health and retain the delicious flavor and aroma which made them popular in the first place," said Steve Snyder, Cargill's Director of Sales and Marketing, Nutraceuticals.

"What we try to do is look at the retail market and create a product solution based on consumer input," said Lee Knudson, *Advantasoy* Product Manager. "This will help our customers be more successful in key product launches. The ready-to-drink tea is one example."

The *AdvantaSoy line* is available in three different forms depending on the application, he explained. Produced using proprietary technology and available in isoflavone concentrations of up to 50%, *AdvantaSoy Clear* has improved solubility, a whiter appearance, and reduced undesirable taste and odor, ideal for beverages and more-attractive food product applications. The product is GRAS for beverages, nutrition bars, yogurt, meal replacement, and confections. *AdvantaSoy Complete Isoflavones* are created using a natural, solvent-free processing technique. The ingredient is a combination of soy protein and isoflavones, ideal for breads, cereals, and meal replacements. *AdvantaSoy Compress*, available in isoflavone concentrations of up to 50%, is formulated for dietary supplements.

"Our soy isoflavones are really next-generation ingredients in the sense that we concentrate ours in a proprietary process from the soy germ," said Snyder. "The first generation of isoflavones was concentrated from the soy protein isolate manufacturing process."

In the future, said Snyder, we'll see soy ingredients that are easier to formulate, with better taste attributes. "Ingredients will be tailored to individual food products."

Improved Flavor and Functional Performance

New soy developments center on improving the flavor and functional performance and developing new ingredient forms to allow use in a wider array of food products. "We have also focused on innovations that contribute unique textures in food products," said Jim Holbrook, Vice President, Food Science Research and Development, The Solae Co. For example, the company's *Supro® XT* proteins, based on soy isolate technology, provide flavor and functional improvements in beverages. The *Alpha®* proteins, based on a revolutionary new manufacturing process, provide improved flavor performance in beverages and a range of dairy alternative products.

Other new offerings include extruded soy nuggets, now delivering protein contents up to 80% protein and providing unique texture and crunch in nutritional food bars and other grain-based foods. "For meat alternatives, we have introduced a range of high-moisture extruded ingredients for use in this application, which provide consumers a more meat-like eating experience," Holbrook said. "We have also introduced a number of products that offer enhanced nutritional attributes, such as soy proteins co-processed with other ingredients, such as calcium phosphate, carbohydrates, and fibers to enhance the nutritional value and functional performance of our ingredients in various food products. We also offer products with guaranteed levels of isoflavones, important health-promoting components found in soy."

Applications that will benefit from Solae's innovations include beverages, nutrition bars, and meat alternatives. "We have recently introduced new technology that makes soy protein more functional in acidic beverages, a big growth area for soy protein today," Holbrook said. "We are looking at both powdered isolate and extruded soy nuggets as technologies we can employ to positively affect shelf life in bars. We are also continuing to innovate with new extruded products and forms for meat alternatives. Additionally, we are very excited about our new *Alpha* technology, based on an innovative new process that delivers very bland-flavored soy proteins. We believe this technology has tremendous potential for future development across a spectrum of new applications."

Better Soy Ingredients

So, in the future, we can expect soy ingredients with improved flavor, texture, color, and mouthfeel. "The food industry will be able to find soy ingredients with very specific functionality, like foaming, whipping, emulsification, solubility, and texturization for specific food applications," said Riaz. "Improved soy ingredients will be available for soy beverages without the chalky flavor. There will be improvement in soybean oil for taste, flavor, and overall quality without the hydrogenation. The food industry will also find soy flour with higher protein levels, through breeding and improved processing techniques."

Expect more great things to come from soy!

REFERENCES

1. Messina, M. and Hughes, C. 2003. Efficacy of soyfoods and soybean isoflavone supplements for alleviating menopausal symptoms is positively related to initial hot flush frequency. J. Medicinal Food 6(1): 1–11.
2. Yamamoto, S., Sobue, T., Kobayashi, M., Sasaki, S., and Tsugane, S. 2003. Soy, isoflavones, and breast cancer risk in Japan. J. Natl. Cancer Inst. 95: 906–913.

Food-Friendly Bugs Do the Body Good

Trillions of bacteria naturally occur in your gut, but don't be alarmed! Many of the bacteria are good and may help protect the body from certain diseases. A number of factors can upset the balance between the levels of good and bad bacteria. However, there is evidence that consuming foods that have "good" bacteria, called probiotics, and food that aid the function of probiotics, called prebiotics, may help maintain a healthy balance of bacteria in the body and help improve certain disease conditions.

"Food-Friendly Bugs"

Our bodies have four lines of defense against infection: skin, mucosal lining, immune system, and gut microflora, sometimes referred to as gut microbiota. Research has shown that adding "friendly" bacteria to your diet will improve the health of your gut microflora, and may help protect both the lining of your intestinal tract and your immune system. An article written by Negendra Shah, associate professor of food science at the School of Life Sciences and Technology, Victoria University of Technology, Australia, in the November 2001 issue of *Food Technology,* highlights the common practice of adding probiotics, similar to bacteria already present in your body, to fermented foods such as yogurt. Probiotics are defined as live microbial food ingredients that have a beneficial effect on human health, when ingested live and in sufficient numbers.

Knowledge of the health benefits of probiotics can be traced back many years when a Nobel Prize winning scientist and director of the Pasteur Institute, Elie Metchnikoff, hypothesized that Bulgarian peasants owed their health and longevity to the consumption of fermented milk products containing lactobacillus, a probiotic bacterium. By 1997, the use of probiotics was becoming well established in Europe, with fermented dairy products accounting for 65 percent of the European "functional food" market. According to an article by Catherine Stanton and colleagues in the *American Journal of Clinical Nutrition* in 2001, health-conscious Americans are realizing the potential health benefits of supplementing their diets with good bacteria and are the fastest growing segment of consumers of probiotic foods.

Different Types of Probiotics

The two most common bacteria added in the production of probiotic foods are lactobacilli and bifidobacteria. According to an article by Fooks and Gibson, published in a supplement of the *British Journal of Nutrition* in 2002, there are numerous species of lactobacilli and bifidobacteria; the main species thought to have probiotic characteristics are *L. casei, B. lactis, L. johnsonii, B. breve, L. bulgaricus, B. animalis, L. rhamnosus, B. infantis, L. reuteri, B. longum,* and *L. acidophilus.*

Today there are more than 70 lactic acid bacteria-containing products worldwide, including sour cream, buttermilk, yogurt, powdered milk, and frozen desserts. According to Shah, more than 53 different types of probiotic milk products are marketed in Japan alone. In an article published in the *American Journal of Clinical Nutrition* in 2000, Belgian expert Marcel Roberfroid states that probiotics have traditionally been consumed as fermented dairy products such as yogurt but have also recently been incorporated into drinks, and in the future may be found in fermented vegetables and meats. They are also being marketed as dietary supplements in tablet, capsule, and freeze-dried preparations.

Health Effects of Probiotics

The health of the gut largely relies on the balance between good and bad bacteria, and probiotics may help the gut prevent an imbalance in which there are too many harmful bacteria. Most of the research on probiotics has been conducted through small clinical studies or epidemiological (observational) studies. This research has shown that probiotics may be promising as treatments for a number of diseases and conditions including: lactose intolerance, diarrhea secondary to antibiotic use or *E. coli* infections, other gastrointestinal infections, vaginal candida (yeast) infections, and lactose malabsorption due to chemotherapy. Research has reasonably well established that probiotics improve the body's ability to resist intestinal infection and improve digestion. Only limited evidence, however, suggests that probiotics have cholesterol-lowering benefits, reduce the risk of cancer, produce vitamins, and reduce the risk of urogenital infections other than candida. Although there is relatively little harm in taking probiotics, more research is necessary to establish a firm basis for using probiotics for specific health benefits.

Prebiotics, The Companion Nutrient

Gut microflora need an environment in which to thrive. Dennis T. Gordon, Ph.D., professor and chair of the department of cereal science at North Dakota State University, explains, "Fermentable dietary fiber is a source of prebiotics and the necessary energy source for our intestinal microbiota." According to an article by Christopher Duggan of Children's Hospital in Boston, Mass., published in the *American Journal of Clinical Nutrition* in 2002, inulin and oligofructose are the two most commonly studied prebiotics. Both inulin and oligofructose are found naturally in many fruits and vegetables as well as in whole-grain foods. They are also widely used commercially to add fiber to foods without adding bulk.

Health Effects of Prebiotics

Most of the research on the potential health benefits of prebiotics has been done in studies with animals or *in vitro* (in a test tube). Studies of inulin have shown that it may have a promising role to play in providing relief from constipation and suppressing diarrhea. Some studies also suggest a possible benefit for reduced risk of osteoporosis through increased calcium absorption, reduced risk of atherosclerosis through decreased cholesterol and triglycerides and improved insulin response, obesity and possibly type 2 diabetes (Roberfroid, *American Journal of Clinical Nutrition,* 2000).

The Lowdown on Consuming Probiotics and Prebiotics

Probiotics and prebiotics are safe to eat and have many positive health

---

Food Sources of Probiotics

- Yogurt
- Buttermilk
- Kefir
- Tempeh
- Miso
- Kim Chi
- Sauerkraut
- Other "fermented" foods

(source:**www.cancer.med.umich.edu/news/pro09spr02.htm**)

---

benefits. Eating a combination of pre- and probiotic foods, or symbiotic foods, those that contain both pre- and probiotics, may provide the most health benefits. Probiotic and prebiotic products are now widely available. Manufacturers formulate their products with different types and amounts of probiotic bacteria. Most work best when refrigerated or vacuum-packed to preserve the freshness of the bacteria.

Currently, there are no established recommended consumption levels of pre- and probiotics for beneficial effects. More research is needed to determine who will benefit most from consumption of those foods, and who should potentially avoid them. For example, as stated by Sanders in an article published in the November 1999 issue of *Food Technology,* immuno-compromised individuals (e.g., young, elderly, patients with AIDS, Crohn's Disease or enteric infection, etc.) should check with their doctor before consuming probiotics and prebiotics. As always, it is important that individuals not self-diagnose any health condition and speak to their healthcare professionals for advice on the nutritional component of any treatment plan

---

Food Sources of Prebiotics

- Oatmeal
- Flax
- Barley
- Other whole grains
- Onions
- Greens (especially dandelion greens, but also spinach, collard greens, chard, kale, and mustard greens)
- Berries, bananas, and other fruit
- Legumes (lentils, kidney beans, chickpeas, navy beans, white beans, black beans, etc.)

(source: **www.cancer.med.umich.edu/news/pro09spr02.htm**)

The Future of Probiotics and Prebiotics

Pre- and probiotics are exciting areas of food and nutrition research; however, more studies are needed to substantiate some of the links between these nutrients and health.

Dr. Gordon sums up the current state of the science by saying, "Probiotics are helping us to not only understand but also improve intestinal health. Emerging research is also revealing an important supporting role for prebiotics." The determination of specific strains of beneficial bacteria may help address various gastrointestinal diseases including Crohn's disease and ulcerative colitis, irritable bowel syndrome, and infections in the stomach and small intestine. Research may also find ways for probiotics to improve tube feedings and infant formula as well as improve the nutritional health of the elderly.

HERBAL LOTTERY

What's on a dietary supplement's label may not be what's in the bottle

JANET RALOFF

Echinacea is a commercial success. The dietary supplement—made from the flowers, stems, and leaves of the purple cone-flower—has become a popular and lucrative over-the-counter cold remedy. It's also one of the few nutraceuticals—natural products with medicinal reputations—that have substantial scientific evidence to support its purported functions: Various studies suggest that echinacea supplements can boost immunity or shorten the duration of colds.

Several years ago, however, Christine M. Gilroy of the University of Colorado Health Sciences Center in Denver was unsure whether to trust data from those experiments because few reports included biochemical proof of which species of purple coneflower had been used. That's important, she notes, because three species—*Echinacea pallida*, *Echinacea purpurea*, and *Echinacea angustifolia*—turn up in supplements "and only the first two have data indicating they might make colds better."

Not Twins—*Echinacea pallida* and *Echinacea purpurea* look different, but manufacturers sometimes swap one for the other in dietary supplements—even though the plants contain different chemicals and may perform differently.

Curious about *E. pallida's* reputed power against colds, Gilroy designed a study and then ordered dried samples from three suppliers. She sent some of each delivery out for analysis of chemicals that were known to distinguish the species and that might even have therapeutic activity.

The data that came back put her study on hold. They showed no batch containing pure *E. pallida*. The one from a bulk whole-saler that supplies herbal-products companies contained almost no *Echinacea* from any species, and what little there was consisted solely of *E. purpurea*. The other batches, acquired directly from coneflower growers, did contain *E. pallida*—but also contaminating plants, including *E. angustifolia*.

Gilroy then turned to 59 commercial echinacea products from local stores. Her team's analyses, reported in the March 24 *Archives of Internal Medicine*, show that none offered con-sumers what had been promised by its label. Six contained no evidence of any echinacea, and 28 failed to contain the specific species that was listed on the box. Some offered echinacea in quantities exceeding or, more often, falling below the quantity on the label, sometimes substantially.

These findings call into question the conclusions of the many earlier studies of echinacea's purported cure for the common cold, says Gilroy. At the least, they suggest that health effects seen with one sample of supplement might not hold for others.

This is just the latest in a string of studies revealing variability in the ingredients of dietary supplements on the market today. Uniform products require consistent ingredients and processes throughout every stage of manufacturing. The troubling findings suggest that many herbal-product makers aren't maintaining adequate quality control.

Several weeks ago, the Food and Drug Administration proposed rules designed to stem quality-control problems in dietary supplements, including nutraceuticals. The agency would mandate so-called good manufacturing practices, or GMPs, in the industry. Under GMPs like those now governing pharmaceuticals, all manufacturers of dietary supplements would have to chemically validate their ingredients and keep stringent records. These would include temperature readings from each batch as it's made and notes about any breakdowns of factory equipment.

However, representatives of the nutraceutical industry say they plan to call for amendments to the proposed FDA rules. They're currently analyzing the hundreds of pages of details before requesting changes. Moreover, any set of standard practices may be severely challenged by the complex makeup of herbal products, several scientists told *Science News*.

"For the most part, with [herbal] supplements, we still don't know what all the active ingredients are," so nobody knows the ideal formulation of most supplements, observes Bill J. Gurley of the University of Arkansas for Medical Sciences in Little Rock.

Says David J. Newman of the National Cancer Institute in Frederick, Md., "The bottom line remains *caveat emptor*," or let the buyer beware.

Beyond Echinacea

There's evidence for poor quality control in the making of many dietary supplements, says Chien M. Wai of the University of Idaho in Moscow. His work focuses on those made from leaves of the maidenhair tree (*Ginkgo biloba L.*). Ginkgo supplements fight memory loss and reinvigorate blood flow in the brain, according to users of the herb.

Scientists have identified five purported active ingredients in ginkgo. In most cases, Wai finds, a product's label describes only how much bulk ginkgo tissue a tablet, powder, or tincture contains without quantifying the active agents. Concentrations of those agents can vary widely in plant tissue.

In 2001, Wai's group reported data showing that, for instance, supposedly equally potent ginkgo supplements could contain anywhere from 0 to almost 4 milligrams of active compounds. Brands varied in which active chemicals dominated them, and some brands exhibited large batch-to-batch variation.

His subsequent studies, Wai says, indicate "the situation is not getting better."

Consumers can't use his team's reports to avoid supplements with weak or erratic ingredients because the researchers haven't published any brand names. Companies challenge any implied criticism of their products, Wai explains, and "we can't afford the time to fight lawsuits."

Gurley has named brands in his published analyses of supplements containing the weight-loss stimulant ephedra and indeed "stirred up a hornet's nest," he notes. It started 3 years ago, when his team first surveyed 20 over-the-counter ephedra products. As Gilroy found with echinacea, the ingredients often didn't match label claims.

Tissues from the *Ephedra sinica* plant, like ginkgo, contain at least five purported active ingredients, which are in the chemical family named alkaloids. Each alkaloid has a different effectiveness as a stimulant, and its concentration varies among individual plants. Most supplements that are labeled with ingredient information claim only to have some specified quantity of mixed ephedra alkaloids—information too general to offer much gauge of potency, says Gurley.

Although one brand that his team tested contained none of the five stimulant alkaloids, most had several, but the amounts varied among brands. When the researchers tested several batches of a brand, some differed in concentration by up to tenfold. Only 13 of the 20 products listed a total quantity of alkaloids on the label; others just listed quantities of the raw source plant. In many cases, Gurley says, those values bore no relation to what was present. His group published its findings in 2000. Since then, the researchers' tests of 130 additional ephedra products found far fewer discrepancies between labels and contents, "although they do still occur," says Gurley.

His team has lately turned to St. John's wort (*Hypericum perforatum*), a possible antidepressant. The researchers are finding a wide range of concentrations of St. John's wort's purported active ingredient, which is called hyperforin. Batch-to-batch hyperforin differences in one supplement brand varied 15-fold.

Gurley acknowledges that some herbal-supplement companies reliably produce what their labels promise. The trick is identifying them, Gurley says, a task beyond the capability of most consumers.

Many Explanations

Quality-control problems in herbal supplements often start with the hundreds of chemicals that plants contain. The type and quantity of these compounds vary in response to the environment in which a plant grew: its soil type and nutrition, water availability, excessive heat or cold, exposure to toxic minerals, degree of shading, and any hybridization.

One team is studying horticulturally triggered variations in several citrus compounds that are regarded as potential nutraceuticals because they've inhibited cancers in laboratory animals. Data collected by Bhimanagouda S. Patil and his colleagues at Texas A&M University in Weslaco show that concentrations of one such chemical—limonin glycoside—peaks midway through the crop's harvest season. So, when it comes to this agent, Patil says, "you must eat two grapefruit in May to get what one picked around Christmas will give you."

He's also been quantifying lycopene, a potential anticancer carotenoid that turns plants red. When his group planted Florida-derived rootstock of Star Ruby grapefruit in Texas, the fruit produced some 50 percent more of this carotenoid than it had in Florida.

Researchers at the University of Newcastle in Ourimbah, Australia, are studying effects of manufacturing techniques on nutraceutical quality. For instance, Douglas L. Stuart and Ron B.H. Wills report that high temperatures reduce concentrations of one of the potential therapeutic agents derived from *E. purpurea*. The scientists report in the March 15 *Journal of Agricultural and Food Chemistry* that drying the plant at 40°C results in one-third more cichoric acid than drying it at 70°C does.

Moreover, Wai's team has shown that whether oil, alcohol, or water is used can effect which chemicals are extracted from a plant. These products can have different potencies.

Even if purported active ingredients make it into a supplement, poor manufacturing techniques can yield tablets that don't effectively release those chemicals, notes Larry L. Augsburger of the University of Maryland in Baltimore.

Working with a synthetic version of melatonin, a hormone that promotes sleep, seems to fight jet lag (*SN: 5/13/95, p. 300*), and maybe even battles cancer (*SN: 10/17/98, p. 252*: http://www.sciencenews.org/sn_arc98/10_17_98/19981017fob.asp), his team showed that tablets don't always release their contents in a timely fashion. Although industry standards for the breakdown of conventional drugs is generally 30 minutes or less, his test-tube studies showed that some commercial melatonin supplements didn't disintegrate or release their contents for periods of 4 hours to more than 20 hours, by which time an ingested tablet may well have been excreted.

Help on the Way?

In the early 1990s, nutraceutical manufacturers feared that FDA would challenge their label claims. Then, the 1994 Dietary Supplement Health and Education Act was passed, permitting the sale of nutraceuticals and other supplements that are nontoxic and make no curative claims.

Immediately following the act's passage, sales of herbal supplements skyrocketed, with many companies regularly reporting up to 11 percent annual growth. But by 2000, U.S. sales started flagging, observes Clare M. Hasler of the University of Illinois at Urbana-Champaign. Reports were emerging of health risks associated with some products, such as ephedra; uncertain efficacy of others; and quality-control problems in the industry.

Because that last item appears to be the easiest for manufacturers to fix, some nutraceutical makers have been voluntarily adopting GMPs of their own design, says Nancy Childs of St. Joseph's University in Philadelphia. These companies tend to be the large prescription-drug manufacturers that have entered the nutraceuticals market in the past half-decade, she adds.

Most nutraceutical makers are far smaller than those companies, notes Kim Smith, an attorney with the National Nutritional Food Association (NNFA) of Newport Beach, Calif. Since 1999, her trade group—which represents many nutraceutical makers with 20 to 500 employees—has provided guidance for developing voluntary GMPs. NNFA also officially supports FDA's March 28 proposal for mandatory GMPs. "It will go a long way toward improving credibility in the industry," Smith says.

However, she adds, small firms could have a hard time paying for stringent FDA-required monitoring and record keeping. The agency estimates that first-year costs for small firms will run about $100,000, with annual costs of $60,000 or so thereafter. In fact, Smith says, her group suspects FDA is substantially underestimating those costs.

Success in complying with mandatory GMPs, Hasler suspects, "is going to sort out the [nutraceutical industry's] major players from the fly-by-night companies and probably put some small players out of business." She adds, " I'm not sure that's a bad thing."

Allen Montgomery, executive director of the American Nutraceuticals Association in Birmingham, Ala., which represents pharmacists and other health professionals, agrees. He says, "I don't know of any other billion-dollar industry that makes ingested products for which [mandatory] GMPs are not in place."

Within the nutraceutical industry generally, Gurley charges, "there are so many bad actors right now, that it's giving the whole industry a bad name."

Fortunately, Montgomery notes, several independent groups—such as the U.S. Pharmacopoeia (USP) of Rockville, Md.—have already begun validating voluntary GMPs for several products. USP is the official standards-setting body for all U.S. medicines and dietary supplements.

Companies that want to carry the USP logo must submit products for a series of stringent tests of such features as a product's purity, potency, and consistency. Also, USP inspectors visit factories to confirm that GMPs are in place, notes Sherrie L. Borden, the organization's spokesperson. "Then we do postmarket surveillance [of a supplement] once a product is on the shelf. It's very rigorous," she notes, "because this mark carries a lot of credibility."

All this sounds comforting, Gurley says, except that pharmaceutical-grade uniformity in herbal products may be amazingly difficult to achieve, and FDA's new rules don't address the complexity of a plant's make-up. Synthetic drugs and vitamins tend to have only one or two well-characterized active ingredients, he explains, while herbal supplements "are a veritable pharmacological Pandora's box."

Indeed, the 48 nutraceuticals that USP recently vetted—all produced under the Nature Made or Kirkland Signature labels—contain only vitamins, minerals, or fish oil—not complex herbal products.

Since plant tissue may contain hundreds of compounds with perhaps dozens of active ingredients, Gurley asks, who knows which of these should be standardized in each product? This "truly daunting" problem would challenge the best pharmaceutical manufacturer, he says, let alone a 30-employee herbal-products company.

Wai and Newman say that they'd like to see the herbal-supplements market develop into a natural-products offshoot of the over-the-counter drug industry. They argue that the best route for making safe and effective nutraceuticals would be to identify each plant's active agents, isolate them for testing in the same kind of trials that conventional pharmaceuticals go through, and then package the proven chemicals in carefully measured doses.

An advantage to this approach for manufacturers, Newman argues, is that unlike an herb, the recipe for a cocktail of natural chemicals is patentable. Thus, it might be market forces after all that bring consistency to the nutraceutical marketplace.

ARE YOUR SUPPLEMENTS SAFE?

Which supplements are safe? Which aren't? Which should you avoid if you're taking blood-thinners or antidepressants?

Don't bother asking the manufacturers...or the government, for that matter. When it comes to herbs and other over-the-counter supplements, you're pretty much on your own.

Seven out of every ten adults in the U.S take vitamins, minerals, herbs, or other supplements, according to a 2002 Harris Poll. Some—calcium, folic acid, glucosamine, and saw palmetto, for example—are beneficial. Others—soy isoflavones, ginseng, ginkgo—may or may not be. And still others—ephedra, usnic acid, kava—can be dangerous.

And *any* supplement can do damage if you take too much or take it in the wrong combinations.

"How many supplement takers suffer adverse reactions, no one really knows," says Christine Haller, a medical toxicologist at the University of California at San Francisco who has analyzed reports on the toxicity of ephedra for the Food and Drug Administration (FDA). (Ephedra, which has been called an "herbal fat burner," was linked to the death of Baltimore Orioles pitcher Steve Bechler last spring.)

"We really can't tell how serious the safety questions are for dietary supplements until we look at these products more carefully," says Mary Palmer, an emergency room physician and toxicologist in Alexandria, Virginia.

Palmer, Haller, and their colleagues recently analyzed nearly 500 calls about bad reactions to supplements that had been phoned in to 11 poison control centers in the U.S. in 1998.[1]

"When I started the study I thought that maybe the safety problems with supplements really were mild and that my worries were unfounded," says Palmer. "I was very surprised to see how serious the adverse reactions really were." A third of them included heart attacks, liver failure, bleeding, seizures, and death.

Prescription medications cause an estimated 100,000 deaths and 2.2 million adverse reactions each year. While the toll from supplements is nowhere near as great, it's far from trivial. For example, more than 20,000 complaints about weight-loss products containing ephedra, including scores of deaths, have been registered during the past decade.

Supplements are regulated so much more loosely than drugs that it's impossible to know how much harm they cause.

"Drugs can be sold only if companies have enough evidence to convince the FDA and panels of independent experts that they're safe and effective and that their benefits justify their risks," says Bruce Silverglade, director of legal affairs at the Center for Science in the Public Interest (publisher of *Nutrition Action Healthletter*).

In contrast, "The dietary supplement market is the Wild West," says Congressman Henry Waxman, a California Democrat and longtime champion of measures to protect consumers' health.

"There are no requirements that a company prove anything about either the safety or the effectiveness of its products before they go to market."

Most people don't realize that.

"About 60 percent of U.S. consumers believe that dietary supplements must be approved by a government agency like the Food and Drug Administration before they can be sold to the public," says Nancy Wong of the Harris Poll.

Not so. Congress made sure of that when it passed the Dietary Supplement Health and Education Act (DSHEA) in 1994. "DSHEA put manufacturers in the driver's seat when it comes to which supplements are sold and what claims can be made for them," notes Palmer.

Before DSHEA, if the FDA questioned a supplement's safety, the manufacturer had to prove that it was safe. "DSHEA shifted the burden of proof," says Silverglade. "With drugs, food additives, and pesticides, it's always up to the manufacturer to prove safety. But thanks to DSHEA, the FDA has to prove that supplements are dangerous."

"Because of DSHEA," says Silverglade, "the FDA has been reduced to regulating by press release."

When the agency considers a supplement unsafe, it typically issues a consumer advisory and then discourages—but doesn't prohibit—companies from continuing to sell the product. How many consumers hear about these FDA advisories? "We don't know," concedes FDA spokesperson Sebastian Cianci. "To find that out would require research we don't have the resources to do."

Bottom line: The FDA can only bark, not bite.

In late 2001, for example, the agency received reports of young adults who developed liver damage or failure soon after starting to use a weight-loss product called Li-poKinetix. (It contained usnic acid, the same substance thought to have destroyed Jennifer Rosenthal's liver a year later.) In response, the agency put out a press release advising consumers to "immediately stop use of LipoKi-netix."

But the FDA didn't ban or suspend its sale. "Given the serious hazard presented by the use of your product," the agency wrote in a letter to the manufacturer, "we strongly recommend that you take prompt action to remove Lipo-Kinetix from the market." (As it happened, the company had already suspended production because it couldn't get a steady supply of one ingredient.) Two years later, anyone can still purchase supplements that contain usnic acid on the Internet.

Consumers are protected from unsafe *drugs* by at least three lines of defense: The law requires manufacturers to test drugs for safety before they're sold, the FDA removes drugs from the marketplace when serious problems become evident, and manufacturers must track and disclose adverse effects, drug interactions, and other safety problems.

But against potentially unsafe *dietary supplements*, consumers are left to fend for themselves. Among the obstacles they face:

No Safety Testing

Pharmaceutical companies have to test their drugs to make sure they don't cause cancer, interfere with reproduction, damage organs, or cause other problems greater than they solve. In contrast, "Supplement companies have no obligation to test their products for safety before they market them," points out Christine Haller of the University of California at San Francisco.

"Some companies do small studies, but certainly not of the magnitude you would need to detect adverse effects," adds toxicologist Mary Palmer. "In many cases, there will be no information at all about a product's safety. But that doesn't mean it's safe."

"The dietary supplement market is the Wild West."

"Supplement manufacturers like to say that their products are safe because they've been used for centuries in other cultures," says Haller. "But traditional use didn't mean taking capsules of herbs day after day, so it was really different from the way we use them now." Continual exposure to concentrated extracts "probably changes the body's response to the herbs," notes Haller. "So these products might become ineffective or even have a detrimental effect."

How can an herb that has been used for centuries still be dangerous? If it causes cancer in, say, one out of every 100 people 20 years after they take it, the increased risk would never be noticed. Yet the government calls some food additives pesticides, and drugs carcinogens if they cause cancer in one out of every *million* people. That's the level that animal studies on those substances are designed to detect.

Supplement manufacturers, on the other hand, don't even have to understand how the body metabolizes their products. If they did, physicians would have learned long ago that St. John's wort can be life-threatening. (It can interfere with HIV drugs and immunosuppressants for transplant patients.)

And if companies had been required to thoroughly research the safety of hydroxycitrate before putting it in weight-loss supplements, they would have learned that the pharmaceutical giant Hoffman-La Roche abandoned the compound in the 1980s because of toxicity problems.

"We dropped hydroxycitrate when we saw that it seemed to cause testicular atrophy and other toxicities in animals," said a Hoffmann-La Roche spokesperson. "We never got as far as testing it in humans."

When told about the potential problems, a spokesperson for the firm that produces one of the two most popular hydroxycitrate formulations sold in the U.S. said, "I'm really, really surprised."

"There's no incentive for supplement companies to study the safety of their products," says Palmer. "It would be nothing but trouble for them, because they have a good deal right now." If anything's going to hurt their sales, "it's going to be safety issues. So why would they go looking for trouble?"

Take usnic acid. It's produced by lichen plants, so it falls within the loose definition of a dietary supplement. You can buy it on the Internet in the form of Usnea Lichen liquid herbal extracts. (We found one company that sells bottles of usnic acid capsules "for experimental research use only and not for human consumption" to anyone who claims to be at least 18 years old.)

Yet usnic acid may have destroyed the livers of at least half a dozen people in the U.S. over the past few years. Apparently that's not enough to motivate the companies that sell it—or the FDA—to investigate its toxicity.

"I don't know anyone else who's working on the toxicity of usnic acid besides me," says Neil Kaplowitz, director of the University of Southern California Research Center for Liver Diseases in Los Angeles.

Underreported Reactions

"Mild symptoms are definitely underreported to physicians and health agencies, and, as a result, there are probably many problems with supplements that are not being described," says toxicologist Christine Haller. A 2001 report by the U.S. Department of Health and Human Services estimated that only about one out of every 100 adverse reactions is reported to the FDA.[2]

EIGHT TO AVOID

**Despite evidence that these eight products can cause serious problems,
most are still available, either over the counter or via the Internet.**

- **Aristolochic acid.** The ingredient in some traditional Chinese medicines is toxic to the kidneys.
- **Chaparral.** In 1992, the FDA advised consumers to "stop taking chaparral immediately" because it can cause hepatitis.
- **Comfrey.** It can cause chronic liver disease.
- **Ephedra.** It has been linked to high blood pressure, strokes, and heart attacks and is 200 times more likely to cause an adverse reaction than all other herbs combined.
- **Kava.** It's a suspect in liver damage that has resulted in 11 liver transplants over the last several years.

- **PC SPES and SPES.** These supplements, which held promise as prostate-cancer fighters, turned out to be frauds. They worked like hormones only because they were spiked with hormones, a blood thinner, an anti-inflammatory, and several other drugs.
- **Tiratricol.** In 2000, the FDA warned consumers not to use weight-loss supplements containing this thyroid hormone, which can cause strokes and heart attacks.
- **Usnic acid.** This "natural" compound (it's found in lichen), which is used in some herbal mixtures, appears to be toxic to the liver.

Sources: Food and Drug Administration (*www.cfsan.fda.gov/%7Edms/ds-warn.html*) and CSPI.

"People are somewhat embarrassed when they have a problem with a supplement that they think maybe they shouldn't have been taking, like one of the weight-loss products," says Haller. "Why tell your doctor if your doctor didn't know you were taking it?"

What's more, people may not make the connection between a bad reaction and a "natural" supplement. And even if people call the consumer complaint number that's on the product label, "manufacturers sometimes don't do anything with those complaints," says Haller.

Troublesome Interactions

"There's competition in the marketplace now to give consumers the most for their dollar by offering combinations of herbs and other ingredients," says Haller. "But combining ingredients, especially herbs, isn't a good idea, because we really don't understand a lot about how they interact."

In their analysis of calls to poison control centers in the U.S., Haller and her colleagues found that multiple-ingredient supplements were more likely than single-ingredient ones to produce severe adverse effects.

No Required Warnings

"About two-thirds of the U.S. public believes that the government requires the labels of dietary supplements to include warnings about potential side effects or dangers," says Nancy Wong of the Harris Poll.

Not so. Unlike drug labels, supplement labels don't have to disclose who shouldn't take the product, what drugs it shouldn't be taken with, or other warnings.

So, for example, beta-carotene supplements labels don't have to disclose who shouldn't take the product, what drugs it shouldn't be taken with, or other warnings.

So, for example, beta-carotene supplements are unlikely to warn smokers that high doses (at least 25 mg, or 42,000 IU) may increase their risk of lung cancer. And zinc supplement labels are unlikely to disclose that too much zinc can compromise the immune system.

Unreported Problems

"The FDA maintains surveillance of prescription drugs by requiring prompt reports from manufacturers of all adverse events brought to their attention," says Arthur Grollman, chair of pharmacology at the State University of New York at Stony Brook.

"But there is no mandatory requirement for manufacturers of supplements to record, investigate, or forward to the FDA reports of adverse effects they might receive," he adds. "Under current regulations, there is no penalty for withholding these reports." Grollman wants Congress to require companies to report safety problems.

For years, Metabolife, the leading manufacturer of weight-loss pills that contain ephedra, denied that it knew of any serious complaints about its products. Then last year, lawyers who were suing the company on behalf of injured consumers learned that Metabolife had, in fact, received more than 13,000 complaints from users.

The Top Ten Supplements: How Safe?

How safe are the 10 most popular herbal supplements? Here's what you need to know. Just keep in mind that most reactions are rare; in some cases they're based on just one or two reports from physicians. Until more research is done, it's probably wise for children and pregnant or nursing women not to take any of these supplements.

Supplement	What Consumers Expect	Reported Reactions	Who Should be Especially Careful	May Interact With
Black Cohosh	To relieve symptoms of menopause.	Mild gastrointestinal distress.	Women who have had breast cancer (in an animal study, black cohosh caused cancer to spread).	No drug interactions known.
Cranberry	To prevent or treat urinary tract infections.	Regular use of cranberry concentrate tablets might increase the risk of kidney stones.	People susceptible to kidney stones.	Antidepressants and prescription painkillers.
Echinacea	To prevent or treat colds or other infections.	Minor gastrointestinal symptoms. Increased urination. Allergic reactions.	People with autoimmune diseases (like multiple sclerosis, lupus, and rheumatoid arthritis). May also trigger episodes of erythema nodosum, an inflammation that produces tender nodules under the skin.	No drug interactions known.
Garlic	To lower cholesterol levels.	Unpleasant breath odor. Heartburn and flatulence.	People who are about to have—or have just had—surgery (garlic thins the blood). Women just before or after labor or delivery.	Blood-thinning drugs like Coumadin (warfarin), heparin, or aspirin. Blood-thinning supplements like ginko or high doses of vitamin E. Chloroxazone, which is used to treat painful muscle conditions. HIV drugs.
Ginkgo Biloba	To improve memory.	Mild headache. Upset stomach. Seizures (possibly caused by contamination with ginkgo seeds, which are toxic).	People with bleeding disorders like hemophilia. People who are about to have—or have just had—surgery. Women just before or after labor or delivery. People with diabetes.	Blood-thinning drugs like Coumadin (warfarin), heparin, or aspirin. Blood-thinning supplements like high doses of vitamin E. The antidepressant trazodone. Anti-diabetes drugs. Thiazide diuretics.
Ginseng	To increase energy and relieve stress.	Insomnia. Menstrual abnormalities and breast tenderness with long-term use.	Women who had had breast cancer (ginseng stimulated the growth of breast cancer cells in test tubes). People with high blood pressure who aren't taking medication to lower it.	Any drug metabolized by the enzyme CYP 3A4 (ask your physician). MAO inhibitor drugs or digitalis. May increase the activity of insulin and oral hypoglycemics and decrease the activity of Coumadin (warfarin) and ticlopidine.
Saw Palmetto	To prevent or relieve the symptoms of an enlarged prostate.	Mild gastrointestinal distress.	People with bleeding disorders like hemophilia. People who are about to have—or have just had—surgery.	Blood-thinning drugs like Coumadin (warfarin), heparin, or aspirin. Blood-thinning supplements like ginkgo or high doses of vitamin E.
Soy Isoflavones	To relieve menopausal symptoms, prevent breast or prostate cancer, and strengthen bones.	None reported.	Women who have had—or are at high risk for—breast cancer (soy isoflavones may increase cell proliferation). Pregnant women. People with impaired thyroid function.	No drug interactions known.
St. John's Wort	To alleviate depression.	Mild gastrointestinal distress. Rash. Tiredness. Restlessness.	People with skin that's sensitive to sunlight. People taking UV treatment. People with bipolar disorder.	Ritalin, ephedrine (found in ephedra), and caffeine. May increase the activity of protease inhibitors (for HIV), digitalis (for high cholesterol), warfarin (blood-thinner), chemotherapy drugs, oral contraceptives, tricyclic antidepressants, olanzapine and clozapine (for schizophrenia), and theophylline (for asthma). May increase sensitivity to sunlight if combined with sulfa drugs, Feldene (anti-inflammatory), or Prilosec or Prevacid (for acid reflux).
Valerian	To induce sleep or relaxation.	May impair attention for a few hours.	People about to operate heavy machinery or drive.	May increase the activity of central-nervous-system depressants like barbiturates (such as Seconal) and benzodiazepines (such as Valium or Halcion).

Source: The Natural Pharmacist, Healthnotes, and CSPI.

Among them were more than 1,000 reports of significant adverse reactions, including 18 heart attacks, 26 strokes, 43 seizures, and five deaths.[3]

An angry FDA has asked the Department of Justice to pursue filing criminal charges against Metabolife officials for lying to the agency.

Unavailable Adverse Reaction Reports

For years, the Food and Drug Administration has been collecting reports of adverse reactions to dietary supplements. But last year the agency pulled the database from its Web site, saying that the information was confusing.

Last June, the FDA installed a new system (the Center for Food Safety and Applied Nutrition Adverse Events Reporting System, or CAERS) to track complaints by consumers and physicians to its MedWatch hotline (800-FDA-1088 or *fda.gov/medwatch/report/consumer/consumer.htm*).

But health professionals and the public can't view the complaints that have been submitted to CAERS.

"We're working on a way to give the public access to this information, but that's at least a year away," says FDA spokesperson Sebastian Cianci. "Until then, you need to file a Freedom of Information Act [FOIA] request to see the information."

That can take months, which is far too long to help people track down what's causing a reaction. And it certainly would have been too long for people like Jennifer Rosenthal, the California mother who paid a steep price for her lesson in supplement safety.

Notes

1. *Lancet 361*: 101, 2003.
2. Department of Health and Human Services, Office of the Inspector General: *Adverse Event Reporting for Dietary Supplements, An Inadequate Safety Valve.* OEI-01-00180, April 2001.
3. Government Accounting Office: *Dietary Supplements Containing Ephedra.* GAO-03-1042T, July 2003.

UNIT 6
Food Safety

Unit Selections

Key Points to Consider

- What are the main causes of food-borne disease?

- What are some of the best methods for avoiding or minimizing disease from contaminated foods?

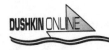 **Links: www.dushkin.com/online/**
These sites are annotated in the World Wide Web pages.

American Council on Science and Health (ACSH)
http://www.acsh.org/food/

Centers for Disease Control and Prevention (CDC)
http://www.cdc.gov

FDA Center for Food Safety and Applied Nutrition
http://vm.cfsan.fda.gov

Food Safety Project (FSP)
http://www.extension.iastate.edu/foodsafety/

National Food Safety Programs
http://vm.cfsan.fda.gov/~dms/fs-toc.html

USDA Food Safety and Inspection Service (FSIS)
http://www.fsis.usda.gov

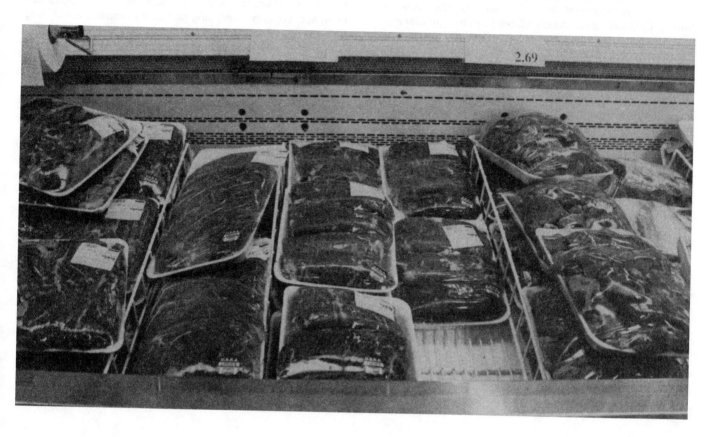

Food-borne disease constitutes an important public health problem in the United States. The U.S. Centers for Disease Control has reported 76 million cases of food-borne illness each year out of which 5,000 end in death. The annual cost of losses in productivity ranges from $20 to $40 billion. Food-borne disease results primarily from microbial contamination but also from naturally occurring toxicants, environmental contaminants, pesticide residues, and food additives.

The first Food and Drug Act was passed in 1906 and was followed by tighter control on the use of additives that might be carcinogenic. In 1958, the Delaney Clause was passed and a list of additives that were considered safe for human consumption (GRAS list) was developed. The Food and Drug Administration (FDA) controls and regulates procedures dealing with food safety, including food service and production. The FDA has established rules (Hazard Analysis and Critical Control Points) to improve safety control and to monitor the production of seafood, meat, and poultry. Even though there have been outbreaks of food poisoning traced to errors at the commercial processing stage, the culprit is usually mishandling of food at home, in a food service establishment, or other noncommercial setting. Surveys show that over 95% of the time people do not follow proper sanitation methods when working with food. The U.S. government, therefore, launched the Food Safety Initiative program to minimize food-borne disease and to educate the public about safe food handling practices. Additionally, for the first time the newest edition of the U.S. government's *Dietary Guidelines* included guidelines for food safety.

Some of the articles in Unit 6 review the need for food safety reforms in public policy because of changes in food production and consumption practices. Others describe the changing scene in what is actually contained in our food including hormones, antibiotics, pesticides, and food-borne microbes. The most common food-borne illnesses come from bacterial infestation of food with bacteria such as *Salmonella, Campylobacter,* hemorrhagic *E. coli,* and *Listeria.* When these bacteria exist along with *Sta-*

phylococcus and *Clostridium botulinum*, they produce toxins that cause illness or otherwise make a big difference on the outbreak. Outbreaks of food poisoning can be very serious and many times even deadly. Where you live and whether you eat at home or outside, makes a big difference on the above outbreaks. But food safety standard have been fraught with inconsistency because there are several Federal agencies with distinct responsibilities for food safety regulation. The need for a sing agency with consistent food safety standards is crucial to ensuring a safe food supply.

The large outbreaks of *E. coli* in the early 1990s prompted food safety reforms that included safe handling labels for raw meat and poultry (USDA) and an active surveillance system (Food Net) or the Centers for Disease Control to assess the effect of food-borne diseases on U.S. citizens and new regulations for meat and poultry processing plants to use standard procedures for sanitation (Pathogen Reduction and Hazard Analysis and Critical Control Points).

How should you enjoy eating healthy without becoming neophobics? People are becoming concerned when they visit the supermarket as to what has been added to their food and how it is going to impact upon their health. Bill Gottlieb carefully reviews whether there are dangers in drinking milk and eating meat that has been produced by dairy cows dosed with growth hormones and antibiotics, eating produce where pesticides have been applied, and consuming genetically modified foods. Suggestions are offered as to what action(s) to take. The most recent scare has involved mercury in fish. Fortunately the consumer has choices to still eat at least two servings of fish per week without increasing intake of mercury.

Finally, the USDA has set the criteria for the need to be met by foods, before they are given the stamp of "certified organic." The National Organic Rule, a product of then years of work by growers, scientists and consumers, defines "organic" as foods that are produced without insecticides, herbicides, chemical fertilizers, radiation, genetic modification, hormones or antibiotics. This has been a breakthrough especially for consumers since it enables them to have a good idea of what is organic and what is not.

AMERICA'S DIETARY GUIDELINE ON FOOD SAFETY: A PLUS, OR A MINUS?

Kathleen Meister

Imagine a delicious, inexpensive convenience food that is low in fat, cholesterol, sodium, and calories—and provides all essential nutrients and dietary fibers in optimum quantities. This may seem the ideal food—but it would be far from ideal if it were contaminated with pathogenic bacteria.

The idea that a food must be microbiologically safe to be healthful may seem obvious. And addressing the issue of microbiological safety might seem integral to any guide to healthy eating. Until this year, however, the U.S. government's principal guide of this sort, the "Dietary Guidelines" document, did not so much as allude to the issue. The 2000 edition gives this issue a distinct Guideline, called "Keep food safe to eat."

WHAT ARE THE DIETARY GUIDELINES?

The Dietary Guidelines, which are issued as a brochure, are official recommendations concerning healthy eating for all Americans who are at least two years old. The document was first published in 1980, and groups of experts have updated it every five years. A draft of the latest edition was released in February 2000.

The Dietary Guidelines affect even Americans who don't know what they are—70 percent of the U.S. population.

The Dietary Guidelines affect even Americans who don't know what they are—70 percent of the U.S. population. They represent a crucial federal policy statement—one that sets the nationwide agenda on food-related issues. Not only do they constitute the basis for federal food and nutrition programs; they are also in extensive educational use by nonfederal groups—

including state and local-government agencies, voluntary organizations, professional associations, and food-industry groups.

FOODBORNE DISEASE

"Foodborne disease" refers to any disease that results from eating food contaminated with a pathogen, most often a bacterium. Such diseases constitute an important public health problem. The U.S. Centers for Disease Control and Prevention (CDC) has estimated that, each year in the U.S., there are 76 million cases of foodborne disease, with 325,000 cases involving subsequent hospitalization and 5,000 ending in death. Moreover, it has been estimated that the annual cost of related decreases in productivity ranges from $20 billion to $40 billion.

But, in the U.S., foodborne disease is almost always preventable. Most cases trace to improper handling of food between its initial production and its ingestion. In 1997 the U.S. government launched the Food Safety Initiative—a program whose goal is to minimize foodborne disease in the U.S. Integral to this program is educating the public about safe food-handling practices.

The emphasis on food safety has increased in recent years. One reason for this is that the proportion of the American population especially vulnerable to foodborne disease, such as the elderly and persons whose immune systems are compromised, has increased. Another is that scientists have become aware that changes in how food is produced and distributed have led to changes in susceptibilities to mishandling and contamination.

Some foodborne-disease hazards have diminished in recent decades in the U.S.—for example, unpasteurized milk, improper home canning, and lack of a home refrigerator. But, meanwhile, the number of centralized, large-scale food-processing operations has increased considerably, and one slip in such an operation can result in the sickening of numerous consumers.

The U.S. Centers for Disease Control and Prevention (CDC) has estimated that, each year in the U.S., there are 76 million cases of foodborne disease . . .

There have been changes in food handling at the end-user level as well. Half of every dollar that American consumers spend is spent on food prepared outside the home. Keeping such foods safe requires measures different from those that apply to dishes prepared at home.

LOOKING OUT FOR NUMBER ONE

Although chemicals can cause foodborne disease, it is most commonly associated with microorganisms. As the food safety Guideline implies, in the U.S. at least, microbial food contamination is far more of a public health problem than is chemical food contamination. Yet many Americans evidently believe the fallacy that manmade additives and pesticides and other such chemicals make their food supply dangerous. The U.S. Food and Drug Administration has ranked diet related hazards in descending order of dangerousness:

1. microbial contamination
2. naturally occurring toxicants
3. environmental contaminants (e.g., metals)
4. nutritional problems (i.e., malnutrition, undernutrition)
5. pesticide residues
6. food additives

By focusing on microbial contamination, the Dietary Guideline called "Keep food safe to eat" facilitates making it center stage in terms of public food-safety education.

THE CONSUMER'S PART IN FOOD SAFETY

The Dietary Guidelines document states: "Farmers, food producers, markets, and food preparers have a legal obligation to keep food safe, but we also need to keep foods safe in the home." For instance, although in the last few years the egg industry has impressively reduced

Salmonella enteritidis contamination of whole chicken eggs, eating raw or undercooked eggs remains somewhat risky. Even the safest food purchase can quickly become unsafe. Foodservice establishments must try to ensure that takeout foods, such as roast chickens or prepared salads, are safe at purchase—but it is in any case incumbent on the buyer to ensure that, within two hours of its purchase, the food is eaten or appropriately refrigerated.

THE ALCOHOL GUIDELINE

Since its introduction, in 1980, the Dietary Guidelines document has called for moderateness in alcoholic-beverage consumption. Three changes in this Guideline, however, are present in the 2000 edition. Two of these are desirable: First, both the 1995 edition and the 2000 edition acknowledge that moderate alcohol consumption may reduce the risk of developing coronary heart disease (CHD), but unlike the previous edition, the 2000 edition states that this holds "mainly among men over age 45 and women over age 55." CHD is rare among young men and premenopausal women. Thus, moderate drinking is associated with lower death rates only among persons who are at least middle-aged.

Second, a mistake in the 1995 edition has been corrected. In that edition a list of "people who should not drink alcoholic beverages at all" included "individuals using prescription and over-the-counter medications." This was an overstatement: Some medications are quite compatible with alcohol. The new edition implies this and advises persons on medication to request "advice about alcohol intake" from their "health care professional."

But one of the three changes present in the 2000 edition is problematic: It states that "even one drink/day can slightly raise the risk of breast cancer." The claim that the positive statistical association of moderate alcohol intake and breast-cancer risk is causal is doubtful. The scientific evidence on this point is not consistent. Moreover, the possibility that this alcohol–cancer association is merely a result of confounders—in this event, non-alcohol related factors accompanying both drinking and the development of cancer—has not been ruled out. In any case, the association is weak, and if it proves causal, it would have to be weighed against the much stronger relationship between alcohol consumption and heart disease in women.

In recent years, several well-publicized outbreaks of food poisoning have been traced to errors at the

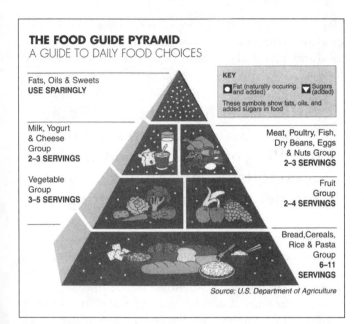

THE FOOD GUIDE PYRAMID
A GUIDE TO DAILY FOOD CHOICES

Fats, Oils & Sweets
USE SPARINGLY

KEY
☐ Fat (naturally occuring and added)   ▽ Sugars (added)
These symbols show fats, oils, and added sugars in food

Milk, Yogurt & Cheese Group
2–3 SERVINGS

Meat, Poultry, Fish, Dry Beans, Eggs & Nuts Group
2–3 SERVINGS

Vegetable Group
3–5 SERVINGS

Fruit Group
2–4 SERVINGS

Bread, Cereals, Rice & Pasta Group
6–11 SERVINGS

Source: U.S. Department of Agriculture

mishandling of food in a foodservice establishment, at home, or in another noncommercial setting, such as a picnic.

While government regulation is crucial to keeping down foodborne disease in the U.S., it has little effect on the committing of food safety mistakes in noncommercial settings. No American governmental agency can pressure households to wash their cutting boards or to refrigerate the food in their doggie bags. The only non-intrusive way to improve food-handling practices in noncommercial settings is to instruct the public on food safety hows and whys. Therein lies the utility of the food safety aspect of the Dietary Guidelines document.

According to government surveys, behavior that is risky in terms of foodborne disease is common among Americans, of whom:

- 50 percent eat raw or undercooked eggs,
- 23 percent eat undercooked hamburger,
- 17 percent eat raw clams or oysters,
- 28 percent leave perishable foods unrefrigerated for more than two hours,
- 26 percent do not wash cutting boards after they have cut raw meat or poultry on them, and
- 20 percent do not wash their hands after they have handled raw meat or poultry.

commercial-processing stage. For example, a large food-poisoning outbreak was traced to an ice-cream mix that had been transported in inadequately disinfected tankers previously used to transport shelled raw eggs. But most cases of foodborne disease in the U.S. result not from errors related to commercial processing, but from the

THE DIETARY GUIDELINES

NOW

The U.S. Department of Agriculture (USDA) and the U.S. Department of Health and Human Services have jointly issued the Dietary Guidelines document every five years since 1980. The 2000 edition differs substantially from the 1995 edition. The number of Guidelines, for example, has increased from 7 to 10:

- Aim for a healthy weight.
- Be physically active each day.
- Let the Pyramid guide your food choices.
- Choose a variety of grains daily, especially whole grains.
- Choose a variety of fruits and vegetables daily.
- Keep food safe to eat.
- Choose a diet that is low in saturated fat and cholesterol and moderate in total fat.
- Choose beverages and foods to moderate your intake of sugars.
- Choose and prepare foods with less salt.
- If you drink alcoholic beverages, do so in moderation.

AND THEN

The statements below represent the 1995 Guidelines.

- Eat a variety of foods.
- Balance the food you eat with physical activity—maintain or improve your weight.
- Choose a diet with plenty of grain products, vegetables, and fruits.
- Choose a diet low in fat, saturated fat, and cholesterol.
- Choose a diet moderate in sugars.
- Choose a diet moderate in salt and sodium.
- If you drink alcoholic beverages, do so in moderation.

Each of the seven messages that amount to the food safety Guideline is consistent with established principles of food handling:

- Clean. Wash hands and surfaces often.
- Separate. Separate raw, cooked, and ready-to-eat foods while storing and preparing.
- Cook. Cook foods to a safe temperature.
- Chill. Refrigerate perishable foods promptly.
- Check and follow the label.
- Serve safely.
- When in doubt, throw it out.

CONTROVERSY OVER THE FOOD SAFETY GUIDELINE

No one can reasonably deny that the message of the food safety Guideline is scientifically well-grounded, but some qualified professionals have objected to the inclusion of this message in the Dietary Guidelines document. Some nutrition scientists say that adding messages on new topics to the document may distract the public from the guide's thrust: discussion of food choices that are better in terms of specific food constituents. For example, the January 25, 2000, edition of *The New York Times* quoted Marion Nestle, Ph.D., of New York

University: "What this has done is shift the focus of the guidelines from food to other factors. The deemphasis on food and increased emphasis on other factors is not a step forward."

> **[M]ost cases of foodborne disease in the U.S. result . . . from the mishandling of food in a food service establishment, at home, or in another noncommercial setting....**

Healthy eating entails many considerations—for example, energy intake versus energy expenditure, intakes of protein and essential nutrients, and intakes of saturated fat. It requires attention to the principles of moderation, variety, and balance. Above all, however, it requires that whatever is eaten be harmless with respect to bacterial and similarly acting pathogens. If it isn't, none of the other factors matter. Thus, the food safety Guideline is perhaps the most fundamental.

KATHLEEN MEISTER, M.S., IS A FREELANCE MEDICAL WRITER AND A FORMER ACSH RESEARCH ASSOCIATE.

Reprinted with permission from *Priorities for Health,* a publication of the American Council on Science and Health (ACSH), 1995 Broadway, 2nd Floor, New York, NY 10023-5860. Visit **www.acsh.org** or **www.prioritiesforhealth.com** to learn more about ACSH.

Safe food from a consumer perspective

Caroline Smith DeWaal[*]

Center for Science in the Public Interest, Noordwijk Food Safety HACCP Forum, USA

Received 8 November 2001; received in revised form 20 April 2002; accepted 22 April 2002

Abstract

Food-safety experts believe that contaminated food causes up to 76 million illnesses, 325,000 hospitalizations and 5000 deaths each year in the US alone. These estimates underline the fact that foodborne-illnesses pose a significant public-health burden. CSPI recommends strengthening the safety of the food supply by setting farm and animal production food-safety standards, by improving Hazard Analysis and Critical Control Points (HACCP) implementation, especially by the US Food and Drug Administration, and finally, by streamlining food-safety policy and regulation. Having several federal agencies with distinct responsibilities for food safety regulation has resulted in inconsistent food safety standards. The US regulatory structure is fragmented and not well equipped to meet current challenges facing the food-safety system. Instead, CSPI calls for a single food safety agency that maximizes allocation of resources resulting in a more rational system of food safety regulation. Legislation establishing a single, independent food-safety agency has been pending in the US Congress since 1997.
@ 2003 Published by Elsevier Science Ltd.

Keywords: HACCP; Consumer; Safety

1. Introduction

CSPI is a non-profit consumer-advocacy organization based in Washington, DC with two offices in Canada. Since 1971, CSPI has been working on nutrition and food-safety issues. We accept no money from the food industry, government, or labor unions. CSPI is supported primarily by over 800,000 subscribers to its *Nutrition Action Health Letter,* the largest circulation health newsletter in North America. CSPI advocates for consumers and we are very attentive to consumer concerns.

The regulation of genetically modified foods (GMOs) is a major concern affecting public policy in Europe. However, the status of GMOs in the US is radically different. Although critics, including environmental organizations, food-safety groups, organic farmers, and religious leaders have raised myriad questions about the safety of GMOs for both the environment and humans, US consumers remain largely unconcerned with the safety of GMOs. GMOs have entered the food supply in the US without becoming or causing a major food safety concern. Unlike the critics of biotech, CSPI believes that these crops have not been shown to cause any health problems, and only minor environmental disturbances, and have in fact yielded major benefits.

However, after watching widespread rejection of GMOs by European consumers, it is clear that GMOs need more oversight to shore up consumer confidence. A consumer attitude survey conducted by the Wirthlin Group, a strategic opinion research and consulting firm in the US, shows that the more controversial GMOs become, the less confident consumers are that they are well informed about the technology. In an opinion poll conducted last spring, the Wirthlin Group found that over 20% of consumers said they were "not at all informed" about biotechnology. In this question, consumers were asked to rank themselves on a scale of zero-to-ten, and 80% of the respondents ranked themselves on the low end of the information scale (Wirthlin Group, 1999, 2000). Clearly, the biotech industry's strategy of withholding information about their products from the public has backfired. We now have a public that feels ill-informed and this puts future acceptance of this new food technology at risk.

While US consumers remain concerned about new technologies and ingredients in their food, the presence of harmful bacteria has become an even greater concern. An annual consumer survey done by the Food Marketing Institute (FMI) documents this trend. From 1993 through 1997, we saw that the number of people who said they were "very concerned" about chemical contaminants such as pesticides declined from 79% to 66%. The

FMI survey first included questions on microbial contamination in 1995. From 1995 to 1997, microbial contamination topped the list of consumer concerns. By contrast, consumers ranking themselves as very concerned about foods produced using bio-technology has hovered around 15% for the same three years (FMI, 2000).

The intense media coverage of food poisoning outbreaks has helped to fuel consumers' growing sensitivity to the issue of microbial contamination of food. Several years ago, CSPI started tracking food poisoning outbreaks, so we could better identify which foods were actually making people sick. Unfortunately, we were unable to obtain complete lists of food poisoning outbreaks from the Centers for Disease Control and Prevention (CDC).

To fill this gap, CSPI began maintaining its own list of food-borne-illness outbreaks that occurred in the US from 1990 to the present. From its humble beginnings, this list now contains over 860 outbreaks. It is the only list of its kind available today. Even so, we believe it represents only a small fraction of the outbreaks that are occurring around the US.

Outbreaks are defined generally as two or more illnesses from a single source. The outbreaks that CSPI has listed were those that could be relatively easily identified, such as highly publicized, novel, or large outbreaks. We also used CDC lists for specific pathogens, such as *Salmonella enteritidis* and *Escherichia coli* 0157:H7 and most recently, CDC has given us a large volume of outbreak data through Freedom of Information requests. Here are our most recent findings:

The foods most likely to be linked to a food poisoning outbreak are: seafood, eggs, beef, and produce. Interestingly, three out of these top four high-risk foods are regulated by the US Food and Drug Administration (FDA).

- 682 outbreaks were linked to FDA-regulated foods, as compared to 179 outbreaks linked to USDA-regulated foods.
- 237 outbreaks were linked to seafood, including mahi mahi, salted whitefish, tuna, buffalo fish, blue marlin, surgeon, grouper, ahi, crab, and shrimp. Of the seafood outbreaks, 41 were linked to shellfish, including oysters, clams, and mussels.
- 170 outbreaks were linked to eggs and egg dishes. Most of the egg-related outbreaks were caused by *S. enteritidis,* a bacterium that can survive in raw or undercooked eggs and egg dishes. Egg dishes involved in several outbreaks include pudding, stuffing, baked ziti, and ice cream made with shell eggs.
- 91 outbreaks were linked to beef, including at least 40 to ground beef. Other types of beef were prime rib, roast beef, corned beef, raw beef, and beef jerky.
- 82 outbreaks were linked to produce, including cantaloupe, tomatoes, strawberries, watermelon, potatoes, scallions, lettuce, raspberries, sprouts, basil, and parsley.
- 52 outbreaks were linked to poultry. *Campylobacter* is the leading bacterial cause of foodborne diarrhea and current data suggest that more individual cases are linked to poultry than to any other food. However, reported outbreaks linked to poultry are not as common as those linked to beef, probably because the illnesses resulting from poultry products are more likely to

occur individually or as part of a family outbreak that is never reported, according to CDC (Griffin, 1999).

- 39 outbreaks were linked to dairy products, including cheese, pasteurized and raw milk, and ice cream.
- 31 outbreaks were linked to pork, including ham and pork sausage.
- 14 outbreaks were linked to game, including venison, bear meat, and cougar meat.
- 10 outbreaks were linked to juices, including apple cider, apple juice, and orange juice.
- Five outbreaks were linked to luncheon meats, such as hot dogs and bologna.
- 130 outbreaks were linked to FDA-regulated foods with multiple ingredients.

Those include salads, baked goods, and soups.

Our outbreak tracking shows that FDAs foods cause four out of every five food poisoning outbreaks, clearly a significant risk. However, FDAs budget for regulating foods is only about one-third of USDAs food inspection budget (Office of Budget & Program Analysis, 2001). In essence, FDA regulates more food with less money. If food-safety resources could be applied on the basis of risk rather than on the basis of historical precedent, it is clear that the food categories regulated by FDA would receive a much greater share of the budget (National Research Council, 1998). This imbalance led CSPI and other consumer organizations to call for the US government to create a single independent food safety agency, so that we could better apply food safety resources to the food safety hazards that are causing the greatest risk to the public.

2. The HACCP solution

To keep up with the changing hazards in our food supply, it is time to change some of the regulatory tools as well. The advent of new systems of preventative controls—so called "HACCP" systems (for Hazard Analysis/Critical Controls Points)—coupled with the expanded use of new technologies have the potential to significantly enhance the safety of food. But these benefits will not be fully realized until the underlying regulatory systems for inspection and technology approvals are modernized as well.

HACCP focuses on preventing foodborne-illnesses by applying science-based controls to food production and has been endorsed by many scientific groups. However, HACCP implementation in the seafood, meat and poultry industries has graphically highlighted the weakness in the fragmented regulatory system in the US.

3. HACCP implementation inconsistent between USDA and FDA

Due to the different regulatory approaches at FDA and USDA, the meat, poultry and seafood HACCP systems share almost as many differences as similarities. For example, while USDA requires both frequent inspection and product testing for meat and poultry products, FDA requires neither for seafood products (Smith De Waal, 1997). That makes seafood HACCP an industry honor system of dubious value and unworthy of public support.

HACCP became a mandatory program for approximately 4000 seafood processors in December 1997 and also for foreign processors that ship seafood to the US (FDA, 1995). The following month, in January 1998, the USDAs Food Safety and Inspection Service (FSIS) began implementing HACCP in the meat and poultry industry, starting with the largest plants (FSIS, 1996). Meat and poultry HACCP implementation was completed in January 2000 (FSIS, 2000a, b). Although both FDA and FSIS began to implement their HACCP programs at about the same time, the results have been very dissimilar.

There have been few surprises with respect to implementing HACCP in meat and poultry plants. Six months after the large plants were brought into the HACCP program, the industry had a 93% compliance rate (Billy, 1998). This past year, even after small plants were brought into the system, compliance increased to 96% (Billy, 1999).

In comparison with meat and poultry plants, the seafood industry has done a dismal job in implementing HACCP. FDA required all seafood processors, both large and small, to develop and implement HACCP plans in December 1997 (FDA, 1995). But data from FDA inspections in 1999—the second year of implementation—showed that only 24% of all seafood firms had fully implemented HACCP plans deemed adequate by FDA (Losikoff, 2000). Thirty percent of the seafood firms inspected in 1999 had inadequate HACCP plans or were failing to properly implement their plans (or both). Sixteen percent of the firms inspected in 1999 failed to have *any* HACCP plan in place, even though FDA inspectors believed they needed a HACCP plan. The remaining 30% of the seafood firms had no HACCP plan, but FDA inspectors did not think that a plan was necessary. (FDAs de facto exemption of nearly one-third of the seafood industry from HACCP requirements stands in stark contrast to FSISs position. In its HACCP final rule, FSIS stated: "FSIS is currently unaware of any meat or poultry production process that can be deemed categorically to pose no likely hazards" (FSIS, 1996).)

FDA and FSIS differ on more than just the applicability of their HACCP programs. Unlike meat and poultry plants, which have statutorily mandated daily on-site inspections by FSIS, FDAs inspections of seafood plants are infrequent—dropping from 3146 inspections in 1998 to 2796 inspections in 1999. That is equivalent to one inspection per year in approximately 70% of seafood firms (Government Accounting Office, 1998).

FDAs failure to enforce the seafood HACCP regulation obscures another critical weakness in the program. FDA failed to mandate any government or industry testing for process verification of the HACCP program. While FSIS requires HACCP verification testing of food samples both by the government and the industry (FSIS, 1996), the FDA made product testing optional. As a result, in many seafood plants, pathogens are not adequately controlled. For example, the FDAs 1999 inspection data showed that 71% of the smoked fish processors, 69% of the vacuum-packed fish industry, and 63% of the cooked, ready-to-

eat seafood firms lacked adequate pathogen controls in their HACCP plans (FDA, 1995).

The meat and poultry HACCP rule, by contrast, has clear tools to evaluate its success, including performance standards for *Salmonella* reduction. This *Salmonella* performance standard is similar to a food safety objective for the government's HACCP program. After two years of product testing in large plants, *Salmonella* contamination has been cut in half in chicken and pork products and has declined substantially in ground beef and ground turkey as well (FSIS, 2000a,b). HACCP performance in small plants has been equally impressive. After one year of testing in small meat and poultry plants, *Salmonella* contamination in ground beef has been reduced by more than 40%, and contamination in chicken by nearly 20% (FSIS, 2000a,b).

This success is further supported by FoodNet data collected by CDC. In the years 1996–1999, the rate of *Salmonella* illness declined from 14.5 cases per 100,000 people to 13.6 cases per 100,000 (Emerging Infections Program, 1999). CDC concluded that this decline "may also reflect disease prevention efforts, particularly for campylobacteriosis and salmonellosis. These efforts include changes in meat and poultry processing in the US mandated by the USDA HACCP rule" (Emerging Infections Program, 1998).

The lessons from the US experience with regulatory HACCP are clear. Without government-enforced performance standards, it is impossible to measure either the relative performance of different processors' HACCP plans or the overall success of the HACCP system to control food-safety hazards. Consumers in the US can be much more confident in the meat and poultry HACCP system, because the industry has complied with the regulation and the government is monitoring its effectiveness using performance standards. In contrast, the seafood industry in the US has a very poor record of compliance with FDAs HACCP regulation, and there is no government testing to monitor its success. Consumers confidence in HACCP will not continue if the weaker model in use in the US seafood industry becomes the prevailing regulatory model. Performance standards enforced by government testing are essential to ensure that HACCP is not just an industry honor system.

Inconsistent HACCP implementation is just one of numerous problems that arise from having several agencies with separate responsibilities for food safety regulation. As the old adage says, "too many cooks can spoil the broth". Other problems include gaps in consumer protections, conflicting public health standards, regulatory redundancies, and slow approvals of new technologies. In addition, gaps in food safety oversight mean that no agency is exercising farm-to-table food safety responsibility. Experience with HACCP implementation shows that coordination between government agencies is not enough. More fundamental reform is needed.

Another area where inadequate government food safety oversight is apparent is on the farm. Bacteria, parasites, and viruses frequently enter the food supply here. Some problems are greatly exacerbated by on-farm practices, especially in the area of animal production.

Reducing pathogens in the food chain starting at the farm level is critical if we hope to reduce foodborne-illnesses in humans. In the past 10 years, outbreaks traced to fruits and vegetables contaminated with hazards normally associated with food animals have become increasingly common. In fact, out of the 865 food poisoning outbreaks in "Outbreak Alert", fruits and vegetables caused nearly 23% of all the illnesses, more than any other single food. The need to address on-farm practices is now undeniable, particularly the problem of manure contamination.

Recent water borne outbreaks indicate that the problems linked to environmental contamination with harmful pathogens are becoming more serious. In the summer of 1999, for example, over 1000 attendees of a New York county fair were sickened by *E. coli* 0157:H7 and two people died (State of New York Department of Health, 1999). The source: unchlorinated water contaminated with manure runoff from a dairy barn (The Orlando Sentinel, 1999).

In May 2000, a similar scenario occurred on a much more frightening scale in a small Ontario, Canada farming community. *E. coli* 0157:H7 literally invaded Walkerton through the town's drinking water. The bacterium sickened 2000 residents and killed seven (Canada News Wire, 2000). The same strain of bacteria responsible for the outbreak was isolated from the cattle near the town, and in particular from a herd next to one of the most contaminated wells (The Globe & Mail, 2000).

Contaminated water is only one problem with livestock manure. Frequently foodborne-illness outbreaks, especially produce outbreaks, are traced to direct manure contamination. For example, in July 1995, over 70 Montana residents were sickened by lettuce contaminated with *E. coli* 0157:H7. The lettuce was most likely from a local farm that used composted dairy manure as fertilizer and kept sheep near the lettuce fields. Another possible source for contamination was irrigation water from a pond fed by streams running through cattle pastures (Ackers, 1998).

Another produce outbreak occurred in 1996 when contaminated lettuce from a small California operation caused a multistate outbreak in which 61 people were sickened, at least 21 were hospitalized and 3 people developed serious complications. Investigators found many potential routes of contamination, but one thing was clear: cattle manure was the problem. Some lettuce was grown in a field where cows had grazed the previous winter. Some irrigation water was drawn from a well located in a cattle pasture. The open processing shed was located less than 100 feed from cattle pens, and lettuce was washed with water from a well-located 20 feet from a cattle pen. In yet another example, 27 people were sickened by *E. coli* 0157:H7 contaminated coleslaw at a Kentucky Fried Chicken fast food restaurant in 1998. Investigators traced the cabbage in the coleslaw back to a farm that had a cow pasture right next to the cabbage patch. The likely source of contamination: fresh manure in the cabbage patch (Belluck & Drew, 1998).

These examples demonstrate that manure contamination is a pervasive problem. While there does not seem to be an easy answer, the solution clearly lies with producers. It is essential that animal producers control manure so that it does not contaminate water and crops. This in turn would minimize the risks associated with foodborne-illness outbreaks that originate on the farm.

In addition to microbial contamination, poor animal production practices have resulted in another problem that Europeans are all too familiar with. Mad cow disease became an international public health concern in 1996 after public health officials in Britain documented that human TSE cases (called a new variant of Creutzfeldt-Jakob disease or nvCJD) were linked to beef consumption, thus showing for the first time that this terrible disease could jump the "species barrier" from cattle to humans (Darnton, 1996).

I certainly do not need to remind you that mad cow disease has now become a safety issue for beef consumers all over Europe. Infected cattle have been discovered in many countries, including France, Portugal, Switzerland, Belgium, Denmark, Liechtenstein, Luxembourg, Netherlands, Germany, and Spain. There are also human cases of nvCJD in France (World Health Organization, 2000). The US has so far escaped the problem largely because we banned the entry of cattle from countries with BSE in 1989 (USDA Actions to Prevent Bovine Spongiform Encephalopathy (BSE), FAS online; http://www.fas.gov/dlp/BSE/aphischron.html).

Mad cow disease not only decimated the British beef industry, it destroyed consumers' faith in the British system for ensuring food safety. It has also shaken European consumers' confidence in government oversight of the food supply. It has led to the revision of food safety laws and creation of new agencies that are responsible for ensuring the safety of the food supply, both in Great Britain and in the European Union.

While the US has not yet suffered from such a devastating crisis in consumer confidence, we are certainly not immune. Weaknesses in our government programs could set the stage for a similar crisis for consumers, a crisis that we would like to see prevented. This is why, we support the creation in the US of an independent food safety agency with responsibility from farm-to-table. Such an agency must be strongly oriented to protecting public health as a means of protecting public confidence. So far, the world is leading the US in the movement to unify food safety functions in government, but not for long, we hope.

Notes

*Tel.: +1-202-332-9110; fax: +1-202-265-9954. *E-mail address:* cspi@cspinet.org (C. Smith DeWaal).

References

Ackers, M. (1998). An outbreak of *Escherichia coli* 0157:H7 infections associated with leaf lettuce consumption. *The Journal of Infectious Diseases, 177,* 1588–1593.

Belluck, P., & Drew, C. (1998). Tracing bout illness to small lettuce farm. *The New York Times,* A1.

Billy, T. J. (1998). *HACCP implementation in small plants—the role of FSIS.* Remarks before the small plant HACCP implementation meeting. Food Safety and Inspection Service.

Billy, T. J. (1999). *FSIS experiences with HACCP.* Remarks before the fisheries council of Canada. Food Safety and Inspection Service.

Canada News Wire (2000). *Office of the Chief Coroner concludes six deaths are related to* E. coli *outbreak in Walkerton;* The Associated Press. (2000). *New regulations coming to Ontario to keep water safer after* E. coli *crisis;* Nelson, M. (2000). *Study targets Walkerton Well.* The London Free Press.

Darnton, J. (1996). Britain ties deadly brain disease to cow ailment. *The New York Times,* A1.

Emerging Infections Program (1998). *FoodNet 1998 Final Report.* Atlanta, GA: Centers for Disease Control and Prevention.

Emerging Infections Program (1999). *FoodNet 1999 Final Report.* Atlanta, GA: Centers for Disease Control and Prevention.

Food and Drug Administration, (1995). Procedures for the safe and sanitary processing and importing of fish and fishery products; final rule. *Federal Register, 60* (242), 65096–65202.

Food Marketing Institute (FMI), (2000). *Trends in the United States— consumer attitudes and the supermarket, 2000.* Washington, DC: The Research Department at FMI.

Food Safety and Inspection Service (1996). Pathogen reduction; hazard analysis and critical control point (HACCP) systems; final rule. *Federal Register, 61*(144), 38806–38989.

Food Safety and Inspection Service. (2000a). *FSIS Reports continued decline of* Salmonella. News release.

Food Safety and Inspection Service. (2000b). *Very small plants successfully implement HACCP.* News release.

Government Accounting Office (1998). *Food safety: Opportunities to redirect federal resources and funds can enhance effectiveness* (p. 8).

Griffin, P. (1999). *Telephone conversation with Chief of Foodborne Diseases, Foodborne and Diarrheal Branch, Division of Bacterial and Mycotic Diseases.* Atlanta, GA: National Center for Infectious Disease, Centers for Disease Control and Prevention.

Losikoff, M. (2000). *Compliance with Food and Drug Administrations seafood HACCP regulations.* Presentation before the International Association for Food Protection.

National Research Council (1998). *Ensuring safe food from production to consumption.* Washington, DC: Institute of Medicine.

Office of Budget and Program Analysis (2001). *U.S. Department of Agriculture 2001 Budget Summary;* Food and Drug Administration. *FY 2001 Congressional Budget Request Table of Contents.*

Smith De Wall, C. (1997). Delivering on HACCP's promise to improve food safety: a comparison of three HACCP regulations. *Food and Drug Law Journal, 52*(3), 331–335.

State of New York Department of Health (1999). *Capital district* E. coli *update—Case numbers as of September 17, 1999.*

The Globe and Mail (2000). *Deadly* E. coli *traced to cattle: this could be the origin of the problem* (p. A1).

The Orlando Sentinel (1999). *More than 1,000 sickened in deadly* E. coli *outbreak* (p. A16).

Wirthlin Group (2000). *U.S. consumer attitudes toward food biotechnology—Wirthlin Group quorum surveys May 5–9, 2000.*

World Health Organization (2000). *Information Fact Sheet. No. 113. Revised December 2000.*

Reprinted from *Food Control*, Vol. 14, No. 2, 2003, pp. 75-79. © 2003 by Elsevier Science, Ltd., Oxford, England.

When science meets the grocery store: The foods you eat are often treated with pesticides, hormones, or antibiotics. What's safe and what isn't?

what **you need** to know before your **next trip** to the **supermarket**

Here's the middle ground where you can enjoy healthy food without becoming a fanatic.

by Bill Gottlieb

What could be simpler than stopping off at the market for a few basic items: a quart of milk, some chicken breasts, salad greens, and a bag of chips? Zip over to the express lane, and with luck, you'll be out in a few minutes. But no sooner have you grabbed a basket and headed down the aisle than questions start to clutch at your mind like thorny weeds.

Should you buy milk from a dairy whose cows were treated with hormones? Should you shell out for free-range chicken that wasn't fed antibiotics and for organic greens that haven't been near pesticides? What if they're tainted with dangerous microbes? And there's the chip dilemma: Most packaged foods now include ingredients from genetically modified crops. Should you skip them?

It's hard enough keeping a watchful eye on your fat and calorie intake, but all these other concerns can turn a quick food run into a marathon.

No evidence shows that milk from hormone-dosed cows increases your risk of developing certain illnesses.

Fortunately, help is at hand. We talked to dozens of people—medical researchers, government officials, consumer advocates, and industry scientists—about the safety of the food you eat every day. Not surprisingly, the experts don't all see eye to eye, and their attitudes range from carefree to cautionary. Yet between the extremes lies a middle ground with a range of reasonable choices.

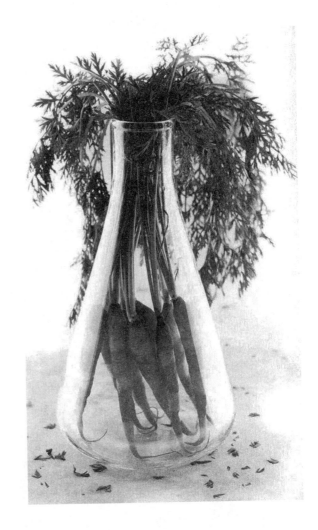

154

Want to enjoy healthy food without becoming a fanatic? Here's what you need to know before your next trip to the supermarket.

hormones in milk and meat

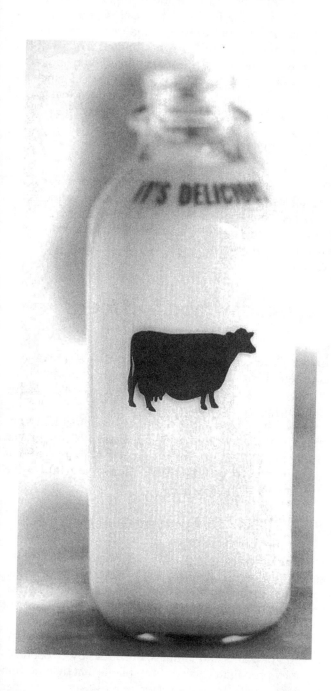

To boost milk output, many American dairy cows are regularly dosed with a synthetic hormone called recombinant bovine growth hormone, which is produced by genetically altered yeast cells. Meanwhile, at least 75 percent of beef cattle are given sex hormones to spur them to grow extra muscle, producing leaner, more tender meat.

Tests of meat and milk sold in U.S. supermarkets reveal minuscule residues of these or related compounds.

IS THERE REALLY ANY DANGER?

Most scientists say the hormones pose no health risk. The milk of hormone-treated cows shows slightly increased levels of a compound called insulin-like growth factor 1. Studies of lab animals show that this compound, which regulates cell growth, may at high levels make the animals more prone to breast, prostate, and colon cancers. In addition, milk from treated cows may show slightly increased levels of thyroid hormone enzymes, which some critics say could result in the disruption of thyroid function in humans. Treated cows' milk has also been shown to have an unusual mix of fatty acids, which may raise the risk of heart disease in milk drinkers. But to date, no one has found that people who drink milk from hormone-dosed cows are any more likely to develop these illnesses.

As for beef, American cattle are routinely given one or more natural or synthetic sex hormones. The government sets rules for their use, requiring tests for residues and prohibiting the sale of meat with amounts that exceed set levels, which generally fall in the range that occurs naturally in the animals. Still, enforcement could be more stringent, and some worry that doses of one often-used hormone—estradiol—may be reaching consumers. Estradiol, a type of estrogen, can play a role in the growth of breast and uterine cancers. Still, there's no evidence that women who regularly eat beef run any extra risk for those diseases.

WHAT YOU CAN DO

If you'd rather drink milk produced without the use of hormones, look for brands that say so on the label. Also, new federal rules specify that dairy products and meat from hormone-treated animals cannot be labeled "organic," so to be extra cautious, shop for organic brands.

pesticides on produce

About 95 percent of all the fruits and vegetables grown in this country are at some stage treated with insecticides or fungicides. Surveys regularly find residues on produce in markets exceeding EPA limits.

IS THERE REALLY ANY DANGER?

For adults, probably not; but for children, possibly. The safety of pesticide residues used to be gauged by research on adults, and few alarms were raised. But a five-year study by the National Academy of Sciences (NAS), published in 1993, showed that although the entire population is exposed to these residues, fetuses, infants, and children run the greatest chance of harm.

Use is almost universal, so it's a good idea to thoroughly wash fruits and vegetables under running water.

Young children are exposed to higher doses than adults because they have smaller bodies and, pound for pound, eat more than their parents do. They also tend to eat the same foods over and over, including more items that contain pesticide residues, like fruit juices. Also, their bodies aren't as efficient at eliminating chemicals. And because their brains are still developing, these realities put them at heightened risk.

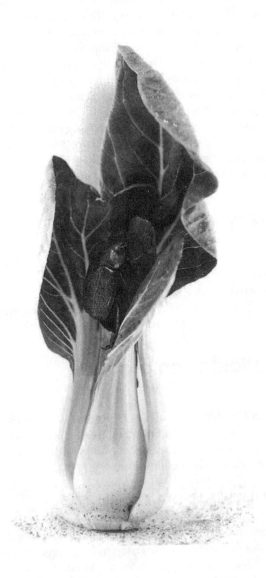

Many of the commonly used pesticides are organo-phosphates, which kill insects by destroying their ner-

vous systems. NAS found they also harm the brains of young rodents—resulting in impaired reflexes, delayed learning, and shortened attention spans. Young children, if overexposed to these pesticides, may be affected in the same way. Farm workers and others who work in close contact with pesticides are at a greater risk for developing a host of health problems, including higher rates of cancer and miscarriages. In 1996, the U.S. Congress unanimously passed a bill to review the risk of pesticides to children, and so far the EPA has limited the use of two common organophosphates, methylparathion and chlorpyrifos. But it may be many years before the agency has an opportunity to review all 600 pesticides that are licensed for use on foods in the United States.

WHAT YOU CAN DO

To play it safe, remember to thoroughly wash fruits and vegetables under running water. To be extra cautious, always peel those with removable skins. And, if your budget allows, buy organic produce or foods available at a farmer's market, which typically have lower pesticide residues.

genetically modified foods

Some 70 percent of all packaged foods now contain certain ingredients—vegetable oils, mainly—produced using biotech methods that allow scientists to splice genetic codes from one species into another. For example, one new variety of corn approved only for animal feed contains bacteria genes that make the plants toxic to insects, ideally permitting farmers to cut back on pesticides. But it has raised worries about risks to people who eat the meat or corn kernels.

IS THERE REALLY ANY DANGER?

There's no evidence that anyone is being harmed by the genetically modified (GM) foods now on the market. However, the method is so new and the possibilities for tinkering so vast that it's impossible to declare all present and future biotech ingredients risk-free.

Scientists have for centuries tampered with the genetic makeup of plants and animals, of course, by crossbreeding or by propagating seeds from plants that by mutation developed new traits—sweeter apples, say, or crisper greens.

But the new technique is different. To create one of these so-called GM crops, scientists trick special viruses called "promoters" into taking up a snippet of DNA from one species, and then attaching it to DNA in cells from another. The modified cells are then grown into plants that have new DNA and new traits. Some people worry that the promoters could infect other plants or animals or develop into harmful new viruses, but so far there's no evidence this has happened.

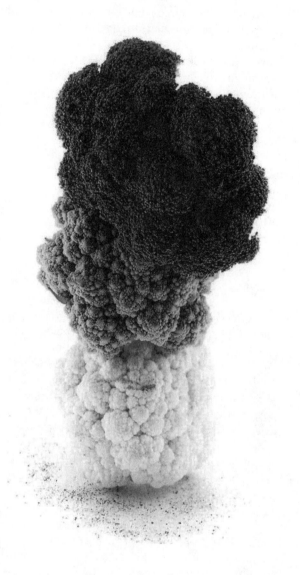

Some worry that genetic tinkering could create dangerous viruses, but thre's no evidence of that happening so far.

It is possible, however, to endow a crop with an unwanted trait. Steve Taylor, Ph.D., head of the University of Nebraska's food science and technology department, tested a new soybean whose protein content had been boosted by the addition of a Brazil nut gene. His studies suggested the modified beans could cause severe reactions in people allergic to the nuts.

Taylor, like most food scientists, takes such findings in stride, noting that after the tests, production of the soybean was stopped. But many people fear that safety testing is inadequate and government rules too lax to keep a public health crisis from someday breaking out.

WHAT YOU CAN DO

Unless you've been actively avoiding them, you probably already eat genetically modified foods and are not in grave danger of harm. But if you prefer not to eat them, start by cutting back on processed foods. Beyond that, shop for 100 percent organic products. Federal rules require them to be free of GM ingredients.

antibiotics in meat

Pigs, chickens, cows—virtually all farm animals—are routinely fed small doses of antibiotics, which make them mature faster, for reasons no one fully understands. The practice has been a boon to farmers, but now it appears to be promoting the development of drug-resistant bacteria.

IS THERE REALLY ANY DANGER?

Your chances of being felled by a resistant bug are very low, but they should not be discounted. Say you accidentally undercook some chicken or ground beef and come down with intestinal distress that lasts several days. It's uncomfortable, but you recover and carry on. Now suppose the bacteria were antibiotic-resistant. That won't matter if, like most people, you're simply waiting out your symptoms. But if you're a person with a weak immune system—you're under 5 years old or over 65, have a chronic disease, or are undergoing chemotherapy—you might not survive, even if you seek medical treatment. "We have patients dying because some of the antibiotics we have are not working," says Stuart Levy, Ph.D., professor of molecular biology and microbiology at Tufts University in Boston, and author of *The Antibiotic Paradox: How Miracle Drugs Are Destroying the Miracle* (Perseus Press, 1992).

People on antibiotics are more prone to foodborne infections because the drugs kill off both bad *and* good bugs in their digestive tracts.

Consider the drugs called fluoroquinolones, used to treat infections of the foodborne microbe *Campylobacter jejuni.* They're also given to poultry to treat respiratory tract disease. A study by researchers from the Minnesota Department of Public Health in Minneapolis found that 14 percent of chickens sold in the state's markets carried fluoroquinolone-resistant campylobacter. What's more, many Minnesotans were being infected, and doctors frequently couldn't treat them with fluoroquinolones.

Though the FDA has on occasion ordered farmers to stop using drugs too similar to those in wide medical use, experts believe the resistance problem is growing.

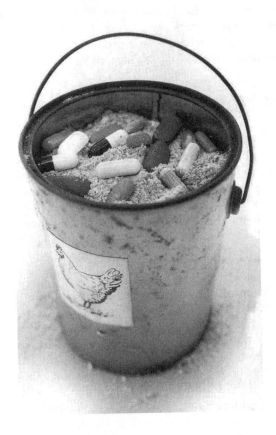

WHAT YOU CAN DO

First, make sure you're doing what you can in the kitchen to cut your chances of falling victim to a foodborne illness. (See "Clean Up Your Act.") Second, take antibiotics only when you really need them. (Many cold sufferers talk their doctors into prescribing the drugs, a gambit that always fails since colds are caused not by bacteria but viruses, which carry on unfazed.) Levy has found that people on antibiotics are more prone to foodborne infections, since the drugs kill off the benign bugs in their digestive tracts, giving the resistant ones a perfect competitor-free environment.

foodborne microbes

At least 80 million Americans suffer a foodborne illness each year, according to the Centers for Disease Control and Prevention. "But I believe that figure is low," says Philip Tierno, M.D., director of microbiology and diag-

clean up your act

Following three simple rules can dramatically cut your risk of getting sick from a foodborne contaminant.

Keep it hot. Cooking is the best way to destroy disease-causing organisms. Use an instant-read food thermometer to make sure you cook all meats thoroughly, following these guidelines:
Beef, lamb, and veal: 145° (rare) to 170 ° (well-done)
Chicken and turkey: 165°
Ground meat: 160° (medium), 170° to 180° (well-done)
Pork: 160° to 170° (reheat ham to 140°)
Casseroles and egg dishes: 160°
Leftovers, reheated: 165°
Keep it cold. Refrigerate perishables as soon as you get them home. Keeping food cold slows or stops the growth of bacteria and viruses. Set the refrigerator at 40°. Never let perishables stay at room temperature longer than two hours—unless, of course, they're whole fruits that need to be stowed in the fridge only after they've been cut or peeled.

Defrost meat in the refrigerator, not on the counter. For safe, rapid defrosting, place the meat in a sealed plastic bag and surround the bag with cool water; the meat will defrost in about 30 minutes.

At picnics, keep meats and other perishables in a closed ice chest in the shade, with cold packs on top of the food. Put out only small amounts of food at a time and, when possible, surround the food with ice.

Keep it clean. The cleaner things are, the less likely you are to get a foodborne illness. Using hot, soapy water, wash and rinse every surface, cutting board, plate, and utensil (including your hands) that touches food before and after each use. This will help eliminate "cross-contamination," when a pathogen is moved from one object to another. For example, if you use a knife to cut up raw chicken, don't rinse the knife and then use it to open a watermelon. This could infect the watermelon with pathogens from the chicken.

Proper hand-washing would eliminate half of all foodborne infections. Be sure to wash your whole hands, not just the palms. And take your time. Most people just give their hands a quick rinse. To be supersafe, scrub continuously through two full choruses of the happy birthday song, about 20 seconds.

nostic immunology at New York University Medical Center in Manhattan. "My estimate is 135 million people, or about half the population of the United States." Most don't even realize their gut-wrenching "stomach flu" is from something they ate, usually microbes on foods such as undercooked ground beef or eggs, mishandled dairy products, or produce tainted by animal waste.

IS THERE REALLY ANY DANGER?

Most sufferers recover completely in several days and without seeing a doctor, but some aren't so lucky. One in every thousand people who has an identified infection by the common foodborne bacterium *Campylobacter jejuni* (usually carried by poultry) will develop Guillain-Barre syndrome, a chronic disease that slowly paralyzes the body from the legs up.

> Most peole don't realize their "stomach flu" is from something they ate, usually microbes on foods such as undercooked eggs, mishandled dairy products, or produce tainted by animal waiste.

Every year, 1,000 or more pregnant women will have a spontaneous abortion after eating a food contaminated with the bacteria *Listeria monocytogenes* (which tend to hang out in soft cheeses like brie, pâtés, rolled and jellied pork, and even hot dogs). Two to 3 percent of those infected with the foodborne microbes salmonella, campylobacter, shigella, or clostridium (which are largely associated with eggs) will get Reiter's syndrome, a fast-developing or "reactive" arthritis of the feet and legs that can become chronic.

Each year an estimated 9,000 of those with a foodborne illness will die from it—typically the very young or old, those with chronic conditions, such as heart disease and diabetes, or others with immune systems crippled by AIDS, hepatitis C, chemotherapy, or immune-suppressing drugs.

WHAT YOU CAN DO

Outbreaks that make the headlines can usually be traced back to restaurants, but the vast majority of foodborne infections start at home, where they're easy to prevent. If you don't do anything else, remember these simple rules: Keep it hot. Or keep it cold. And always keep it clean.

Bill Gottlieb is the author of Alternative Cures (Rodale, 2000).

Unforgettable Foods:
WHAT'S MOST LIKELY TO MAKE YOU SICK

By David Schardt

If today is an average day in the United States, 13 people will die from food poisoning. Another 200,000 will get sick for a few days. And several thousand more may begin to suffer reactive arthritis, paralysis, or other symptoms that can last for months or years.

Which foods cause the outbreaks that sicken the most people? "Fruits and vegetables top the list," says Caroline Smith DeWaal, director of food safety at the Center for Science in the Public Interest (which publishes *Nutrition Action Healthletter*).

CSPI has just issued the fifth edition of *Outbreak Alert*, a tally of food poisoning outbreaks in the U.S. since 1990 in which the food sources have been identified. (The Centers for Disease Control and Prevention—CDC—declares an outbreak when at least two people who eat the same contaminated food get sick. Since 1990, 2,472 outbreaks have sickened 90,355 people.)

"About half of the fruit-and-vegetable outbreaks were caused by salads, berries, raw sprouts, and lettuce," notes DeWaal. "Four out of every ten produce outbreaks were the result of bacteria, viruses, and other pathogens that are commonly found in meat and poultry," she adds. That means that the fruits and vegetables were probably contaminated in the fields with tainted water or manure.

"Contamination is a good reason to buy only pasteurized fruit juices and to wash your fruits and vegetables under running water," says DeWaal. "It's not an excuse to eat fewer fruits and vegetables."

Second on the foods-most-likely-to-make-you-sick list: poultry. A new *Consumer Reports* analysis found *Salmonella* or *Campylobacter* in about half of the whole fresh chickens it purchased at supermarkets nationwide. And some of the bacteria were resistant to human antibiotics. If you become ill after eating chicken contaminated with antibiotic-resistant bacteria, you may get sicker and stay sick longer.

"The only way to protect yourself is to avoid contaminating kitchen counters and utensils when handling raw poultry and to always cook your poultry thoroughly," says DeWaal. That means making sure it reaches at least 170°F in the breast and 180°F in the other parts or in the whole bird.

Then there are beef and eggs, which are neck-and-neck in the dubious race for third place on the Food Poisoning Hit Parade.

"Use a meat thermometer to make sure you cook your burgers to at least 160° F and your steaks and roasts to at least 145°F," says DeWaal. "That will kill harmful bacteria." You also need to thoroughly cook your eggs and any dishes made with eggs.

Location, Location

Where you live figures into how likely you are to get food poisoning, according to the CDC.

"We found substantial variations in the rate of *Campylobacter*, *Salmonella*, and *E. coli* infections in the states we studied," says the CDC's Fred Angulo. Angulo is chief of Foodnet, a network that keeps track of foodborne illnesses in nine states.

In the year 2000, for example, California residents were six times more likely to suffer a *Campylobacter* infection than Tennessee residents. "That probably reflected greater rates of *Campylobacter*-contaminated poultry in California," says Angulo.

Bugs to Go

Where you eat can also affect your risk. "Consuming food prepared outside the home is associated with an increased risk of foodborne illness," says Angulo.

The CDC estimates that people who ate chicken out in 1998 and 1999 were twice as likely to get sick with a *Salmonella* infection than people who ate chicken only at home.

What's more, people who ate hamburgers at non-fast-food restaurants were ten times more likely to become infected with *E. coli* O157:H7 than people who ate hamburgers only at home.

"We don't know why," says Angulo. People might be more likely to report restaurant outbreaks, or there might be more opportunities for food or utensils to touch a contaminated surface in a restaurant kitchen.

On the other hand, "major fast-food restaurant chains have strict standards for the presence of bacteria like *E. coli* and *Salmonella* in the ground beef they buy from their suppliers," says Angulo. Also, production is more mechanized at fast-food chains, so it's easier to cook every burger to a temperature that kills *E. coli*.

For a list of the major food bugs and toxins and the symptoms they cause, see "The Dirty Dozen."

THE DIRTY DOZEN				
Bug	Major Symptoms	Foods that Have Caused Outbreaks	How Soon it Typically Strikes	How Soon it Typically Ends
Campylobacter (bacteria)	diarrhea (can be bloody), fever, abdominal pain, nausea, headache, muscle pain	undercooked poultry, unpasteurized (raw) milk, contaminated water	2 to 5 days	2 to 10 days
Ciguatera (toxin)	*within 2 to 6 hours:* abdominal pain, diarrhea, general pain and weakness, nausea, temperature reversal (hot things feel cold and cold things feel hot), tingling, vomiting *within 2 to 5 days:* slow heartbeat, low blood pressure	large reef fish like barracuda, grouper, red snapper, and amberjack	2 hours to 5 days	days to months
Clostridium botulinum (bacteria)	vomiting, diarrhea, blurred vision, double vision, difficulty swallowing, muscle weakness that spreads from the upper to the lower body	home-canned foods, improperly canned commercial foods, herb-infused oils, potatoes baked in aluminum foil, bottled garlic	12 to 72 hours	days to months (get treatment immediately)
Cyclospora (parasite)	fatigue, frequent protracted bouts of diarrhea	imported berries, contaminated water, lettuce	1 to 11 days	weeks to months
E. coli O157:H7 (bacteria)	severe diarrhea that is often bloody, abdominal pain, vomiting (usually accompanied by little or no fever)	undercooked beef, unpasteurized (raw) milk or juice, raw produce, salami, contaminated water	1 to 8 days	5 to 10 days (get treatment immediately, especially for a child or elderly person)
Hepatits A (virus)	diarrhea, dark urine, jaundice (yellow "whites" of the eyes), flu-like symptoms	shellfish, raw produce, foods that are not reheated after coming into contact with an infected food handler	15 to 50 days	2 weeks to 3 months
Listeria (bacteria)	fever, muscle aches, nausea, diarrhea (pregnant women may have mild flu-like symptoms; can lead to premature delivery or still-birth)	fresh soft cheeses, unpasteurized (raw) or inadequately pasteurized milk, ready-to-eat deli meats and hot dogs	9 to 48 hours for gastrointestinal symptoms, 2 to 6 weeks for infections in the blood, brain, or uterus	days to months (get treatment immediately)
Norwalk virus	nausea, vomiting, large-volume watery diarrhea	poorly cooked shellfish, ready-to-eat foods touched by infected food handlers, salads, sandwiches	24 to 48 hours	24 to 60 hours
Salmonella (bacteria)	diarrhea, fever, abdominal cramps, vomiting	eggs, poultry, unpasteurized (raw) milk or juice, cheese, raw produce	1 to 3 days	4 to 7 days
Scombrotoxin (toxin)	flushing; rash; burning sensation in skin, mouth, and throat; dizziness, hives, tingling	fresh tuna, bluefish, mackerel, marlin, mahi mahi	1 minute to 3 hours	3 to 6 hours
Vibrio parahaemolyticus (bacteria)	watery diarrhea, abdominal cramps, nausea, vomiting	undercooked or raw seafood	2 to 48 hours	2 to 5 days
Vibrio vulnificus (bacteria)	vomiting, diarrhea, abdominal pain, bacteria in the blood, wounds that become infected	undercooked or raw shellfish (especially oysters), other contaminated seafood	1 to 7 days	2 to 8 days (get treatment immediately)

Source: Adapted from *Diagnosis and Management of Foodborne Illnesses, A Primer for Physicians* (www.cdc.gov/mmwr/preview/mmwrhtml/rr5002a1.htm), by the American Medical Association, the Centers for Disease Control and Prevention, the Food and Drug Administration, and the U.S. Department of Agriculture.

CERTIFIED ORGANIC

STAMP OF APPROVAL: New government rules will define 'organic.' The sale of these fruits, veggies and snack foods has soared, but we still aren't sure what good they do. Here's a guide to how purer products affect the health of our families and the planet.

BY GEOFFREY COWLEY

OTTO KRAMM USED TO COME home from work at night and warn his toddlers to keep their distance until he'd bathed and changed his clothes. He wasn't just trying to keep them clean. As a vegetable farmer in California's Salinas Valley, Kramm spent his days covered in pesticides, herbicides and fungicides, and he worried about their effects on young children. "I didn't know what was on my clothes," he says, "or how it might affect the kids 15 years down the road." The more he thought about it, the less he liked the feeling. So in 1996, Kramm did something radical. He bought into a farm that was being cultivated organically. "It was scary," he says. "I couldn't fall back on the tools I'd always used to fight the pests and the weeds." But he worked out a new relationship with the soil and ended up not only cleaner but more prosperous. Today Kramm has 6,000 acres on three farms. The nation's largest organic-produce distributor, Earthbound Farm, is buying up everything he can grow. And he's never off-limits to his kids.

Organic farms are still sprouts in a forest of industrial giants. They provide less than 2 percent of the nation's food supply and take up less than 1 percent of its cropland. But they're flourishing as never before. Over the past decade the market for organic food has grown by 15 to 20 percent every year—five times faster than food sales in general. Nearly 40 percent of U.S. consumers now reach occasionally for something labeled organic, and sales are expected to top $11 billion this year. Could dusty neighborhood co-ops sell that many wormy little apples? Well, no. That was the old organic. The new organic is all about bigger farms, heartier crops, better distribution and slicker packaging and promotion. Conglomerates as big as Heinz and General Mills are now launching or buying organic lines—and selling them in mainstream supermarkets.

What exactly are consumers getting out of the deal? Until now, the definition of "organic" has varied from one state to the next, leaving shoppers to assume it means something like "way more expensive but probably better for you." Not anymore. As of Oct. 21, any food sold as organic will have to meet criteria set by the United States Department of Agriculture. The National Organic Rule—the product of 10 years' deliberation by growers, scientists and consumers—reserves the terms "100 percent organic" and "organic" (at least 95 percent) for foods produced without hormones, antibiotics, herbicides, insecticides, chemical fertilizers, genetic modification or germ-killing radiation. Food makers who document their compliance will qualify for a new USDA seal declaring their products "certified organic." "This really signifies the start of a new era," says Margaret Wittenberg of the Whole Foods supermarket chain. "From now on, consumers will get a very solid idea of what is organic and what is not."

Yet for all the clarity they provide, the standards say nothing about what's worth putting in your shopping cart. "This is not a food-safety program," says Barbara Robinson, the USDA official overseeing the effort. "We're not saying that organic food is safer or better than other kinds of food." How, then, should we read the new label?

Does "certified organic" tell us anything worth knowing about a chicken breast or a candy bar? Are organically grown grapes more nutritious than conventional ones? And is organic agriculture a viable alternative to modern factory farming? These are complicated, politically charged questions, but they're questions worth asking ourselves—both as consumers and citizens.

When the counterculture embraced organic food and farming in the early '70s, the motivation was more philosophical than practical. Maria Rodale, whose family runs the pro-organic Rodale Institute in Kutztown, Pa., sees the current boom as evidence that people are still "expressing their values about the environment and even spirituality and politics through the food choices they make." Market research suggests she's about 26 percent right. When the Hartman Group of Bellevue, Wash., surveyed consumers two years ago, only one in four cited concern about the environment as a "top motivator" for buying organic food. Flavor was a bigger concern, cited by 38 percent as reason enough to pay a premium of 15 percent or more. Sophisticated chefs have responded in droves, many now serving only fresh, seasonal food from small local growers. "The difference is huge," says Peter Hoffman, owner of New York's Restaurant Savoy and chairman of the Chefs' Collaborative. "When people taste asparagus or string beans grown in richly composted soil, they can't get over the depth and vibrancy of the flavor."

To most consumers, though, organic means healthier. Fully 66 percent of the Hartman Group's respondents cited health as a "top motivator"—as will almost any shopper on the street. "Buying an apple that has poison on it, even if you wash it you don't know how much has come off," says Wendy Abrams, a suburban Chicago mother with four kids at home. Abrams buys organic milk and stocks her pantry with Newman's Own pretzels and raisins on the theory that anything organic is less likely to harbor cancer-causing chemicals. "There have been six cases of cancer on my street," she says. "It's just weird."

All of these folks—market analysts refer to them as "true naturals," "connoisseurs" and "health seekers"—seem happy with their purchases. But are they getting what they're seeking? It's hard to argue with the connoisseurs, and not just because they know what they like. A tomato grown on a vast commercial plot is bred less for taste than for durability, notes Bob Scowcroft of the nonprofit Organic Farming Research Foundation. It has to resist disease and ship well. Organic growers, with their smaller harvests and their reliance on nearby markets, can plant delicate heirloom strains and give the fruit more time on the vine. "They pick it when it's ripe," says Marion Cunningham, author of "The Fannie Farmer Cookbook." "No one goes around picking organic fruits when they're as hard as little rocks."

Managed property, organic farms can match conventional ones for productivity, and beat them during drought conditions.

The health seekers may have common sense on their side, but no one has found a way to determine whether people eating well-balanced organic diets are healthier than those eating well-balanced conventional ones. No one denies that nonorganic produce contains pesticide residues that would be toxic at high doses. Nor is there any question that children (because of their size) consume those residues in higher concentrations than adults. But there is still no evidence that pesticides cause ill health at the doses found in food, or that people who eschew them come out ahead. Technological optimists find it ludicrous that anyone would fret over pesticide residues when the hazards of foodborne bacteria are

so much clearer. *E. coli* is "perhaps the deadliest risk in our modern food supply," says Dennis Avery of the Hudson Institute—"and its primary hiding place is the cattle manure with which organic farmers fertilize food crops." So wash your produce, but don't let it scare you. Organic or conventional, fruits and vegetables are the best fuel you can put in your body.

Dangerous bacteria are even more common in animal products, but the organic program is not a germ-control initiative. Under the new guidelines, meat and dairy labeled organic must come from creatures that are raised on organic grains or grasses, given access to the outdoors and spared treatment with growth hormones and antibiotics. Experts agree that by spiking animal feed with antibiotics, conventional farmers are speeding the emergence of drug-resistant bacteria. Buying organic is one way to vote against that practice. But in terms of your own health, you'll profit more from holding back on animal products than by eating organic ones. In one study, Danish research found that organic chickens were actually more likely than conventional ones to carry campylobacter, a pathogen that can cause severe diarrhea.

So organic food is tastier and more appealing, but not demonstrably better for you. If you're shopping with only yourself in mind, maybe you'll save your money. But if you pause to think about what you're buying into with every food purchase, organic goods start to look like a bargain. Our current agricultural system took off in the years following World War II, when farmers discovered that chemical fertilizers could force higher yields out of tired soil—and that pesticides could clear croplands of competing species. As farmers saw what the new chemicals made possible, American agriculture was transformed from a rural art into a heavy industry dominated by large corporations growing single crops on vast stretches of poisoned soil.

As any ecologist might have predicted, the new approach was hard to sustain. A small, varied farm can renew itself endlessly when managed with care. Last year's bean stocks help nourish next year's cantaloupes, and a bad year for tomatoes may be a good year for eggplant. As they lost sight of those lessons, the factory farmers grew ever more dependent on chemicals. Insects died off conveniently at

first. But each application of insecticide left a few heart survivors, and within a few generations whole populations were resistant. Today, says Scowcroft, "we're applying three times as much chemical as we were 40 years ago to kill the same pests." It's not just insects. Conventional farmers now use herbicides to kill weeds, fungicides to kill fungi, rodenticides to kill field mice and gophers, avicides to kill fruit-eating birds and molluscicides to kill snails. Strawberry growers now favor all-purpose fumigants such as methyl bromide. "You inject it into the soil and put a tarp over it," says Monica Moore of the Pesticide Action Network of North America. "It kills everything from mammals to microbes. It's a complete biocide."

These practices may not be poisoning our food, but there is no question they're killing off wildlife, endangering farmworkers and degrading the soil and water that life itself depends on. Pesticides now kill 67 million American birds each year. The Mississippi River dumps enough synthetic fertilizer into the Gulf of Mexico to maintain a 60-mile-wide "dead zone" too choked with algae to support fish. And soil erosion threatens to turn much of the world's arable land into desert. "Conventional agriculture still delivers cheap, abundant food," says Fred Kirschenmann of the Leopold Center for Sustainable Agriculture in Ames, Iowa. "But when you factor in the government subsidies and the environmental costs, it gets very expensive. We're drawing down our ecological capital. At some point, the systems will start to break down."

Can organic agriculture save the day? Not if it's just a boutique alternative. But as demand grows, more and more farmers are taking a leap backward—and landing on their feet. They're discovering they can enrich the soil and manage some pests simply by rotating their crops. They're learning that they can often control insects with other insects—or lure them away from cash crops by planting things they prefer. Well-run organic farms often match conventional ones for productivity, even beat them when water is scarce. Creating a sustainable food supply may well require advanced technology as well as ecological awareness. But an organic ethic could be the very key to our survival.

With ANNE UNDERWOOD
and KAREN SPRINGEN

Hooked on fish?
There might be some catches

Health-conscious people eat it three, even four times a week. But farm-raised fish and worries about mercury contamination are churning the waters.

The advantage of eating fish has become one of those health-advice truisms, ranking right up there with getting exercise and eating fruits and vegetables. "Studies show that fish consumption lowers your risk of… "—you can fill in the blank, although the evidence remains strongest for heart disease.

The topic has spawned plenty of research. We recently did a quick computer search of the medical literature for fish-consumption studies. Within minutes we found research papers on stroke in American women, prostate cancer in Swedish men, Alzheimer's disease in French seniors, and leptin (an appetite hormone) levels in Tanzania. Not surprisingly, all came out swimmingly for the fish eaters.

Farm vs. Wild

The glowing health reports have whet the American appetite for fish, and the millions of pounds of farm-raised fish produced each year help meet that demand. In addition to farm-raised catfish, salmon, and trout, we now have tilapia, striped bass, sturgeon, and walleye on the menu and at the store. In Australia, they've started tuna "ranching"— catching the fish in large nets and herding them into pens for several months of feeding.

Dilemmas abound. Farming fish makes a healthy food less expensive for consumers. The added supply almost certainly eases overfishing of dwindling stocks of some species. But some environmental groups are critical, especially of salmon operations on the West Coast, and want consumers to boycott farm-raised salmon. They say the "floating feedlots" harm fragile marine environments. There's also an argument that raising carnivorous fish like salmon is wasteful of natural resources because it takes several pounds of wild

What is it about fish?

When you eat carbohydrates (sugar or starch) or protein, your body shows little respect for the artistry of those molecules. It tears them apart and reassembles them to suit its own purposes. Carbohydrates and protein— they're just fodder.

But it's different with fat. Some gets roughed up during digestion and metabolism. But some gets through more or less intact, becomes part of our cell membranes, and thus has considerable say-so over how cells behave. We are the fat that we eat.

Fish is a special food because it contains two important varieties of *long-chain omega-3* fats that you won't find anywhere else in a conven-

tional diet. *Long-chain* refers to the number of carbon atoms, *omega-3* to a position of a certain chemical bond that puts a 45-degree kink in that chain. Both attributes determine how a fat molecule is going to fit into cell membranes and what it's going to do once it gets there.

As it turns out, long-chain omega-3 fats in fish are just the sort of fat molecules that any healthy cell should gladly welcome into its membranes. One of them, *eicosapentaenoic acid*, manages to displace molecules that could otherwise give rise to active prostaglandins, leukotrienes, and other inflammatory compounds. And inflammation seems to be a root cause of many diseases. *Eicosapentaenoic acid* also seems to be the

omega-3 with the most pronounced cardiac benefits.

The other main omega-3 in fish is *docosahexaenoic acid* (DHA). It's important to brain and vision development in infants and is added to infant formulas.

Sometimes there's some confusion about where the *alpha-linolenic acid* in walnuts, flaxseed oil, and soy products fits in. It's also an omega-3 fat, but has fewer carbon atoms and therefore isn't a long-chain omega-3. Being shortchanged those few carbon atoms makes a difference because alpha-linolenic acid doesn't have as many health benefits as the more carbonblessed omega-3s in fish.

fish like herring or anchovy to produce a pound of salmon. The industry says it has responded by cutting back on antibiotics, switching to low-phosphorous feeds that make fish waste less polluting, and experimenting with soy and other vegetable-based feeds.

Nutritional Issues

Coddled and cooped up, farm fish tend to be anywhere from two to five times fattier overall than wild fish, although the fat content of wild fish varies tremendously depending on the season and where the creature is in its reproductive cycle. That extra fat means more calories. But fattier (oilier) fish also tend to have more of the omega-3 fats that are the main reason fish is such a health food. (*See sidebar.*) A meal of an oily fish like bluefish will give you twice as many omega-3s as a like-sized serving of halibut, and four times as many as farmed catfish.

So farm-raised fish—simply because they're fattier—tend to have more omega-3s than wild fish. But actual comparisons become complicated. Both the amount and type of fat in farmed fish depend on their feed, particularly the type of oil (fat) it contains.

When we looked up the omega-3 content of farmed and wild Atlantic salmon in a nutritional database compiled by the United States Department of Agriculture (USDA), they were the same. But wild Atlantic salmon is scarce and not commercially available very often. A more realistic comparison is farmed Atlantic with other wild salmon species. And according to the USDA database, wild coho salmon, for example, contains half the amount of omega-3s as farmed Atlantic salmon.

Researchers at Oregon Health & Science University have made their own comparisons. So far, their tests haven't shown any difference in the omega-3 content of farmed and wild salmon, according to Dr. William E. Connor, one of the researchers. But when they tested catfish, the omega-3 content of the wild fish was much higher than the farmed.

Fish Feed

Fish feeds vary tremendously with the species. There is also continual ex-

perimentation with, for example, different sorts of enzymes to make the fish metabolize feed more efficiently and thus grow faster. British scientists announced last year that they had successfully added *pheromones* to feed to make it more appetizing. Red coloring in the form of synthetic carotenoids is added to salmon feed to give the flesh that rosy color that consumers have come to expect.

For consumers, the oil content of the feed is a key issue because it influences omega-3 levels. Currently, most of the oil used for fish feed comes from small fish like herring and menhaden—and it's rich in omega-3s. But the industry is worried about dwindling supplies and rising costs and thus interested in plant-based alternatives. Researchers at the University of Stirling in Scotland have published several studies showing that replacing fish oil with plant-derived substitutes is feasible, but, not surprisingly, a high proportion of plant oil significantly reduces the omega-3 content of salmon.

Omega-3 and mercury content of select fish

Omega-3 fats (grams in 3-oz. serving)*		Mercury (parts per million)**	
Atlantic salmon, farmed	1.8	Tilefish	1.45
Anchovy	1.7	Swordfish	1.00
Sardines	1.4	Shark	0.96
Rainbow trout, farmed	1.0	King mackerel	0.73
Coho salmon, wild	0.9	Tuna (fresh and frozen)	0.32
Bluefish	0.8	Halibut	0.23
Striped bass	0.8	Mahi mahi	0.19
Swordfish	0.7	Tuna (canned)	0.17
Tuna, white, canned	0.7	Catfish	0.07
Halibut	0.4	Salmon	Not detectable
Catfish, channel, farmed	0.2	Tilapia	Not detectable

*SOURCE: USDA NUTRIENT DATABASE

**SOURCE: FDA

Some experts we talked to said feed makers are more likely to switch from fish to vegetable (soy) sources of protein, not fat. For one thing, some species—notably salmon, trout, and steelhead—need omega-3 oil to flourish. The industry also has an interest in preserving the reputation of fish as a healthy food, which means keeping the omega-3 levels as high as possible.

As for farm vs. wild taste, we defer to the palate of Roger Berkowitz, CEO of Legal Sea Foods, a chain of seafood restaurants based in Boston. He says that wild fish, especially salmon, has a gamier, more intense flavor. It's also more expensive. Berkowitz says farm-raised flounder has foundered because of poor taste and texture.

Mercury Contamination

But an even bigger worry these days is that the fish we're urged to eat for health may contain some very unhealthy contaminants, particularly mercury. Most research suggests that if the mercury in fish causes harm, the danger is primarily to the developing nervous systems of children, although studies have suggested a link between mercury and the atherosclerosis that underlies heart disease. Last spring, the FDA advised pregnant women and all women of childbearing age not to eat any shark, swordfish, king mackerel, and tilefish because of their high mercury content, and to limit consumption of all fish to 12 ounces (about two servings) per week. Harvard researchers recently published a study in the *New England Journal of Medicine* showing that Americans who eat more fish have higher levels of the metal in their bodies (more specifically, in their toenails), although they don't believe the levels cause harm. No one is recommending routine mercury testing. But the contaminant does seem to pose a damned-if-you-do, damned-if-you-don't problem for people who want to eat a lot of fish for health reasons. Mercury tends to accumulate in the food chain: the higher on the chain, the greater the concentration of mercury. But species rich in omega-3 fats also tend to be the food chain's higher-ups, including swordfish, mackerel, and tuna.

The FDA is correct to take a better-safe-than-sorry approach to mercury in fish. But consider the risks and benefits. The amount of mercury you're exposed to by occasionally eating swordfish and mackerel is very small. Besides, you have other choices. Salmon, for example, is high in omega-3s and so far has tested very low for mercury. Smaller tuna are used for canning, so apart from all that mayonnaise, eating a tunafish sandwich, a couple times per week isn't a major hazard.

In November 2002, the American Heart Association re-emphasized its recommendation that all adults should eat at least two servings of fish per week because of the cardiovascular benefits. The association takes the position that for adult men and older women not having children, any risk from mercury is offset by the advantages.

So you can have your fish and enjoy it, too. Eating fish remains one of the better health bets out there.

UNIT 7

World Hunger and Malnutrition

Unit Selections

Key Points to Consider

- How extensive is global malnutrition and infection?

- What are some of the causes of global malnutrition?

- What sort of role will genetically modified food have in feeding people in developing countries?

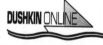 **Links: www.dushkin.com/online/**
These sites are annotated in the World Wide Web pages.

Population Reference Bureau
http://www.prb.org
World Health Organization (WHO)
http://www.who.int/en/
WWW Virtual Library: Demography & Population Studies
http://demography.anu.edu.au/VirtualLibrary/

The cause of malnutrition worldwide is poverty. The United Nations Food and Agriculture Organization (FAO) determined that a body mass index (BMI) (body weight divided by the square root of height) of 18.5 is indicative of chronic energy deficit in adults. Approximately 840 million people are malnourished in the developing world: Asia has the largest number of them and children under 5 years of age are the most susceptible. Infectious disease kills approximately 10 million children each year. Thus, the director general of FAO launched, in 1994, a Special Programme for Food Security (SPFS) for low-income food-deficit countries (LIFDCs), which was endorsed by the World Food Summit held in Rome in 1996. They pledged to increase food production and access to food in LIFDCs so that the number of malnourished people would be reduced by half. They set goals to increase sustainable agricultural production within the cultural, political, and economic millieu of each country to improve access to food, increase the role of trade, and deal effectively with food emergencies.

Malnutrition is also the main culprit for lowered resistance to disease and infection and death, especially in children. The malnutrition-infection combination results in stunted growth, lowered mental development in children, and lowered productivity and higher incidence of degenerative disease in adulthood. This directly affects the economies of developing countries. The 2002 report of the Food and Agriculture Organization of the United Nations entitled "The State of Insecurity in the World 2002" describes the relationship between mortality rates, life expectancy, and hunger, especially among malnourished children in developing countries, and highlights how infectious diseases are often fatal for malnourished children. Over two billion people globally suffer from micronutrient malnutrition, frequently called "hidden hunger." Vitamin A, iron, iodine, zinc, folate, selenium, and Vitamin C deficiencies are especially critical for growing children and women of childbearing age. Food fortification and supplementation and the promotion of home gardens, community fish ponds, and poultry production can alleviate "hidden hunger." Additionally, partnerships between the public and private sectors may prove valuable in combating malnutrition.

Nutrient deficiencies magnify the effect of disease and result in more severe symptoms and greater complications of a disease. For example, vitamin A deficiency leads to blindness in about 250,000–300,000 children annually and also exacerbates the symptoms of measles. Iron deficiency, which is widespread among pregnant women and those in the childbearing years in developing countries, increases the risk of death from hemorrhage in their offspring and reduces physical productivity and learning capacity. Finally, iodine deficiency causes brain damage and mental retardation. It is estimated that 1.5 billion people are at risk for iodine deficiency disorders (IDD). Even though there is malnutrition in the U.S. this is a result of too much of the wrong food. Government programs such as WIC, the School Lunch and Breakfast Program, provide high-calorie, high saturated-fat and cholesterol foods, a major factor for the obesity epidemic.

Biotechnologist believe that genetically modified (GM) foods such as rice that is fortified with beta-carotene, iron and zinc may not only help feed the world, but also eradicate nutritional deficiencies. Additionally, GM foods may decrease damage to crops from pests, viruses, bacteria, and drought. Yet it seems too good to be true. If farmers cannot afford to grow GM crops or afford to buy the food, if the infrastructure for transport and distribution is not available, the same products may never reach the consumers. Since the safety of humans and the efficacy for the environment of GM corps has not been adequately studied, the Union of Concerned Scientists believe that genetic engineering is by no means the panacea for hunger. Additionally, the potential of GM foods to cause allergies is real. It is so real that the U.S. EPA gathered scientists from Universities and Government laboratories in a workshop to discuss strategies to "Assess the Allergenic Potential of GM Foods." Since GM foods have not been tested on humans, scientists have no hazard identification plans or do not know the basic science that may underlie these allergies.

While scientists are attempting to find ways to be prepared for outbreaks of GM food allergies, GM foods are invading the market and contaminating non-GM crops with the ultimate goal to flood the market so that the consumer will have no choice but buy them. Because of lack of a research of GM foods on human health, even though Afrikaners in some African countries are starving, their leaders prefer to let GM corn rot in storage areas than feed it to their citizens.

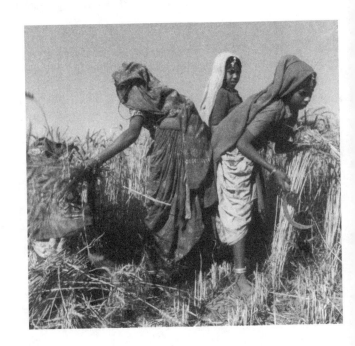

Undernourishment around the world

Hunger and mortality

MILLIONS OF PEOPLE, including 6 million children under the age of five, die each year as a result of hunger. Of these millions, relatively few are the victims of famines that attract headlines, video crews and emergency aid. Far more die unnoticed, killed by the effects of chronic hunger and malnutrition, a "covert famine" that stunts their development, saps their strength and cripples their immune systems.

Where prevalence of hunger is high, mortality rates for infants and children under five are also high, and life expectancy is low (see map and graphs). In the worst affected countries, a newborn child can look forward to an average of barely 38 years of healthy life (compared to over 70 years of life in "full health" in 24 wealthy nations). One in seven children born in the countries where hunger is most common will die before reaching the age of five.

Not all of these shortened lives can be attributed to the effects of hunger, of course. Many other factors combine with hunger and malnutrition to sentence tens of millions of people to an early death. The HIV/AIDS pandemic, which is ravaging many of the same countries where hunger is most widespread, has reduced average life expectancy across all of sub-Saharan Africa by nearly five years for women and 2.5 years for men.

Even after compensating for the impact of HIV/AIDS and other factors, however, the correlation between chronic hunger and higher mortality rates remains striking. Numerous studies suggest that it is far from coincidental. Since the early 1990s, a series of analyses have confirmed that between 50 and 60 percent of all childhood deaths in the developing world are caused either directly or indirectly by hunger and malnutrition.

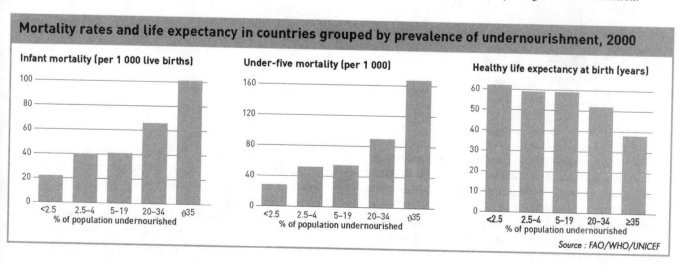

Mortality rates and life expectancy in countries grouped by prevalence of undernourishment, 2000

Infant mortality (per 1 000 live births)

Under-five mortality (per 1 000)

Healthy life expectancy at birth (years)

% of population undernourished

Source : FAO/WHO/UNICEF

Correspondence between high rates of chronic hunger and childhood mortality, 2000

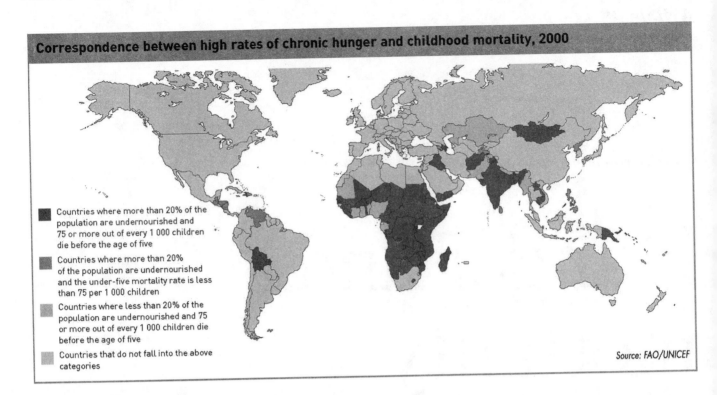

■ Countries where more than 20% of the population are undernourished and 75 or more out of every 1 000 children die before the age of five

■ Countries where more than 20% of the population are undernourished and the under-five mortality rate is less than 75 per 1 000 children

■ Countries where less than 20% of the population are undernourished and 75 or more out of every 1 000 children die before the age of five

■ Countries that do not fall into the above categories

Source: FAO/UNICEF

Hunger and child mortality

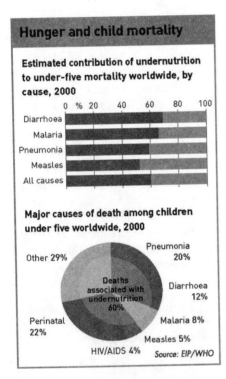

Estimated contribution of undernutrition to under-five mortality worldwide, by cause, 2000

Diarrhoea
Malaria
Pneumonia
Measles
All causes

Major causes of death among children under five worldwide, 2000

Other 29%
Pneumonia 20%
Deaths associated with undernutrition 60%
Diarrhoea 12%
Perinatal 22%
Malaria 8%
Measles 5%
HIV/AIDS 4%

Source: EIP/WHO

Proportion and number of underweight children, 1997–99

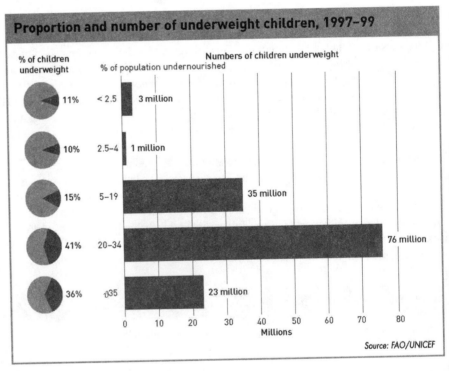

% of children underweight
% of population undernourished
Numbers of children underweight

11%	< 2.5	3 million
10%	2.5–4	1 million
15%	5–19	35 million
41%	20–34	76 million
36%	≥35	23 million

Source: FAO/UNICEF

Relatively few of those deaths are the result of starvation. Most are caused by a persistent lack of adequate food intake and essential nutrients that leaves children weak, underweight and vulnerable.

As might be expected, the vast majority of the 153 million underweight children under five in the developing world are concentrated in countries where the prevalence of undernourishment is high (see graph above).

Even mild-to-moderate malnutrition greatly increases the risk of children dying from common childhood diseases. Overall, analysis shows that the risk of death is 2.5 times higher for children with only mild malnutrition than it is for children who are adequately nourished. And the risk increases sharply along with the severity of malnutrition (as measured by their weight-to-age ratio). The risk of death is 4.6 times higher for children suffering from moderate malnutrition and 8.4 times higher for the severely malnourished.

Common diseases often fatal for malnourished children

Infectious diseases are the immediate cause of death for most of the 11 million children under the age of five who die each year in the developing world. But the risk of dying from those diseases is far greater for children who are hungry and malnourished.

The four biggest killers of children are diarrhoea, acute respiratory illness, malaria and measles. Taken together, these four diseases account for almost half of all deaths among children under the age of five. Analysis of data from hospitals and villages shows that all four of these diseases are far more deadly to children who are stunted or underweight.

In the case of diarrhoea, numerous studies show that the risk of death is as much as nine times higher for children who are significantly underweight, the most common indicator of chronic undernutrition. Similarly, underweight children are two to three times more likely to die of malaria and acute respiratory infections, including pneumonia, than well-nourished children.

Lack of dietary diversity and essential minerals and vitamins also contributes to increased child and adult mortality. Iron deficiency anaemia greatly increases the risk of death from malaria, and vitamin A deficiency impairs the immune system, increasing the annual death toll from measles and other diseases by an estimated 1.3–2.5 million children.

Improving nutrition to save lives

The weight of evidence clearly argues that eliminating hunger and malnutrition could save millions of lives each year. That conclusion has been confirmed by a study that examined factors that had helped reduce child mortality during the 1990s. Topping the list were the decline in the proportion of children who were malnourished and lacking access to adequate water, sanitation and housing.

Undernourishment around the world

Undernourishment, poverty and development

T HE WORLD FOOD SUMMIT (WFS) in 1996 set the goal—to reduce the number of hungry people in the world by half before the year 2015. Four years later, that goal was echoed in the first of the Millennium Development Goals (MDGs), which set targets of reducing by half both the proportion of people who suffer from hunger and the proportion living on less than US$1 per day.

These targets are closely related; neither can be achieved without the other, and achieving both is essential to success in reaching the rest of the MDGs.

Poverty and hunger—mutual causes, devastating effects

Measures of food deprivation, nutrition and poverty are strongly correlated (see graphs). Countries with a high prevalence of undernourishment also have high prevalences of stunted and underweight children. In these countries, a high percentage of the population lives in conditions of extreme poverty. In countries where a high proportion of the population is undernourished, a comparably high proportion struggles to survive on less than US$1 per day.

Undernourishment, poverty and indicators for other Millennium Development Goals: 1995–2000

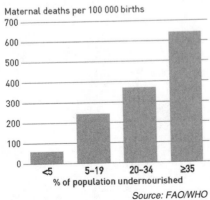

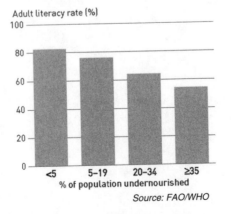

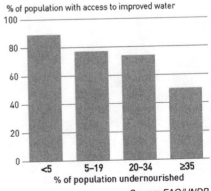

Hunger impacts other Millennium Development Goals

Goal	Selected indicators	Impact of hunger
Achieve universal primary education	• net enrolment ratio • literacy rate	• reduces school attendance • impairs cognitive capacity
Promote gender equality	• ratio of girls to boys in primary education	• may reduce school attendance more for girls
Reduce child mortality	• under-five mortality rate	• associated with 60 percent of child deaths
Improve maternal health	• maternal mortality rate	• greatly increases risk of maternal death
Combat HIV/AIDS, malaria and other diseases	• HIV prevalence among pregnant women • death rates associated with malaria	• spurs migratory labour that increases spread of HIV • multiplies child death rates from two- to three-fold
Ensure environmental sustainability	• proportion of land area covered by forest	• leads to unsustainable use of forest lands and resources

While poverty is undoubtedly a cause of hunger, hunger can also be a cause of poverty. Hunger often deprives impoverished people of the one valuable resource they can call their own: the strength and skill to work productively. Numerous studies have confirmed that hunger seriously impairs the ability of the poor to develop their skills and reduces the productivity of their labour.

Hunger in childhood impairs mental and physical growth, crippling the capacity to learn and earn. Evidence from household food surveys in developing countries shows that adults with smaller and slighter body frames caused by undernourishment earn lower wages in jobs involving physical labour. Other studies have found that a 1 percent increase in the Body Mass Index (BMI, a measure of weight for a given height) is associated with an increase of more than 2 percent in wages for those toward the lower end of the BMI range.

Micronutrient deficiencies can also reduce work capacity. Surveys suggest that iron deficiency anaemia reduces productivity of manual labourers by up to 17 percent. As a result, hungry and malnourished adults earn lower wages. And they are frequently unable to work as many hours or years as well-nourished people, as they fall sick more often and have shorter life spans.

Hunger and the poverty of nations

Widespread hunger and malnutrition impair economic performance not only of individuals and families, but of nations. Anaemia alone has been found to reduce GDP by 0.5–1.8 percent in several countries (see graph). Studies in India, Pakistan, Bangladesh and Viet Nam estimated conservatively that the combined effect of stunting, iodine deficiency and iron deficiency reduced GDP by 2 to 4 percent. Recent calculations by FAO suggest that achieving the WFS goal of reducing the number of undernourished people by half by the year 2015 would yield a value of more than US$120 billion. That figure reflects the economic impact of longer, healthier, more productive lives for several hundred million people freed from hunger.

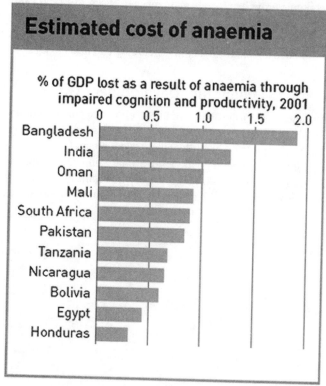

Estimated cost of anaemia

% of GDP lost as a result of anaemia through impaired cognition and productivity, 2001

Source: World Bank

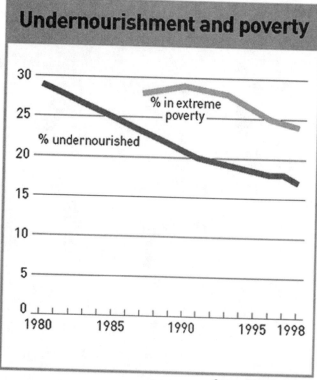

Undernourishment and poverty

Source: FAO/World Bank

Nobel Prize-winning economist Robert Fogel has pointed out that hungry people cannot work their way out of poverty. He estimates that 20 percent of the population in England and France was effectively excluded from the labour force around 1790 because they were too weak and hungry to work. Improved nutrition, he calculates, accounted for about half of the economic growth in Britain and France between 1790 and 1880. Since many developing countries are as poor as Britain and France were in 1790, his analysis suggests reducing hunger could have a similar impact in developing countries today.

A key to Millennium Development Goals

Evidence clearly shows that failure to eliminate hunger will undermine efforts to reach the other MDGs as well (see box, "Hunger impacts other Millennium Development Goals").

Hopes for achieving universal primary education and literacy, for example, will be thwarted while millions of hungry children suffer from diminished learning capacity or are forced to work instead of attending school. Low birth weight, protein energy malnutrition, iron deficiency anaemia and iodine deficiency are all linked to cognitive deficiencies. Hunger also limits school attendance. In Pakistan, a relatively small improvement in height for age increased school enrolment rates substantially: 2 percent for boys, 10 percent for girls. This steep increase for girls suggests one way in which reducing hunger would also accelerate another of the MDGs—promoting gender equality.

Data and analysis confirm that reducing hunger and malnutrition could have a decisive impact on reducing child mortality, improving maternal health, and on combating HIV/AIDS, malaria and other diseases.

Towards the Summit commitments

Confronting the causes of malnutrition: the hidden challenge of micronutrient deficiencies

OVER 2 BILLION PEOPLE worldwide suffer from micronutrient malnutrition, often called "hidden hunger". Their diets supply inadequate amounts of vitamins and minerals such as vitamin A, iron, iodine, zinc, folate, selenium and vitamin C. Deficiencies usually occur when the habitual diet lacks diversity and does not include sufficient quantities of the fruits, vegetables, dairy products, meat and fish that are the best sources of many micronutrients.

Vitamin A and mortality, 1992

A World Health Organization study concluded that an improved vitamin A nutriture could prevent 1.3 to 2.5 million deaths each year among children aged six months to five years in the developing world.

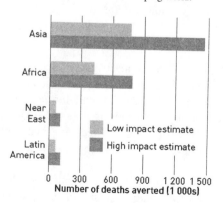

Source: WHO

Micronutrients are essential for human growth and development as well as normal functioning. The three most common forms of micronutrient malnutrition are deficiencies of vitamin A, iodine and iron. In developing countries, deficiencies of micronutrients often are not present in isolation but exist in combination (see map).

Children and women are the most vulnerable to micronutrient deficiencies—children because of the critical importance of micronutrients for normal growth and development, women because of their higher need for iron, especially during childbearing years and pregnancy.

"We will implement policies aimed at . . . improving . . . access by all, at all times to sufficient, nutritionally adequate and safe food . . ."

Between 100 and 140 million children suffer from vitamin A deficiency. That figure includes more than 2 million children each year afflicted with severe visual problems, of whom an estimated 250 000 to 500 000 are permanently blinded.

Lack of vitamin A also impairs the immune system, greatly increasing the risk of illness and death from common childhood infections such as diarrhoea and measles (see graph).

Prevalence of micronutrient deficiencies in developing countries

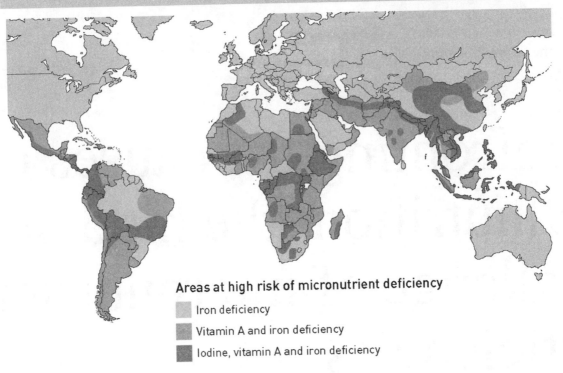

Areas at high risk of micronutrient deficiency

Iron deficiency

Vitamin A and iron deficiency

Iodine, vitamin A and iron deficiency

Source: USAID

Dietary diversification reduces vitamin A deficiency

Home gardens boost consumption of micronutrient-rich food

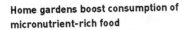

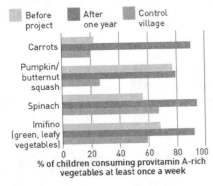

Before project   After one year   Control village

Carrots

Pumpkin/ butternut squash

Spinach

Imifino (green, leafy vegetables)

0 20 40 60 80 100

% of children consuming provitamin A-rich vegetables at least once a week

A home gardening programme focusing on production and consumption of vegetables rich in vitamin A and its precursor, beta carotene, has been successfully demonstrated by the Medical Research Council of South Africa in a mountainous, rural village in KwaZulu-Natal.

Prior to the programme, the diet of children in the village consisted mainly of maize porridge, bread and rice. The lack of variety and vitamin-rich foods resulted in high incidence of vitamin A deficiency. The programme changed that by promoting cultivation of vegetables, such as carrots, pumpkins and spinach, that are rich in beta carotene and by teaching villagers, especially women, the importance of including them regularly in their diet.

After only one year, the percentage of children consuming vitamin-A rich vegetables had increased significantly. And the increased diversity in their diets led to measurable improvements in vitamin A status.

Source: Faber et al.

The most devastating consequence of iodine deficiency is reduced mental capacity. Some 20 million people worldwide are mentally handicapped as a result of iodine deficiency, including 100 000 born each year with irreversible brain damage because their mothers lacked iodine prior to and during pregnancy.

Iron deficiency and the anaemia it causes are the most widespread of all forms of micronutrient malnutrition. Anaemia results in fatigue, dizziness and breathlessness following exertion.

Children with anaemia are less able to concentrate and have less energy for play and exploratory behaviours. In adults, anaemia diminishes work capacity and productivity by as much as 10–15 percent. And for pregnant women, anaemia substantially increases the risk of death in childbirth, accounting for up to 20 percent of maternal deaths in Asia and Africa.

The three main strategies for reducing micronutrient deficiencies are dietary diversity and food fortification along with supplements.

Most micronutrient deficiencies could be eliminated by modifying diets to include a greater diversity of nutrient-rich foods. Promoting home gardens, community fish ponds, and

Biofortification increases nutrient content of staple foods

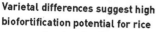

Varietal differences suggest high biofortification potential for rice

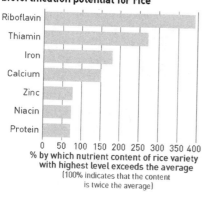

% by which nutrient content of rice variety with highest level exceeds the average
(100% indicates that the content is twice the average)

Source: FAO

Both conventional plant breeding techniques and genetic engineering can be used to develop varieties of staple food crops that are enriched with essential minerals.

"Golden rice" offered proof that biotechnology can produce both nutrients and controversy. Golden rice owes its colour and its name to beta carotene, introduced by transplanting genes from daffodils and bacteria. Critics have charged that the enriched rice will not provide enough beta carotene to satisfy vitamin A requirements. But supporters argue that it could provide 15 to 20 percent of daily requirements and significantly reduce the incidence and severity of vitamin A deficiency, particularly if consumed in conjunction with other nutrient-rich foods.

Conventional plant breeding also holds promise for enhancing the nutrient content of staple foods. Varieties of crops differ considerably in the quantities of nutrients that they contain (see graph). Advances in plant breeding techniques and biotechnology may make it possible to cross varieties that are relatively rich in micronutrients with high-yielding varieties preferred by farmers.

Iodine deficiency disorders

Access to iodized salt, 1995–98

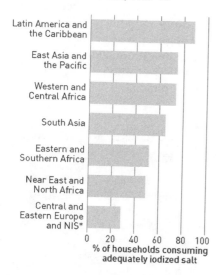

% of households consuming adequately iodized salt

NIS = newly independent states   *Source: FAO*

Iodine deficiency disorder (IDD) is particularly prevalent in the mountainous regions of the world.

The areas with the most severe deficiencies include the Himalayas, the Andes, the European Alps and the vast mountains of China. IDD is also common in frequently flooded lowlands. In both mountains and flooded areas, iodine that is naturally present in the soil is leached away, reducing the iodine content in locally grown crops.

Iodization of salt has virtually eliminated IDD in the mountainous regions of industrialized countries in Europe and North America. Three-quarters of the countries in the developing world have enacted legislation for iodizing salt, mostly over the past 15 years. More than two-thirds of households now get adequately iodized salt. But access varies considerably (see graph). Increasing access to iodized salt and improving quality control of its iodine content hold the key to eliminating iodine deficiency worldwide.

livestock and poultry production can contribute to increasing dietary diversity, while improving food supplies and incomes at the same time (see box on dietary diversification).

Another important food-based strategy is food fortification. The most successful of these initiatives is fortification of salt with iodine (see box). Other micronutrients can also be supplied to populations by enriching widely consumed foods such as milk and flour. In addition, recent advances in crop breeding and biotechnology have heightened the prospects for "biofortification"—developing crops with higher concentrations of micronutrients (see box).

Supplementation involves treating and preventing micronutrient deficiencies by administering capsules, tablets, syrups or other preparations. This medical approach is the method of choice when the deficiency is severe and life-threatening or when access to regular intake of the deficient micronutrient is limited. Use of high-dose vitamin A supplements can reduce mortality from acute measles by up to 50 percent.

Successful campaigns to eliminate micronutrient deficiencies often combine all of these strategies. Vitamin A intake, for example, can best be increased over the long term by adding nutrient-rich foods to the diet and fortifying staple foods, while providing supplements to high-risk groups in vulnerable areas.

AGRICULTURAL POLICIES AND PROGRAMS CAN IMPROVE FOOD SECURITY

The objectives of agricultural policy and production should be to increase food consumption among poor households, generate sustainable livelihoods, and improve the nutritional content of food, not simply to produce crops and livestock. Therefore, agricultural policy must be concerned about improving access to land, agricultural inputs and knowledge, and income, particularly for women.

In many eastern, southern and central African (ECSA) countries, aggregate food supplies are adequate, but chronic and severe malnutrition persists. Many small and medium-sized farmers—who comprise 30–80 percent of the labor force in the region—continue to engage in subsistence production because they lack the skills, tools, and infrastructure to increase their yields. Yet, new promise for improving the output of smaller-scale producers exists, increasing rural incomes, tapping new farm markets, *and* spreading the cultivation of new staple food crops that are naturally rich in key vitamins and minerals.

HOUSEHOLD FOOD SECURITY

Food security refers to the availability, accessibility, and affordability of safe, balanced, and nutritious food through production, distribution, purchase, or exchange at the household level and implies sufficient food for a normal, healthy life for each and every member of the household. Households get food through their own production, by gathering wild food, as gifts from the community, by spending income or assets, and through migration.

The availability of food at the household level is essential for im-proving nutrition, but is not sufficient. In fact, various non-food factors affect households' ability to translate access to food into nutrition including health and disease, habitat and environment, and the quality and composition of its diet. In fact the household's overall well-being is a product of its food and nutritional security. This concept of overall household "livelihood security" is illustrated in on the next page.

AGRICULTURAL TRENDS IN THE ECSA REGION

Causes of household food insecurity include low agricultural productivity combined with fluctuations in food supply, low incomes, insecure livelihoods, financial shocks (such as death of livestock), war, theft, civil conflict, illness and death.

The multi-dimensional nature of household food security partly explains why in many ECSA countries, malnutrition and poverty exist even in times of high agricultural productivity.

Insufficient Food Production

The recent record of food production in Africa has been dismal. From 1980 to 1990, Africa's population grew by 3 percent each year, while agricultural production, growing at just 1.8 percent annually, lagged far behind. With the increase in total population,

and the stagnation of the rates of malnutrition (at 30 percent over the last decade), the aggregate number of malnourished children has increased significantly. This extreme and growing gap between the production and the demand for food highlights the need for increased agricultural production so as to adequately feed the populations of the ECSA region.

Zimbabwe has been lauded as a food-secure country with a surplus for export, particularly because its agricultural policies have emphasized domestic self sufficiency as well as regional food security. However, 25 percent of the children under 5 are chronically malnourished (stunted). Studies have shown that most of the food production comes from small geographic areas; commercial farms and resettlement areas, which are not involved in this food production, have high rates of malnutrition. Therefore even if a surplus of food exists most of the time, these households lack sufficient income to buy enough food to eat.

It is clear that increasing food production is only one dimension of the problem. It is equally important to ensure that all families have *access* to food at all times, either by increasing at-home food production, or increasing their income in order to purchase food.

Components of Household Livelihood Security

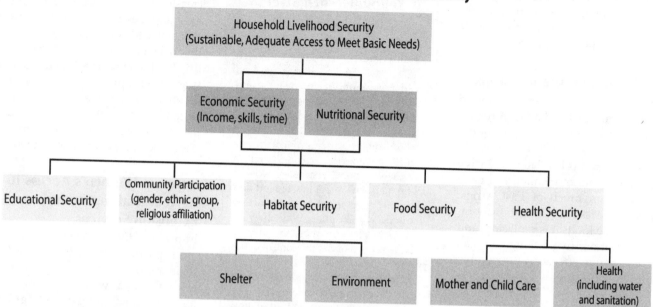

Source: Adapted from Frickenbarger TR, McCaston MK, "The household livelihood security concept" special issue on Food Security and Community Members. Food, Nutrition, and Agriculture 22, 1998. p.31.

Inadequate Attention to Women

Although countries in the ECSA region recognize the importance of women in agricultural production, there is little being done to overcome the various constraints that limit their productivity as the main producers and gatekeepers of family welfare.

Women account for 70–80 percent of household food production in much of the region, but generally lack access to resources such as credit and land, technology, and knowledge.

Women's lack of access to such critical resources makes their labor much less productive than men's (although their agricultural productivity equals that of men when they are given access to the same resources). Women therefore must work long hours to generate subsistence levels of food production, leaving them less time to care for their children or themselves. The aggregate impact of these discrepancies is enormous in terms of lost agricultural and economic production, increased household food and nutritional insecurity, and, ultimately, decreased maternal and child health and survival.

Promotion of Cash Crops

Encouraging the production of cash crops, especially for export, has been a major trend in countries in the region. This can serve as a double-edged sword in terms of its effects on household food and nutritional security. On the one hand, improved production techniques can spill over and help raise productivity in the food crop sector. On the other hand,

In the early 1990's, gains from traditional exports (tea and coffee) from **Kenya** decreased significantly and the production of flowers and luxury vegetable production as non traditional exports (NTEs) to help repay the trade deficit was encouraged. As large amounts of water were required to irrigate these flowers, traditional farmers were deprived of water for their crops, local food production decreased, and food prices skyrocketed. This NTE promotion has contributed to the increase in Kenya's unemployment rate, (as traditional farmers and pastoralists were forced to sell their land or migrate into towns), as well as an increase in malnutrition, social disintegration, and increased crime.

production of cash crops can reduce nutrition if the income generated is not used to purchase food and if land and labor is taken away from food production. For example, food prices may increase if local production falls, and household food security may be reduced when women's labor is used to generate income from cash crops rather than food, because women rarely control how such income is spent. This has been the scenario in several countries in the region.

Food Losses

The commitment by African governments to reducing food losses has been repeated in recent OAU Summits, but this problem has remained largely unresolved. Food losses affect the amount of food available and contribute to the increase of food prices to a level most households can not afford. Food losses occur at various stages: while growing in the field before harvesting, during storage in the post-harvest stage, during transportation, during storage by the trader, while processing, and in the consumer's home. The benefits of reducing food losses range from increasing food and incomes and reducing land under cultivation (to prevent soil erosion). Improving storage, particularly in homes, can reduce food losses by 10–20 percent in many areas.

Production of Inferior Crops

The production of inferior crops in several countries in the ECSA region has increased over the years. For example cassava, which can grow in poor soils, and is less labor intensive than sorghum and millet, has been promoted in much of East Africa. However, cassava is nutritiously inferior to the foods it is replacing, and its promotion, in the long run, can have negative effects on the population's nutrition status.

APPROACHES THAT WORK

Integrate Strategies

In general, agricultural policy best promotes food and nutritional security when it is integrated into an overall, multisectoral strategy. For example, horticultural and agricultural extension services should be complemented by nutrition education and beneficial land-use regulations.

Balance Food for Export and Food for Domestic Consumption

Policy makers should ensure that agricultural policies focus on assuring sufficient production for their countries. In addition, great attention should be paid to the economic, social and environmental consequences of export diversification.

Involve Women in Planning and Implementing Agricultural Projects

Because women have primary responsibility for producing, processing, and cooking food for members of their household, interventions should target activities under women's control—for example, introducing improved varieties of crops traditionally cultivated by women (on land un-

---

New Orange- and Yellow-Fleshed Sweet Potatoes in Kenya

Sweet potatoes are widely cultivated and, following maize, are a staple food in many countries in eastern and southern Africa. The orange-fleshed varieties can be easily cultivated year-round in many areas and have proven to be drought-resistant. Furthermore, sweet potatoes are considered a "women's crop," because women plant them on small plots of land and generally keep much of their harvest for home consumption. When they do sell some of their crops, the income tend to remain under the control of the women producers.

This was the case in Kenya, where the orange-fleshed sweet potatoes were recently introduced into several villages in the western part of the country, the primary sweet potato-producing region of the country. The goal was to increase the dietary intake of vitamin A among children, and so villagers were taught new recipes for using the sweet potatoes (particularly for weaning foods for young children). They were also trained to process and market sweet potato-based foods to generate income. Moreover, many of the women producers used the home visits by project fieldworkers to review nutrition lessons and reconcile these with their cultural beliefs and practices.

---

der their control) and providing education and technology for better food storage and preparation.

Safeguard Women's Land Rights

This can be achieved through nondiscriminatory registration and titling, as well as the inclusion of women as sole or joint beneficiaries in land reform programs and can have a positive impact on household livelihood security.

Produce Traditional, Nutritious Foods

Measures to expand production and consumption of traditional foods such as roots, tubers, pulses, and legumes

---

can be particularly effective. Many traditional foods serve as staples, and increasing their production can improve food supplies for groups particularly vulnerable to undernutrition. Most traditional foods also are well adapted to the local environment and provide year-round supplies. Furthermore, traditional crops are often produced, processed, and marketed by women, and increasing their production can increase the incomes of these women.

Improve Women's Access to Agricultural Inputs and Extension Services

Improving tools, resources and services, particularly for women, is key to increasing the adoption of new technologies as well as reaching adequate productivity gains in agriculture. These include new varieties of seed for crop diversification, fertilizer, labor saving technologies and tools, and knowledge about more ecologically sustainable practices.

Increase Income-Generating Opportunities

Creating off-farm employment can improve living standards for many members of a community. Small farmers tend to spend additional income on locally produced goods and services, and women tend to use their income to provide improved nutrition, education, or health care for members of their household.

Improve Drying and Storage Techniques

This can not only improve the *supplies* of food for these groups; they can also improve the *quality* of foods by preserving the micronutrient content and preventing production of toxins and bacteria.

Encourage Traditional Gardening

Home and community gardening improves household food security by providing direct access to food that can be harvested, prepared, and fed to the family on a regular, even daily, basis. The practice is ancient and widespread, even in urban areas.

For example, in 1991, 67% of households in Tanzania's capital, Dar es Salaam, gardened. Poor people garden on small patches of land; the landless use containers or school and community gardens.

Traditional gardening uses few resources and low-cost technology. The gardens can be adapted to reflect local growing conditions, resource availability, and customs and traditions.

Provide Extension Services that Link Agriculture and Nutrition

Agricultural programs must be supported by health and nutrition education and by extension services to assist in cultivation, harvest, and processing of food. Agricultural extension workers therefore need training to improve the links between agricultural production and improved food consumption.

Involve the Community

Including men and other community members in activities to improve the production and consumption of wholesome foods can help spur behavior change at the household level. School students, especially girls, should also be taught skills to improve basic health, nutrition, and food security at the household level.

From *Nutrition Beliefs: Linking Multiple Sectors for Effective Planning and Programming,* September 1999. The preparation and ditribution of this brief was funded by the United States Agency for International Development (USAID), Bureau for Africa, Office of Sustainable Development, through the SARA Project managed by the Academy for Educational Development (AED).

Too Much Food for the Hungry

Federal programs are contributing to obesity among the poor

By Douglas J. Besharov

In the summer of 1967, as a civil rights worker in the Mississippi Delta, I saw American starvation and malnutrition up close. Children there were sick and emaciated because their families lacked money to buy food. Since then, we have seen massive expansions of federal food aid for the poor. We now spend $18 billion annually on food stamps, $8 billion on school breakfasts and lunches, and $5 billion on WIC, the Special Supplemental Nutrition Program for Women, Infants and Children.

Today, the central nutritional problem facing the poor—indeed, all Americans—is not too little food, but too much of the wrong food.

But despite a striking increase in obesity among the needy, federal feeding programs still operate under their nearly half-century-old objective of increasing food consumption.

Few experts are willing to say that federal feeding programs are helping to make the poor fat, although the evidence points in that direction. But I know of no one who thinks those programs are doing much to help fight this growing public health problem.

Being overweight is not simply a matter of aesthetics. The growing girth of Americans is a major health catastrophe. Overweight people are three times more likely to have coronary artery disease, two to six times more likely to develop high blood pressure, more than three times as likely to develop *Type 2* diabetes, and twice as likely to develop gallstones as people of normal weight. Obesity, of course, is more serious, causing an estimated 50 to 100 percent increase in the risk of premature death.

About 65 percent of all Americans are overweight, and nearly half of those are obese. The best estimates place the rates for the poor at 5 to 10 percentage points higher. Adolescents from needy families are twice as likely to be overweight.

Yet today, low-income families have access to more free or low-cost food than ever before, and many can be enrolled in all three federal feeding programs at the same time, plus Temporary Assistance for Needy Families, a welfare program that pays out $12 billion a year.

> Federal rules dating back to 1946 require a disproportionate number of calories in school lunches and breakfasts, assuming that needy children will not get much dinner. By the time participants get home from school, they've already eaten 58 percent of their appropriate calorie level.

CONSIDER FOOD STAMPS, THE LARGEST of the programs. In 2002, it is serving about 20 million people a month, providing up to $465 per month for a household of four. On the theory that the poor would be tempted to use food money for other things, the government designed food stamps as coupons (now largely using a credit card-like system) that can be used in grocery stores.

Food stamps work as intended, raising calorie consumption by as much as 10 per-

cent more than if recipients were given cash, according to Department of Agriculture studies. It's like buying tickets for a set number of rides before entering an amusement park. The tendency is to buy more tickets than one needs and, rather than throw away the unused ones, take those extra rides before leaving. Like the tickets, unused food stamps can't be turned in for cash. So they are used for food that recipients wouldn't otherwise buy.

If we want people to consume food more wisely, the remedy seems simple enough: Give them cash instead of food stamps, and let them make their own decisions about how much to buy. The same Agriculture Department studies have demonstrated that "cashing out" food stamps is more convenient for the poor and does not result in unhealthful diets or mismanagement of family finances. Recipients continue to get well above the recommended levels for most nutrients.

The school lunch and breakfast programs, serving almost 28 million lunches and more than 8 million breakfasts on an average day, also lead to overconsumption. Federal rules dating back to 1946 require a disproportionate number of calories in those meals, assuming that needy children will not get much dinner. Schools are required to provide 25 percent of the Recommended Dietary Allowance (RDA) of calories for breakfast and 33 percent for lunch, so by the time participants get home from school, they've already eaten 58 percent of their appropriate calorie level. That leaves for dinner and snacks only 42 percent, or about 950 calories for the average student—the equivalent of a roasted chicken breast, mashed potatoes, green beans, low-fat milk and a half-cup of ice cream for the rest of the day and evening. Try telling that to a child who would also like to have an after-school or bedtime snack.

What's more, the levels of fat and saturated fat in school lunches exceed the lunch program's own standards by about 10 percent. Successive administrations have tried to reduce the fat content of the meals, but with only modest success. Much of the problem stems from portion size, the kinds of foods served and poor cooking practices. In keeping with federal rules, most schools provide lunches that have one meat, two fruits or vegetables, one bread or grain product, and milk. Preparing tasty and healthful meals in school-sized quantities requires a level of proficiency beyond that of the frequently low-paid staff found in many cafeterias.

Large, fattening school meals might have made sense decades ago, but the federal government now gives low-income families other sources of food as well. The time is long overdue for allowing schools to provide smaller and simpler meals.

WIC, too, is designed as if other federal feeding programs did not exist. It provides food vouchers and counseling to more than 7 million children and mothers each month. The free monthly food packages are worth about $120 for infants and post-partum mothers, and about $35 for each child from ages 1 through 4.

WIC's popularity among service providers is based largely on its generous package of formula, enriched juice and fortified cereal for infants, guaranteeing that they get sufficient nutrients. The other WIC food packages are heavily tilted toward high-calorie, high-cholesterol food-stuffs. The monthly package for 1- to 4-year-olds, for example, is 9 quarts of fruit juice, 36 ounces of cereal (hot or cold), 24 quarts of whole or reduced-fat milk, 2 to 2.5 dozen eggs, and about a pound of peanut butter, dried beans or dried peas.

A food package like that makes sense only if it is the family's major source of food, which almost certainly is not the case.

It would be better to use the package to introduce low-income families to more healthful foods, such as fruits and vegetables.

But it is WIC's nutritional counseling program that is the biggest disappointment. In addition to food packages, the program is supposed to provide nutritional advice. In practice, counselors spend an average of about 15 minutes with mothers every three months, hardly enough to make any real difference, particularly because many other topics must be covered during those sessions, including—pursuant to congressional mandate—voter registration. WIC programs cannot increase the time spent with young mothers because federal rules establish a strict percentage of funding for the food packages and the counseling sessions.

ADVOCATES ARE STILL PUSHING TO get more families on WIC. But nearly 50 percent of all newborns are already enrolled in the program, whose eligibility guidelines are quite lenient. Instead of increasing the number of families in the program, WIC should pay more attention to the problems of overweight and obesity. More funds should go toward providing intensive counseling about preparing more healthful food and for actual cooking instruction. Some WIC programs already do that, but almost always with non-WIC funds. Because they can't afford to use WIC money for those purposes, local WIC programs must raise money some other way—through grants from local foundations, for example—in order to provide meaningful help.

Although there is still some real hunger in America, it is found predominantly among people with behavioral or emotional problems, such as drug addicts and the dysfunctional homeless.

That is no secret to senior policymakers and food advocacy groups. In 1998, for example, then-Agriculture Secretary Dan Glickman said that "The simple fact is that more people die in the United States of too much food than of too little,

and the habits that lead to this epidemic become ingrained at an early age."

WHAT, THEN, IS PREVENTING THE modernization of federal feeding programs? Of course, various industry groups have a vested interest in the continuation and expansion of feeding programs, and they are adept at lobbying Congress. For farm and dairy interests, for example, the programs are a way to get the government to purchase surplus commodities. And for unions, localities and individual grantees, the programs represent jobs and financial aid. But those vested interests alone are not powerful enough to stymie reform.

Ironically, it is liberal advocacy groups that have thwarted reform of the programs, for, to make the case for change, one must first accept that hunger has largely disappeared from America. I want to be careful here, because I have friends in such organizations and I know them to be completely dedicated to what they see as the best interests of the poor.

But they seem to believe that admitting any weaknesses in federal feeding programs would make those programs vulnerable to budget cuts. How else to explain their periodic press releases about growing hunger, and their silence about overeating? Perhaps the advocates are correct to fear financial repercussions, but it makes them the main protectors of the status quo.

America's growing weight problem has many causes, primarily less exercise and more eating. Federal feeding programs may be only one part of the problem, but they urgently need to be part of the cure.

Douglas Besharov is the Joseph J. and Violet Jacobs scholar at the American Enterprise Institute for Public Policy Research and a professor at the University of Maryland's School of Public Affairs. Peter Germanis helped prepare this article.

The Promise of Biotechnology in Addressing Current Nutritional Problems in Developing Countries

Abstract

To meet the nutritional needs of a rapidly growing world population, which is likely to reach 8 billion by 2030, 50% more food grains with higher and more stable yields must be produced. Biofortification is considered the most effective way to increase micronutrient intakes. It is low cost and sustainable and does not require a change in eating habits or impose recurring costs. A research project to improve the iron and zinc content of rice was initiated at the International Rice Research Institute in 1992. Several experimental lines of rice with increased iron and zinc content have been produced. In another experiment rices with β-carotene have been produced. Other experimental efforts aim at raising the micronutrient content in wheat, maize, cassava, sweet potatoes, and beans. Maize with improved amino acid balance is being grown in several African countries.

Key words: Biotechnology, nutrition, biofortification, micronutrient malnutrition

Gurdev S. Khush

Access to a healthy diet is a fundamental right of every human being, yet 800 million people, mostly in the developing world, go to bed hungry every night. Furthermore, micronutrient deficiencies, which affect 3 billion people, hinder the development of human potential and the social and economic development of nations.

Access to food depends on income. Currently, more than 1.3 billion people in the world are extremely poor, with incomes of less than US$1 per person per day, and another 2 billion are only marginally better off [1]. Thus, investments in employment generation are as important as investments in food production.

The malnutrition problem is further exacerbated by increases in the world population, which is likely to reach 8 billion by 2030. Most of this increase (83%) will take place in the developing world, whose share of the global population is projected to increase from 78% in 1995 to 83% in 2020. To meet the challenge of feeding an ever-increasing population and alleviating protein–energy malnutrition, we will have to produce 50% more food grains. To meet this challenge, we will need crop varieties with higher and more stable potential yields. Conventional plant-breeding as well as biotechnology techniques will be employed to develop crop varieties with higher yields and greater resistance to diseases and insects.

Tackling Micronutrient Malnutrition

In addition to protein–energy malnutrition, deficiencies of minerals and vitamins affect a high proportion of the world's poor. Deficiencies of iron, zinc, iodine, and vitamin A are most acute. An estimated 2 billion people in the world are iron deficient. At least 400 million are deficient in vitamin A, 100 million of whom are young children. As many as 3 million children die annually as a result of vitamin A deficiency [2]. One billion people live in iodine-deficient regions, and many of them suffer from iodine-deficiency disorders, including goiter, cretinism, lower intelligence, and increased prenatal mortality [3]. Zinc deficiency, which is thought to be widespread, can lead to retarded growth, depressed immune function, anorexia, dermatitis, skeletal abnormalities, and child mortality if prolonged [4]. Furthermore, zinc deficiency has been linked to underutilization of vitamin A. Even in developed countries, micronutrient deficiencies affect a significant number of people. Taken together, micronutrient deficiencies affect a far greater number of the world's population than does protein–energy malnutrition [5].

Intervention programs for alleviating micronutrient malnutrition include supplementation, food fortification, education, and biofortification. Fortification programs have been successful in reducing malnutrition in specific situations, for example, fortification with iodine through the use of iodated salt.

However, for iron, zinc, and vitamin A, fortification and supplementation programs are expensive, incur ongoing costs, and are unlikely to reach all of those at risk. Moreover, such intervention programs have often been suspended for economic, political, or logistical reasons [6].

One approach to solving the problem of micronutrient deficiencies is to persuade people to make their diets more nutritious. However, attempts to change eating behavior are generally unsuccessful. It is often difficult for poor people to make dietary changes using local food. These attempts require a lot of input, constant follow-up, and education. When they are scaled up, they rarely work, so they tend not to be sustainable.

Under these limitations, biofortification is considered the most effective way to tackle micronutrient malnutrition. This strategy for supplying micronutrients to the poor in developing countries involves making staple foods eaten by the poor more nutritious by using conventional plant breeding and biotechnology. This strategy is low cost and sustainable, and it does not require a change in eating habits and does not impose the recurring costs that accompany food supplementation and fortification.

Increasing the Mineral and Vitamin Concentration of Staple Crops

The main concern about the potential benefits of using mineral- or vitamin-dense staple crops is whether the increased concentrations will in fact result in significant increases in bioavailable minerals and vitamins and, consequently, improve the nutritional status of malnourished populations. For this to happen, vulnerable groups have to consume the improved varieties of staple crops in sufficient quantities.

Even more important, the net amounts of bioavailable nutrients they ingest must be greater than those in traditional crops. For example, the main sources of iron for impoverished populations are staple cereals and starchy roots, tubers, and legumes, but most of the iron ingested from these sources has low bioavailability. It is estimated that cereals contribute up to 50% of iron intake in households from lower socioeconomic groups [7]. For zinc, the contribution from plant sources can be as high as 80%. This means that doubling the iron and zinc density of food staples could increase the total intake by at least 50%. The main problem, however, is that diets based on plant staples usually contain large amounts of phytic acid [6], which inhibits iron and zinc absorption. Thus, crop-improvement strategies should aim at increasing the level of micronutrients, on the one hand, and reducing the amount of phytic acid, on the other.

Improving the Amount and Bioavailability of Iron and Zinc

A research project to develop improved rice varieties with high iron and zinc content was initiated at the International Rice Research Institute (IRRI) in 1992. Considerable variation in both iron and zinc was observed in the rice germplasm. Iron concentrations ranged from 6.3 to 24.4 mg/kg, with a mean value of 12.2 mg/kg. For zinc, the range was 15.3 to 58.4 mg/kg [8].

Efforts are under way to develop improved rice germplasm with elevated levels of iron and zinc. Crosses between traditional varieties and high-yielding varieties have produced progenies with both high yield and high micronutrient levels. For example, an improved breeding line, IR68144, has both a high concentration of iron in grain (about 21 mg/kg) and a high yield potential. Milled rice of this variety is being used in human feeding trials to determine the bioavailability of the iron [8].

A genetic engineering approach has been successfully applied to raise the iron content of rice. Goto et al. transferred the soybean ferritin gene into the Kita-ake rice variety through transformation [9]. The iron content of the transgenic seeds was as much as threefold greater than that of untransformed seeds. Similarly, Lucca et al. introduced the ferritin gene from the common bean into rice, and the transgenic lines had twice as much iron as controls [10]. Mutants of barley, maize, and wheat with low amounts of phytate are available and may be employed to develop varieties of these crops with improved iron bioavailability.

Ortiz-Monasterio found a fourfold variation between the lowest and highest concentrations of iron and zinc in the grains of several hundred wheat accessions [11]. Studies at the International Center for Tropical Agriculture showed that certain varieties of common bean had 60% to 80% more zinc than other widely grown varieties. Breeding efforts are under way to incorporate high levels of zinc into improved varieties [12].

Improving the Vitamin A Content of Crops

β-carotene, a precursor of vitamin A, does not occur naturally in the endosperm of rice. Therefore, populations that derive most of their calories from rice suffer from vitamin A deficiency. The poor people in many Asian countries (Vietnam, Laos, Cambodia, Myanmar, Bangladesh, and India) derive more than 60% of their calories from rice.

Ye et al. introduced two genes from daffodil (*Narcissus pseudonarcissus*) and one gene from a bacterium (*Ervinia uredovora*) into rice variety Taipei 309 through genetic engineering [13]. Ten plants had a yellow endosperm (because of the presence of β-carotene), had a normal vegetative phenotype, and were fully fertile. Taipei 309 was used to introduce the β-carotene biosynthetic pathway, which is easy to transform. However, Taipei 309 is no longer cultivated. IRRI has started a project with the aim of introducing the genes for β-carotene production into widely grown improved varieties through transformation as well as through conventional hybridization techniques. It is anticipated that improved rice varieties containing β-carotene will become available during the next two to three years.

Strong carotenoid pigmentation was present in older wheat varieties used for bread. However, during the twentieth century, market demand drove wheat breeding to focus on the production of wheat varieties for white flour. The pigmented-type wheat varieties can be brought back into breeding programs if desired. There also are high β-carotene maize types (yellow maize) that are high yielding. However, in many cultures, consumers prefer white maize, which lacks carotenoids and is nutritionally inferior. Education programs should be undertaken to popularize the use of yellow maize.

Cassava is an important staple food for 50 million poor people. Genetic variation in cassava roots for β-carotene content is high. Orange-colored roots have 9 to 10 times more β-carotene than white roots. There is thus an obvious advantage in popularizing the use of orange-colored varieties of cassava.

An action research project was recently implemented by the Kenya Agricultural Research Institute in Nairobi in collaboration with the International Potato Center in Lima, Peru. Orange-fleshed varieties of sweet potatoes that were both high yielding and rich in β-carotene were introduced to women farmers. The orange-fleshed sweet potatoes, both when eaten alone and when consumed as ingredients in processed foods, were highly acceptable to both producers and consumers. Using standard methods of analysis, it was demonstrated that their increased consumption contributed to the alleviation of vitamin A deficiency in case study households [14]. In sub-Saharan Africa, sweet potatoes are an important source of calories for poor people, but most of the sweet potato varieties grown there have white flesh and therefore lack β-carotene. The introduction of orange-fleshed sweet potatoes should receive priority.

Improving the Amino Acid Balance

A human diet derived from cereal grains is deficient in some of the 10 essential amino acids, especially lysine, that are required for normal growth and development. Natural variation in the maize germplasm was exploited to develop quality protein maize (QPM) at the International Maize and Wheat Improvement Center (Mexico). The opaque 2 gene was incorporated into improved maize germplasm, and it doubled the amount of lysine and tryptophan. QPM maize varieties have been released in several countries and are now grown on almost 1 million hectares, and the area under QPM maize cultivation is also increasing.

Biotechnology approaches are also being used to enhance the lysine content of rapeseed (canola), corn, and soybean. The introduction of two bacterial genes for dihydrodipicolinic acid and aspartokinase enzymes encoded by the *dapA* gene from *Corynebacterium* and the *lysC* gene from *Escherichia coli* led to a fivefold increase in lysine in canola, corn, and soybean [15]. Similarly, the amino acid profile and total protein content of potato were improved through the introduction of the *AmA1* gene from *Amaranthus hypochondriacus* [16].

Conclusions

The use of biotechnology is proving to be important in improving germplasm to alleviate the malnutrition that affects almost half of the world's people. Linking agriculture and nutrition to promote dietary change and improve nutritional status can generate wide social as well as economic benefits.

The author is affiliated with the International Rice Research Institute, Los Baños, Laguna, Philippines.

References

1. World Bank. Word development report 1997. New York: Oxford University Press, 1997.
2. Sommer A. Vitamin A status, resistance to infection and childhood mortality. Ann NY Acad Sci 1990; 587:17–23.
3. Hetzel BS. Iodine deficiency: an international public health problem. In: Brown ML, ed. Present knowledge in nutrition, 6th ed. Washington, DC: International Life Sciences Institute, 1990: 308–13.
4. Cousins RJ, Hempe JM. Zinc. In: Brown ML, ed. Present knowledge in nutrition, 6th ed. Washington, DC: International Life Sciences Institute, 1990: 251–60.
5. Chandra RK. Micronutrients and immune functions. Ann NY Acad Sci 1990; 587: 9–16.
6. Gibson RS. Zinc nutrition and public health in developing countries. Nutr Res Rev 1994; 7: 151–73.
7. Bouis H. Plant breeding: a new tool for fighting micronutrient malnutrition. J Nutr 2002; 132: 491–4.
8. Gregorio GB, Senadhira D, Htut H, Graham RD. Breeding for trace mineral density in rice. Food Nutr Bull 2000; 21: 382–6.
9. Goto F, Yoshihara T, Shigemoto N, Toki S, Takaiwa F. Iron fortification of rice seed by the soybean ferritin gene. Nature Biotechnol 1999, 17: 282–6.
10. Lucca P, Hurrell R, Potrykus I. Genetic engineering approaches to improve the bioavailability and level of iron in rice grains. Theor Appl Genet 2001; 102: 392–7.
11. Ortiz-Monasterio I. CGIAR micronutrient project. Update No. 3. Washington, DC: International Food Policy Research Institute, 1998.
12. Beebe S, Gonzalez AV, Rengifo J. Research on trace minerals in common bean. Food Nutr Bull 2002; 21: 387–91.
13. Ye X, Al-Babili S, Kloti A, Zhang J, Lucca P, Beyer P, Potrykus I. Engineering the provitamin A (β-carotene) biosynthetic pathway into (carotenoid free) rice endosperm. Science 2000; 287: 303–5.
14. Hagenimana V, Low J. Potential of orange-fleshed sweet potatoes in raising vitamin A intake in Africa. Food Nutr Bull 2000; 21: 414–8.
15. Falco SC, Guida T, Locke M, Mauvais J, Sanders C, Ward RT, Webber P. Transgenic canola and soybean seeds with increased lysine. Biotechnology 1995; 13: 577–82.
16. Chakraborty S, Chakraborty N, Datta A. Increased nutritive value of transgenic potato by expressing a nonallergenic seed albumin gene from *Amaranthus hypochondriacus*. Proc Natl Acad Sci USA 2000; 97: 3724–9.

Assessment of Allergenic Potential of Genetically Modified Foods: An Agenda for Future Research

Speakers and participants in the workshop "Assessment of the Allergenic Potential of Genetically Modified Foods" met in breakout groups to discuss a number of issues including needs for future research. These groups agreed that research should progress quickly in the area of hazard identification and that a need exists for more basic research to understand the mechanisms underlying food allergy. A list of research needs was developed. *Key words:* biotechnology, food allergy, genetically modified food, hazard identification, research needs. *Environ Health Perspect* 111: 1140–1141 (2003). doi:10.1289/ehp.5815 available via *http:/dx.doi.org/*[Online 19 December 2002].

MaryJane K. Selgrade,[1] Ian Kimber,[2] Lynn Goldman,[3] and Dori R. Germolec[4]

Potential benefits that may be derived from biotechnologies involving genetically modified organisms could be enormous. Potential risks of allergenicity possibly associated with their use will likely be manageable, provided appropriate information is available to decision makers. At the end of the workshop "Assessment of the Allergenic Potential of Genetically Modified Foods," speakers and participants met in small groups to discuss information needs. Five groups considered the following key issues: *a*) use of human clinical data, *b*) animal models to assess food allergy, *c*) biomarkers of exposure and effect, *d*) sensitive populations, *e*) dose-response assessment, and *f*) postmarket surveillance. The groups were asked to consider two general questions: On the basis of current information, what can we do to assess the potential allergenicity of genetically modified food, and what do we need to know to improve this process, i.e., what are the most critical research needs? The first question is the topic discussed in another article in this mini-monograph (Germolec et al. 2003). The research needs are the topic of this article. Just as research provided the tools to generate genetically modified food, it can also provide the tools needed for effective safety evaluation and risk assessment/management.

Regulatory problems are rarely stated in scientific terms. The problem in this case is we wish to avoid inadvertently introducing an allergenic protein into the food supply. One task for this workshop was to translate this problem into research needs. Because there is a sense of urgency to develop tools for hazard identification, much of the conversation revolved around the short-term research required to develop test methods for this purpose. This discussion focused largely on the potential allergens and how to distinguish these from other proteins. However, it was recognized also that more long-term (basic) research is needed on the characteristics of food allergens, allergic disease, and the mechanisms underlying susceptibility to food allergy. This discussion considered more broadly the factors leading to allergic sensitization, including the nature of the allergen, and how genetics, life stage, and other environmental influences might affect susceptibility.

Hazard Identification: Immediate Needs

Research needed to improve hazard identification fell into three categories: development of animal models, identification and characterization of food allergens, and establishment of well-defined clinical serum banks. All were deemed important to improve the Food and Agriculture Organization of the United Nations/World Health Organization (FAO/WHO) decision tree (FAO/WHO 2001) or to replace it with a better approach. Also discussed was the need to improve human skin test technology for incorporation in a decision tree. Animal models are needed that could be used not only for hazard identification purposes but also to determine relative potency, to derive sensitization and elicitation thresholds, and to define the conditions under which tolerance (failure to develop an allergic response to potential food allergens) is induced. Identification, characterization, purification, and banking of food allergens (and nonallergens) are needed for two reasons: to provide positive (and negative) controls for animal and serum bank tests and for use in defining the characteristics that confer on food proteins the ability to induce allergic sensitization, that is, to establish structure-activity relationships. Serum from clinically well-defined allergic individuals needs to be banked for use in

Table 1. Summary of research needs.

Hazard identification
- Development, evaluation, and validation of animal models
- Establishment of clinically well-defined banks of human serum containing antibodies to allergens
- Improved human skin test technology
- Identification, purification, and banking of both known protein allergens and proteins believed not to be allergenic
- A systemic approach to recording adverse events (case studies)
- Definition of relative potency and thresholds for sensitization and the elicitation of allergic reactions
- Development, refinement, standardization, and validation of test protocols

Basic mechanistic
- Development of animal models of allergic disease
- Studies of the qualitative and quantitative relationships between antigen-specific IgE and overt disease
- Investigation of the influence of route, duration, timing, and nature of exposure on the development of sensitization
- Studies of the factors that contribute to susceptibility to food allergy
- Investigation of the mechanisms underlying food allergy
- Investigation of potential windows of vulnerability during development
- Identification of unique situations that cause children or other individuals to be at greater risk
- Epidemiology to establish the incidence of food allergy and whether it is changing
- Studies of the potential role of non–IgE-mediated reactions in food allergy

screening proteins of unknown allergenicity. Development of proteomic approaches to screen potential allergens (specific IgE on a chip) was also suggested as a research need. Characterization of allergens and development of serum banks require a systematic process for recording adverse events and obtaining informed consent for use of serum obtained in epidemiologic and experimental studies. Once developed, all tests for hazard identification will require standardization and validation—no small task. These research needs are summarized in Table 1.

Basic Mechanistic Research

Appropriate animal models (not necessarily the same as those used for hazard identification) and human clinical and epidemiologic studies are needed to assess the correlation between antigen-specific IgE and clinical disease and to investigate the influence of the route, duration, and nature of exposure on the development of sensitization. An important research need is to investigate the mechanisms underlying food allergy, including the development of and failure to develop oral tolerance, and identification of possible windows of vulnerability during immune development (including *in utero* and during lactation) or unique exposure conditions that might place children at greater risk. The mechanisms underlying the development of tolerance to ingested antigens, whether by passive (anergy) or active (suppressor cells) processes, are poorly understood and may be crucial to understanding what makes a protein allergenic and what makes an individual susceptible. The contributions of *in utero* exposure, gut immaturity, and exposure via breast milk to children's risk of sensitization also need to be determined. Studies (possibly using tansgenic mice) are needed to assess the heritable factors that contribute to susceptibility to food allergy. Epidemiology is needed to determine whether the incidence of food allergy in the industrialized world, like the incidence of other types of allergic disease, is increasing.

The natural history of non–IgE-mediated food allergies (although somewhat beyond the scope of this current workshop) was also considered an important long-term research need. Questions were raised as to whether certain foods were associated with this type of allergy and whether IgE is a reasonable surrogate marker in this instance or if other biomarkers would be more appropriate. The context in which food is presented, including the matrix, concomitant infections, and other sources of gut inflammation, also deserves further attention with respect to both IgE- and non–IgE-mediated food allergies. Basic mechanistic research needs are summarized in Table 1.

Recommendations

In summary, there was consensus that research should progress quickly in the area of hazard identification to improve or replace the FAO/WHO decision tree. Support was particularly strong for the development, standardization, and validation of appropriate animal model(s) for this purpose. It was also generally agreed that there is much we do not know about the development of food allergies, and that more basic research in this area would help us to control the risks more effectively and efficiently. More work is needed than any one funding organization is likely to be able to support. Therefore, it is recommended that there be significant coordination between these organizations and an integrated approach to tackling this problem. Open and free exchange of information as it becomes available is needed to facilitate these research endeavors

[1]National Health and Environmental Effects Research Laboratory, Office of Research and Development, U.S. Environmental Protection Agency, Research Triangle Park, North Carolina, USA; [2]Syngenta Central Toxicology Laboratory, Alderley Park, Macclesfield, Cheshire, United Kingdom; [3]Johns Hopkins University Bloomberg School of Public Health, Baltimore, Maryland, USA; [4]Laboratory of Molecular Toxicology, National Institute of Environmental Health Sciences, Research Triangle Park, North Carolina, USA

References

FAO/WHO. 2001. Evaluation of Allergenicity of Genetically Modified Foods. Report of a Joint FAO/WHO Expert Consultation of Allergenicity of Foods Derived from Biotechnology, 22–25 January 2001, Rome, Italy. Available: http://www.fao.org/es/esn/gm/allergygm.pdf [accessed 11 September 2002)

Germolec DR, Kimber J, Goldman L, Selgrade MJK. 2003. Key issues for the assessment of the allergenic potential of genetically modified foods: breakout group reports. Environ Health Perspect 111: 1131–1139.

From *Environmental Health Perspectives,* June 2003. Printed by the National Institute of Environmental Health Sciences.

Seeds of Domination

Don't want GMOs in your food? It may already be too late.

By Karen Charman

Americans have been eating genetically engineered foods every day for several years, though many remain unaware of that basic fact. Consequently, the question of whether our food should be manipulated with genes from foreign species may already be moot.

Walter Fehr is an agronomist and director of the Office of Biotechnology at Iowa State University. He says genetically engineered varieties of staple crops like corn and soybeans have contaminated seed stocks all the way to the "breeder seed," the purest version of a crop variety. If breeder seed contains material from genetically modified organisms, or GMOs, all the seeds and plants that descend from that stock will contain GMOs as well. According to Fehr, transgenic contamination of breeder and other seed stocks "happens routinely."

That shocks Theresa Podoll, executive director of the Northern Plains Sustainable Agriculture Society (NPSAS), an organization that represents 350 organic farmers throughout the Upper Midwest and Canada. Podoll is intimately familiar with the problems GMOs are causing organic farmers, but she is astounded to hear somebody within the biotech establishment admit that transgenic contamination goes all the way to breeder seed.

Podoll points out that the nation's agricultural universities, the so-called land-grant institutions, are charged with safeguarding the public seed stocks. "If research with transgenic crops at land-grant facilities makes contamination of the seed stocks a forgone conclusion, why are they doing transgenic research?" she asks. "To gamble all our crops' genetic resources to do research on a questionable technology that is in its infancy is unconscionable."

Genetically engineered crops were first commercially planted just seven years ago. Ninety-nine percent of the world's estimated 145 million acres of genetically modified crops are planted in four countries: Argentina, Canada, China and the United States. Four crops—canola, corn, cotton and soybeans—that are altered to tolerate herbicides or produce pesticides make up most of these plantings.

From the beginning, the U.S. Food and Drug Administration deemed biotech food "substantially equivalent—that is, no different from food produced by conventional breeding methods, which can only occur between members of the same or closely related species. This classification does not require long-term food-safety testing. Such tests have never been done on GMO crops.

However, in order to breach the natural barriers between species and make foreign genes function in their new homes, bioengineers use genes from viruses and bacteria, as well as genes resistant to antibiotics needed to treat human diseases. The public health implications of this genetic manipulation are unknown. The technology also raises concerns about the creation of toxic substances and allergens that have never been part of the human diet. For these reasons, the British Medical Association and other scientists have called for a worldwide moratorium on GMO crops until safety questions are answered.

Fehr's conclusions are not based on comprehensive research documenting the extent of transgenic contamination in the public seed stocks held by Iowa State or other public agricultural institutions, though such an effort is now underway at his university. However, the problem of GMO contamination became "obvious," he says, when Europe raised concerns about receiving bioengineered soybeans and corn after the first commercial harvest of transgenic crops in 1996. "From that point on, the whole issue of contamination has been at the forefront of our thinking."

Fehr is not the only one who acknowledges the transgenic contamination of seed stocks. The Grain Quality Task Force at Purdue University also notes that "whenever new genetic material is introduced into the agricultural crop mix, trace contamination of non-target crops is unavoidable."

That's because wind and insects carry genetically engineered pollen far and wide. According to Kendall Lamkey, a corn breeder at Iowa State, the traits of GMO crops are dominant because there is nothing in a non-transgenic receptor plant's genome to counter the introduced foreign genes.

Contamination also occurs when GMO seeds fall into non-transgenic fields from farm equipment previously used on a gene-altered crop. Researchers are not required to use separate equipment for GMO varieties that are already commercialized; and because of the cost and trouble of keeping them separate from everything else, Fehr says, they don't. "If you're growing both GMO and non-GMO and running them through the same equipment and cleaning facilities," he says, "you can be assured that there's going to be contamination."

For years, Podell and her organization have been raising concerns about contamination from transgenic research plots at North Dakota State University, their local land-grant institution. In 2001, NPSAS learned that a research plot of wheat engineered to resist Roundup, Monsanto's best-selling herbicide, had been planted at North Dakota State next to the foundation seed stocks for Coteau wheat, which is popular among organic growers.

Foundation seed stocks, which are grown directly from breeder seed, form the genetic basis for any given crop variety. They are "the seed for the seed" that farmers buy and plant. Genetically modified wheat—like Monsanto's "Roundup Ready"—is not approved for human consumption, yet North Dakota State told the NPSAS via e-mail that "there can be no guarantee that GMO DNA has not been introduced" into any wheat varieties grown at its research stations.

Last March, the NPSAS delivered a petition with more than 1,600 signatures from farmers and consumers to North Dakota State officials, demanding that transgenic crops not be planted or handled where conventional seeds were bred, grown, cleaned or stored. The petition also went to three other land-grant institutions: South Dakota State University, the University of Minnesota and Montana State University.

In May, Fred Cholick, dean of the College of Agriculture and Biological Sciences at South Dakota State, acknowledged the problem and told NPSAS that protocols were in place to prevent transgenic contamination. The protocols include testing to make sure seed stocks and conventional varieties are GMO-free. However, Cholick also said more than 80 percent of his university's soybean varieties were already transgenic. He ended his letter with this disclaimer: "As a biologist, I also realize that genetic systems are not perfect."

Minnesota and Montana State officials say they understand the need to keep seed varieties pure and are following procedures to do so. But they didn't spell what steps they were taking, nor did they agree to NPSAS's demand to halt work on genetically engineered crops in facilities that also contain foundation seed stocks.

North Dakota State, however, did agree last year to use separate, designated equipment for harvesting transgenic research plots. While this is a positive step, it only applies to crop varieties not yet approved for commercial release. Dale Williams, who's in charge of seed stocks at the university, defends the protocols and says that even if foundation seed stocks are contaminated by GMOs, "it's not that much of a problem."

The university's foundation seed stocks are now routinely tested for GMOs, and so far none have turned up in any of the samples. But relying on tests from seed samples is not foolproof. John Lukach, a research manager at the university, points out that to be absolutely sure GMOs aren't present, every single seed would need to be tested. Further, some commonly used testing methods can only detect GMOs at a contamination level of about 10 percent.

If transgenes are detected, Williams says, North Dakota State could produce new foundation stocks from breeder seed (assuming it isn't already contaminated) or take, say, 100 randomly selected seed samples from the foundation plots, test them, and, if they are free of GMOs, use that seed to produce another foundation crop. Kendall Lamkey, the corn breeder from Iowa State, says either of those strategies could work, but he doubts either would be employed for contamination with GMOs that are already approved—like Roundup Ready soybeans.

In fact, last autumn two lots of North Dakota State foundation seed stocks for Natto soybeans, a non-GMO variety, were found to be contaminated with Roundup Ready genes. Williams says the contamination occurred in the winter of 2000 when the seeds were sent down to Chile. (In the winter, breeder seed and foundation seed stocks are typically sent to nurseries in warmer climates.) The contamination wasn't discovered until after the seed was brought back and grown out at a North Dakota State seed farm—and then not until after some of the seed had been distributed to growers of registered and certified seed, who sell to organic and other farmers.

Theresa Podoll says that the university had promised that any foundation seed stocks found to be contaminated with GMOs would be destroyed. But in November, Williams told North Dakota's *Grand Forks Herald* that since Roundup Ready soybeans are "not regulated"—that is, they are approved for human consumption—"small amounts of it, or tolerances of amounts, are allowed in most markets."

But GMOs are not allowed in organic food. The widespread transgenic contamination of organic crops threatens the very existence of organic grain producers throughout the Midwest, a situation that speaks volumes about mainstream agriculture's deep-seated bias against non-industrial farming systems. In *The Last Harvest*, Paul Raeburn writes that for decades, organic farming was "dismissed as the work of zealots," and that USDA scientists—many of whom are stationed at land grant universities—historically looked upon organic production systems as "gardening" and "irrelevant to modern agriculture."

By contrast, industrial agriculture has enjoyed enormous benefits. These included the close working relationships between the land-grant universities and agribusiness corporations like Monsanto, massive public subsidies for commodity crops, and weak environmental and public health laws that permit widespread pollution of air, water, soil and food with chemicals and fertilizers used in industrial agriculture.

Despite the uneven playing field, the success of organic farming has made it impossible to ignore. With consistent growth in retail sales of 20 percent a year since 1990, organics are the fastest-growing sector in the food industry. When given a

Down on the Biopharm

The GMO contamination issue is about to get a lot more dangerous with the introduction of transgenic crops that produce pharmaceutical and industrial compounds. Some of the products being tested include a protein for an experimental AIDs vaccine, herpes treatment, contraceptives and cancer drugs. Since 1991, more than 300 field trials of such crops have taken place in the open environment, most over the past three years. Corn, which is wind pollinated and therefore spreads its traits easily, is the crop of choice of biopharming.

While land-grant universities are working with pharma crops on their premises, it's difficult to know exactly what they are doing. Biotech companies also contract with individual farmers to grow pharma crops. To grow the plants in the open environment, farmers must have permits issued by the USDA's Animal Plant Health Inspection Service (APHIS). But the USDA won't reveal the exact location of biopharming test plots or, in most cases, what compound the plants are engineered to produce. This information is considered "confidential business information."

In July, Genetically Engineered Food Alert, a coalition of environmental and consumer groups, released a meticulously researched report by Friends of the Earth policy analyst Bill Freese outlining the risks that biopharming poses to consumers, farmers, food manufacturers and the environment. Transgenic contamination of food crops and the potential for dangerous health consequences like allergic reactions or the creation of toxic substances in the food top the list.

Last autumn, the issue came to a head when food manufacturers made public their concerns about food crops being used for biopharming. In response, the Biotechnology Industry Organization (BIO), a trade association and lobbying group, put out a short-lived voluntary policy announcing that their members would not be permitted to grow pharma crops in the heart of the corn belt. But after pressure from Iowa politicians complaining that their state should not be excluded from the opportunity to take part in a potentially high economic bonanza, BIO rescinded its policy.

In November, federal regulators announced that the Texas-based company ProdiGene had contaminated 500,000 bushels of soybeans destined for the food supply with pharmaceutical corn the company had grown in the same field the previous year. The contamination occurred when corn plants sprouted from seed left in the field. Although APHIS inspectors saw the corn plants and told the farmer to remove them before the soybean field was harvested, that didn't happen.

The pharma corn was harvested along with the soybeans and sent to a grain elevator in Aurora, Nebraska, where it was mixed in with 500,000 bushels. ProdiGene was fined $250,000 and had to assume liability for the $3 million worth of soybeans that had to be destroyed. Two months earlier, ProdiGene had to burn 155 acres of a neighbor's corn crop in Iowa because of suspected contamination of that corn from pollen from the company's pharma corn.

In September, the Food and Drug Administration issued draft guidelines advising biotech companies what to include in their pharma crop permit applications. Although FDA "strongly recommends" that biotech companies have tests available that can detect the presence of pharma crop transgene in the raw food crop, the agency doesn't require it. Without those tests, it may be difficult, if not impossible, to catch biopharm contamination of food or feed crops.

"This technology moves so fast," says Theresa Podoll of the Northern Plains Sustainable Agriculture Society, "it's almost impossible to keep up with."

choice, increasing numbers of people show with their purchases that they want their food produced in an environmentally friendly manner. Food manufacturers have taken notice, and large conglomerates now own the major organic food companies.

Still, GMO contamination is reaching crisis portions in the organic-farming community. "Organic producers can no longer produce organic corn," says NPSAS president Janet Jacobson, an organic farmer in North Dakota's northeast corner. "I don't know any organic farmers that can grow canola, because there's so much GMO canola around. There are also organic farmers who have had soybeans rejected because they were contaminated with GMOs."

Transgenic contamination is now so rampant that the FDA prohibits organic food manufacturers from labeling their products "GMO-free."

In Canada, a group called the Saskatchewan Organic Directorate (SOD) last year filed a lawsuit on behalf of all certified organic producers in the province, seeking millions of dollars in damages from Monsanto and Aventis, another biotech corporation (which was recently purchased by Bayer), for the loss of the organic canola market due to GMO contamination. Canola is pollinated by insects, and SOD claims the companies knew, or ought to have known, when they introduced bioengineered canola that it would spread and contaminate the environment and neighboring farmers' fields. SOD is also seeking an injunction against the introduction of transgenic wheat.

Unlike conventional agriculture, which relies on chemical pesticides and synthetic fertilizers to be able to produce one or two crops year after year, organic agriculture can only work by growing a diversity of crops in rotation around the farm. Crop rotations enable organic farmers to control pests and weeds and manage diseases, while also building soil fertility. With corn, soybeans and canola already gone from organic crop rotations on the northern plains, SOD President Arnold Taylor says the loss of wheat would be catastrophic. The introduction of GMO wheat would likely spell the end of organic farming on the northern prairie.

Organic farmers aren't the only ones who have suffered from the introduction of biotech crops. Consumers overseas, particularly in Europe, have emphatically rejected GMOs. Dan MacGuire, a policy analyst with the American Corn Growers Association, says economic analysis of USDA data reveals that the introduction of biotech corn is directly responsible for a roughly 30 cent per bushel drop in corn prices. With returns to farmers at their lowest level in decades, and well below the cost of production, he says farmers cannot afford this further cut.

Conventional farmers and the folks who distribute commodity corn already incurred huge losses because StarLink corn, a biotech variety not approved for human consumption, found its way into more than 300 food products—including Taco Bell taco shells—in 2000 and 2001. The StarLink incident prompted expensive recalls and a massive legal quagmire that will take years to resolve. StarLink contamination is still an issue; in December, Japanese officials detected it in a shipment from the United States.

Rejection of GMOs in foreign markets and the contamination debacle have made transgenic wheat the subject of raging debate and political infighting in North Dakota. Wheat is North Dakota's No. 1 industry, indirectly generating some $4 billion a year. Half of the crop is exported, and buyers in eight of its 11 main export markets have said they don't want transgenic wheat. Many have warned that they'll go elsewhere if GMO wheat is planted because of the likelihood of transgenic contamination. As a result, most farming organizations in North Dakota have called for a moratorium on the commercial release of Roundup Ready wheat until there are assurances that export markets won't evaporate. So far, powerful Republicans in the state Senate have blocked such a measure.

Some supporters have indicated that the biotech industry may be deliberately contaminating the food supply with GMOs so that alternatives to bioengineered food no longer exist. In January 2001, food industry consultant Don Westfall told the *Toronto Star*: "The hope of the industry is that over time the market is so flooded that there's nothing you can do about it. You just sort of surrender."

Last April, Dale Adolphe, executive director of the Canadian Seed Growers Association, told Canadian canola growers at their annual meeting that despite growing public opposition and new regulations, the increasing acreage of bioengineered crops may eventually end the debate. Adolphe told *The Western Producer*, a Canadian agricultural paper, "It's a hell of a thing to say that the way we win is don't give the consumer a choice, but that might be it."

Perhaps the biotech industry has already won.

Some Africans prefer hunger to a diet of gene-altered corn

Text by Danna Harman

For 24 days, the crew of the Liberty Grace saw nothing but endless Atlantic Ocean, a handful of whales, thousands of dolphins, and each other. The hum of engines buzzed in their ears constantly. The wind hammered them as they took long shifts on deck.

On the three-week journey from Louisiana to the ports of East Africa, the ship's chief engineer learned to play the electric piano. Capt. John Codispoti got through some Tom Clancy paperbacks, and the cook perfected his chili-dog recipe.

But no one thought much about the cargo—50,000 tons of genetically modified (GM) corn being taken to help some of the 14.5 million hungry men, women, and children facing food shortages in Southern Africa.

"Sometimes I wonder about the hungry people out there and this corn we are shipping in," says Mr. Codispoti. "But we never see them, so it's hard to imagine."

What also may be hard for this American crew to imagine is that other shipments of corn—genetically modified, just like the corn in countless US products—is rotting in storehouses in Zambia while the people there go hungry. Zambian President Levy Mwanawasa has rejected US corn because he believes that it poses health risks to his people.

While science has yet to prove any health problems caused by GM corn, misinformation has clouded the debate. Now many hungry Africans don't know what to think of it.

Radios, but no batteries

There are no paved roads in Shangombo, Zambia. Just miles upon miles of dirt paths crisscrossing the dry savanna. Villagers farm or fish in the swamps by day, and sit around their thatched huts in the evenings, swatting mosquitoes as hot days turn into cool nights.

Neither electricity nor phone lines run here. Visitors are rare, and most of those fortunate enough to own radios have no money to buy batteries. Yet, somehow, everyone here has heard something of the debate about genetically modified corn raging in the capital, Lusaka, some 500 bumpy miles away.

Information, however, is often confused. Farmer Victor Bwalia heard that GM corn makes women infertile. His neighbor told him. Meanwhile, Amroando Dandola, who makes flip-flops, thinks it infects people with HIV/AIDS. That is what his grandfather, Augustine, thinks, too.

"It is bad. That is for sure," says Richwell Nalumwe, a fisherman who can't feed his family. "We heard that in the Southern Province some people who ate it are now suffering. Plenty, plenty problems over there."

After two years of drought, people here are hungry. Boys dive for mancada roots in the swamp. Men and women go into the forests looking for nuts and berries to boil. Countrywide, according to the World Food Program (WFP), 2.9 million Zambians are in need of food aid. Some 250 tons of it, more than half of which were donated by the US, were headed for Zambia when Mr. Mwanawasa decided, in mid-August, to reject it.

Genetically modifying crops involves splicing genes from one organism into an unrelated crop in order to insert traits such as insect resistance or drought tolerance. The US, as well as other large grain-producing countries such as Argentina, Canada, and China, has begun using this technology extensively in recent years. Most Americans eat GM food every day.

But the technology is contentious. Some say it's so new that the health risks are unknown. Others say that if planted, GM crops could potentially infect a country's native crops and cause problems down the road.

Mwanawasa will not accept GM food, he explained, because if cross-pollination does occur, it could hurt future exports to Europe, where GM foods are prohibited or require special labeling. "We may be poor and experiencing severe food shortages, but we aren't ready to expose our people to ill-defined risks," he told journalists in Lusaka.

The crackling sound of weevils

On Aug. 12, two truckloads of US corn set off from Lusaka to Shangombo. Each village in the district had little sheds built for the expected food.

But it never came. Catholic Relief Services, a nongovernmental organization and the WFP's implementing partner in the region, received its new directions over the radio. One truck was ordered back to the capital. The other, carrying a few hundred bags of corn, unloaded its precious cargo directly into a locked storage room. There it stayed, watched by two guards with strict instructions not to distribute it.

The villagers gathered around, looked at the locked-up corn, and shook their heads. The district administrator, himself confused about the situation, traveled to the provincial capital Mongu to find out what was going on. A week later he returned, adamant that the GM corn should not be consumed, and yet no more enlightened as to the reasons.

Humphry Katumwa is the storage manager in Senanga. He looks after a warehouse filled to the ceiling with the US-donated corn. If he puts his ear up close to the bags, he can hear crackling sounds. It's weevils, eating away.

"Since it was decided this was not fit for human consumption, it has just been sitting here," he says. "Maybe we will be told to give it to refugees." Some 130,000 Angolan and Congolese in refugee camps in Zambia are still being fed GM food. "When locals come and cry to me about hunger, I tell them this is not good for you. It's just for Angolans," he says.

"It's a strange story. I don't know what is going on," says Richard Nkhoma, coordinator of the Shangombo food-receiving committee. "This one comes, gives some instructions. That one says, 'No'—gives different instructions." Sometimes, he admits, he feels like opening the gates of the small warehouse and letting the people "steal" the food. "I feel too sorry for them," he says. In October, villagers from Mumbwa, 30 miles west of Lusaka, took more than 500 bags of GM corn.

Zambia is the only country to reject the food aid outright, but Zimbabwe, Malawi, Lesotho, and Mozambique all expressed concern over the imports. When those countries finally decided to accept the aid, it was on condition that it would only be distributed after milling so as to prevent people from planting the seeds and risking cross-pollination.

Leaving with hands empty

The WFP, which has reassured Zambia and other countries that GM food is safe to eat, nonetheless maintains the position that it will not force any country to accept the donations and will do everything possible to bridge the food gap by substituting other food for the US donated GM corn. But this is no easy task.

"It is the right of every government to reject the corn, but we cannot then replace that fully with different food," says Gerard Van Dijk, the WFP country director in Malawi. "More than 70 percent of our donations come from the US." With growing food crises in Ethiopia and Eritrea, and with only 37 percent of its Southern African appeal met, the WFP says that finding additional donor sources will be difficult.

On the outskirts of the Shangombo district sits a tiny village called Natakoma. The food committee here, hearing that aid was coming, built a special holding hut. These days, Sapu Phebbian, the committee coordinator, stands outside the hut and faces the hungry with empty hands. Every day the elderly, sick, and frail from the surrounding villages show up to see if the food has arrived. They walk here. Wait. Shoo the flies away from their eyes and mouths. Place their hands atop their heads to shield themselves from the sun. And walk home with nothing. "The problem is with the GM poison," says Phebbian. "It shortens human life. I would not eat it—for I could die."

Educational Success Depends on Adequate Nutrition

Better nutrition enhances school enrollment, attendance, and performance, especially for girls. Success in education leads to greater economic productivity in the medium term and to improved health and nutrition for future generations. Formal and non-formal schools also provide opportunities to teach nutrition education and to target nutritional interventions at school-age children most in need.

Better nutrition enhances school enrollment, especially for girls, When children are weakened by poor nutrition and ill health, their capacity to learn is diminished, and they may be forced to end their schooling early or never enroll in school at all.

Conversely, a lack of access to basic education is one cause of malnutrition. Girls and women who face discrimination in education may lack the skills for productive employment and the knowledge that can help them support the health and nutrition of their families.

For many children, schools also can be a haven from the economic, social, and civil problems that affect their households and communities. Schools can provide children opportunities for learning and creativity that they would otherwise lack by providing them with physical safety, clean water, good sanitation, health care, nutritious food, and food supplements. Schools can also equip children with life skills to overcome other problems that may threaten their health and well-being later in life.

School-based treatment of children is especially cost-effective. Schools often provide social services that reach many children at risk for malnutrition or poor health, and they generally provide more effective community outreach than health facilities or clinics.

Girls who stay in school tend to have their first child later in life than those who leave school earlier, and simply delaying childbearing brings myriad benefits to future generations in terms of lower birth rates, better birth outcomes, and improved child health. Furthermore, female literacy is positively associated with reduced infant mortality (see graph).

Malnourished children enter school later, miss more days of school, have difficulty paying attention and concentrating, and drop out earlier.

Causes and Effects

The relationships between nutrition and education are numerous and complex. Several forms of malnutrition increase the risks and severity of illness for children, which affect their ability to attend school and learn.

Protein-Energy Malnutrition (PEM)

Stunting (low height for age) is a primary indicator of chronic malnutrition. It is also an indicator of poor school performance in developing countries. Children who are stunted during their preschool years enroll in school later. Moreover, taller children score higher on tests in arithmetic, reading, spelling, and verbal ability.

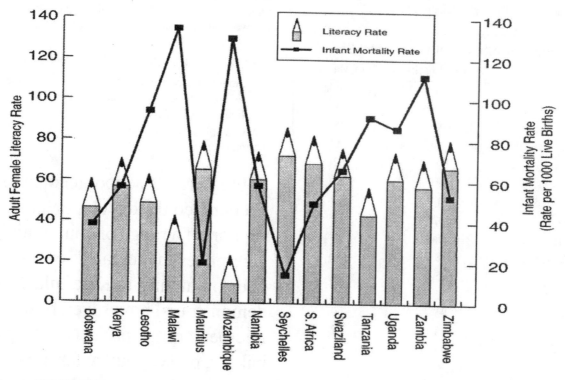

Female Literacy and Infant Mortality in ECSA Countries

Sources: UNICEF, SOWC, 1998 & 1999

Micronutrient Malnutrition

Micronutrient deficiencies are linked to poor school performance throughout childhood. Even moderate vitamin A deficiency can cause vision problems that make it difficult for children to participate in school. More severe vitamin A deficiencies cause mental retardation that can preclude a child from attending school altogether.

Deficiencies of both iodine and iron impair cognitive development and influence children's school attendance and performance. For example, children in Malawi who received iodine supplements showed significantly increased IQs (21 points, on average), and the increase was even greater when they were given iron supplements too.

Helminthic Infection

Parasitic infection, especially hookworm, delays psychomotor development. More severe infection leads to PEM and iron deficiency, which further reduces the chances for the child to attend or succeed in school.

On a global scale, the long-term loss of mental capacity, educational achievement, and economic and social productivity attributable to malnutrition is staggering: over 225 million children under age 5, or nearly 40 percent of all children in this age group, suffer from moderate to severe stunting. In eastern, central, and southern Africa (ECSA), the figure ranges from one-third to one-half.

Approaches that Work

Use school-based programs to implement key health and nutrition interventions. Targeting nutrition interventions to school-age children can help reverse some, though not all, of the ill effects of poor nutrition during infancy and early childhood. The task requires a multisectoral effort that involves parents, communities, nutrition and health workers, and educators.

Focus on Improving School Performance

Improving school children's health and nutrition can improve educational effectiveness. For example, South Africa's Integrated Nutrition Program has been shown to increase children's concentration and decrease absenteeism. The program includes school-based feeding programs, micronutrient supplementation activities, and nutrition education.

Increase Girls' School Enrollment

In many ECSA countries, primary school enrollment of girls lags slightly behind that of boys (see table). In most cases, the gap widens in secondary school. Increasing girls' enrollment and, especially, keeping them in school delays their first birth, increases their marriage age, and improves their lifetime earnings and overall health.

School feeding programs may help keep girls in school. For example, girls' enrollment increased in Ghana when they were given extra food rations take home in addition to their meals at school. Other strategies include ensuring their safety and privacy at school, establishing schools close to home, increasing the number of female teachers, and making school hours more flexible to accommodate work demands on girls.

School Enrollment of Girls, 1990-95

Country	Female Enrollment (% of Male)	
	Primary	Secondary
Botswana	103	105
Kenya	100	78
Lesotho	114	143
Malawi	90	62
Mauritius	99	99
Mozambique	71	63
Namibia	102	120
Seychelles	no data	99
South Africa	98	115
Swaziland	95	101
Tanzania	97	78
Uganda	85	59
Zambia	93	62
Zimbabwe	97	80

SOURCES: UNICEF, SOWC, 1998.

Giving girls a greater awareness of their opportunities for the future can help lengthen and improve their school careers. This can also help improve their self-esteem and give them a sense of empowerment, which in turn reinforces other long-term benefits of education, such as delayed child rearing, better health, and improved income-earning potential.

Teach Health and Nutrition Skills

Integrating nutrition and health messages into the teacher-training curriculum can positively influence health-related attitudes and behaviors among students and their families. The curriculum can include nutrition, family planning and reproductive health, and services to help postpone first births. Teaching today's young people the skills they need to lead healthier lifestyles can lower their risks of a range of preventable diseases and can improve the health of future generations.

Target the non-formal education-sector

Schools and institutions outside the formal sector should be targeted for the dissemination of key nutrition messages, particularly to women. These include literacy training schools, youth and womens' associations, as well as other training institutions.

Involve the Community

School-based community nutrition programs can effectively deliver both preventive and curative services. These include health and nutrition education, family planning, and micronutrient supplementation, and such curative services as deworming and first aid.

South Africa's school feeding program encouraged the development and support of a range of community-based enterprises that created jobs. In fact, one community in KwaZulu-Natal demonstrated how seven basic microenterprise projects—a piggery, bakery, dairy, poultry farm, vegetable garden, and sewing club—can provide a solid nutritional and economic basis for most every rural community.

Address high-priority problems in a cost-effective manner:

- **Mass application of deworming medications:** Treating all school children helps eliminate any stigma or shame.
- **Delivery of micronutrients, particularly iron and iodine:** Vitamin A capsules cost about 2 cents per dose, and only two to three doses are needed per year per child. A single annual dose of iodine costs just 32 cents, and a year's worth of iron folate tablets costs less than 10 cents per child.
- **Treatment of injuries and routine health problems:** Treating cuts and injuries can prevent infections, and treating other diseases (where feasible) can help slow their spread in the wider community.

From *Nutrition Briefs*, October 1999, pp. 1-3. © 1999. Nutrition Briefs: Linking Multiple Sectors for Effective Planning and Programming. Academy of Educational Development (AED), Support for Analysis and Research in Africa (SARA) Project; Commonwealth Regional Health Community Secretariat for East, Central and Southern Africa; funding provided by United States Agency for International Development, Bureau for Africa, Office of Sustainable Development (USAID/AFR/SR). Reprinted by permission.

Glossary

Absorption   The process by which digestive products pass from the gastrointestinal tract into the blood.

Acid/base balance   The relationship between acidity and alkalinity in the body fluids.

Amino acids   The structural units that make up proteins.

Amylase   An enzyme that breaks down starches; a component of saliva.

Amylopectin   A component of starch, consisting of many glucose units joined in branching patterns.

Amylose   A component of starch, consisting of many glucose units joined in a straight chain, without branching.

Anabolism   The synthesis of new materials for cellular growth, maintenance, or repair in the body.

Anemia   A deficiency of oxygen-carrying material in the blood.

Anorexia nervosa   A disorder in which a person refuses food and loses weight to the point of emaciation and even death.

Antioxidant   A substance that prevents or delays the breakdown of other substances by oxygen; often added to food to retard deterioration and rancidity.

Arachidonic acid   An essential polyunsaturated fatty acid.

Arteriosclerosis   Condition characterized by a thickening and hardening of the walls of the arteries and a resultant loss of elasticity.

Ascorbic acid   Vitamin C.

Atherosclerosis   A type of arteriosclerosis in which lipids, especially cholesterol, accumulate in the arteries and obstruct blood flow.

Avidin   A substance in raw egg white that acts as an antagonist of biotin, one of the B vitamins.

Basal metabolic rate (BMR)   The rate at which the body uses energy for maintaining involuntary functions such as cellular activity, respiration, and heartbeat when at rest.

Basic four   The food plan outlining the milk, meat, fruits and vegetables, and breads and cereals needed in the daily diet to provide the necessary nutrients.

Beriberi   A disease resulting from inadequate thiamin in the diet.

Beta-carotene   Yellow pigment that is converted to vitamin A in the body.

Biotin   One of the B vitamins.

Bomb calorimeter   An instrument that oxidizes food samples to measure their energy content.

Buffer   A substance that can neutralize both acids and bases to minimize change in the pH of a solution.

Calorie   The energy required to raise the temperature of one gram of water one degree Celsius.

Carbohydrate   An organic compound composed of carbon, hydrogen, and oxygen in a ratio of 1:2:1.

Carcinogen   A cancer-causing substance.

Catabolism   The breakdown of complex substances into simpler ones.

Celiac disease   A syndrome resulting from intestinal sensitivity to gluten, a protein substance of wheat flour especially and of other grains.

Cellulose   An indigestible polysaccharide made of many glucose molecules.

Cheilosis   Cracks at the corners of the mouth, due primarily to a deficiency of riboflavin in the diet.

Cholesterol   A fat-like substance found only in animal products; important in many body functions but also implicated in heart disease.

Choline   A substance that prevents the development of a fatty liver; frequently considered one of the B-complex vitamins.

Chylomicron   A very small emulsified lipoprotein that transports fat in the blood.

Cobalamin   One of the B vitamins (B_{12}).

Coenzyme   A component of an enzyme system that facilitates the working of the enzyme.

Collagen   Principal protein of connective tissue.

Colostrum   The yellowish fluid that precedes breast milk, produced in the first few days of lactation.

Cretinism   The physical and mental retardation of a child resulting from severe iodine or thyroid deficiency in the mother during pregnancy.

Dehydration   Excessive loss of water from the body.

Dextrin   Any of various small soluble polysaccharides found in the leaves of starch-forming plants and in the human alimentary canal as a product of starch digestion.

Diabetes (diabetes mellitus)   A metabolic disorder characterized by excess blood sugar and urine sugar.

Digestion   The breakdown of ingested foods into particles of a size and chemical composition that can be absorbed by the body.

Diglyceride   A lipid containing glycerol and two fatty acids.

Disaccharide   A sugar made up of two chemically combined monosaccharides, or simple sugars.

Diuretics   Substances that stimulate urination.

Diverticulosis   A condition in which the wall of the large intestine weakens and balloons out, forming pouches where fecal matter can be entrapped.

Edema   The presence of an abnormally high amount of fluid in the tissues.

Emulsifier   A substance that promotes the mixing of foods, such as oil and water in a salad dressing.

Enrichment   The addition of nutrients to foods, often to restore what has been lost in processing.

Enzyme   A protein that speeds up chemical reactions in the cell.

Epidemiology   The study of the factors that contribute to the occurrence of a disease in a population.

Essential amino acid   Any of the nine amino acids that the human body cannot manufacture and that must be supplied by the diet, as they are necessary for growth and maintenance.

Essential fatty acid   A fatty acid that the human body cannot manufacture and that must be supplied by the diet, as it is necessary for growth and maintenance.

Fat   An organic compound whose molecules contain glycerol and fatty acids; fat insulates the body, protects organs, carries fat-soluble vitamins, is a constituent of cell membranes, and makes food taste good.

Fatty acid   A simple lipid—containing only carbon, hydrogen, and oxygen—that is a constituent of fat.

Ferritin   A substance in which iron, in combination with protein, is stored in the liver, spleen, and bone marrow.

Fiber   Indigestible carbohydrate found primarily in plant foods; high fiber intake is useful in regulating bowel movements, and may lower the incidence of certain types of cancer and other diseases.

Flavoprotein   Protein containing riboflavin.

Folic acid (folacin)   One of the B vitamins.

Fortification   The addition of nutrients to foods to enhance their nutritional values.

Fructose   A six-carbon monosaccharide found in many fruits as well as honey and plant saps; one of two monosaccharides forming sucrose, or table sugar.

Galactose   A six-carbon monosaccharide, one of the two that make up lactose, or milk sugar.

Gallstones   An abnormal formation of gravel or stones, composed of cholesterol and bile salts and sometimes bile pigments, in the gallbladder; they result when substances that normally dissolve in bile precipitate out.

Gastritis   Inflammation of the stomach.

Glucagon   A hormone produced by the pancreas that works to increase blood glucose concentration.

Glucose   A six-carbon monosaccharide found in sucrose, honey, and many fruits and vegetables; the major carbohydrate found in the body.

Glossary

Glucose tolerance factor (GTF) A hormone-like substance containing chromium, niacin, and protein that helps the body to use glucose.

Glyceride A simple lipid composed of fatty acids and glycerol.

Glycogen The storage form of carbohydrates in the body; composed of glucose molecules.

Goiter Enlargement of the thyroid gland as a result of iodine deficiency.

Goitrogens Substances that induce goiter, often by interfering with the body's utilization of iodine.

Heme A complex iron–containing compound that is a component of hemoglobin.

Hemicellulose Any of various indigestible plant polysaccharides.

Hemochromatosis A disorder of iron metabolism.

Hemoglobin The iron-containing protein in red blood cells that carries oxygen to the tissues.

High-density lipoprotein (HDL) A lipoprotein that acts as a cholesterol carrier in the blood; referred to as "good" cholesterol because relatively high levels of it appear to protect against atherosclerosis.

Hormones Compounds secreted by the endocrine glands that influence the functioning of various organs.

Humectants Substances added to foods to help them maintain moistness.

Hydrogenation The chemical process by which hydrogen is added to unsaturated fatty acids, which saturates them and converts them from a liquid to a solid form.

Hydrolyze To split a chemical compound into smaller molecules by adding water.

Hydroxyapatite The hard mineral portion (the major constituent) of bone, composed of calcium and phosphate.

Hypercalcemia A high level of calcium in the blood.

Hyperglycemia A high level of "sugar" (glucose) in the blood.

Hypocalcemia A low level of calcium in the blood.

Hypoglycemia A low level of "sugar" (glucose) in the Blood.

Incomplete protein A protein lacking or deficient in one or more of the essential amino acids.

Inorganic Describes a substance not containing carbon.

Insensible loss Fluid loss, through the skin and from the lungs, that an individual is unaware of.

Insulin A hormone produced by the pancreas that regulates the body's use of glucose.

Intrinsic factor A protein produced by the stomach that makes absorption of B_{12} possible; lack of this protein results in pernicious anemia.

Joule A unit of energy preferred by some professionals instead of the heat energy measurements of the calorie system for calculating food energy; sometimes referred to as "kilojoule."

Keratinization Formation of a protein called keratin, which, in vitamin A deficiency, occurs instead of mucus formation; leads to a drying and hardening of epithelial tissue.

Ketogenic Describes substances that can be converted to ketone bodies during metabolism, such as fatty acids and some amino acids.

Ketone bodies The three chemicals—acetone, acetoacetic acid, and betahydroxybutyrie—that are normally involved in lipid metabolism and accumulate in blood and urine in abnormal amounts in conditions of impaired metabolism (such as diabetes).

Ketosis A condition resulting when fats are the major source of energy and are incompletely oxidized, causing ketone bodies to build up in the bloodstream.

Kilocalorie One thousand calories, or the energy required to raise the temperature of one kilogram of water one degree Celsius; the preferred unit of measurement for food energy.

Kilojoule See Joule.

Kwashiorkor A form of malnutrition resulting from a diet severely deficient in protein but high in carbohydrates.

Lactase A digestive enzyme produced by the small intestine that breaks down lactose.

Lactation Milk production/secretion.

Lacto-ovo-vegetarian A person who does not eat meat, poultry, or fish but does eat milk products and eggs.

Lactose A disaccharide composed of glucose and galactose and found in milk.

Lactose intolerance The inability to digest lactose due to a lack of the enzyme lactase in the intestine.

Lacto-vegetarian A person who does not eat meat, poultry, fish, or eggs but does drink milk and eat milk products.

Laxatives Food or drugs that stimulate bowel movements.

Lignins Certain forms of indigestible carbohydrate in plant foods.

Linoleic acid An essential polyunsaturated fatty acid.

Lipase An enzyme that digests fats.

Lipid Any of various substances in the body or in food that are insoluble in water; a fat or fat-like substance.

Lipoprotein Compound composed of a lipid (fat) and a protein that transports both in the bloodstream.

Low-density lipoprotein (LDL) A lipoprotein that acts as a cholesterol carrier in the blood; referred to as "bad" cholesterol because relatively high levels of it appear to enhance atherosclerosis.

Macrocytic anemia A form of anemia characterized by the presence of abnormally large blood cells.

Macroelements (also macronutrient elements) Those elements present in the body in amounts exceeding 0.005 percent of body weight and required in the diet in amounts exceeding 100 mg/day; include sodium, potassium, calcium, and phosphorus.

Malnutrition A poor state of health resulting from a lack, excess, or imbalance of the nutrients needed by the body.

Maltose A disaccharide whose units are each composed of two glucose molecules, produced by the digestion of starch.

Marasmus Condition resulting from a deficiency of calories and nearly all essential nutrients.

Melanin A dark pigment in the skin, hair, and eyes.

Metabolism The sum of all chemical reactions that take place within the body.

Microelements (also micronutrient elements; trace elements) Those elements present in the body in amounts under 0.005 percent of body weight and required in the diet in amounts under 100 mg/day.

Monoglyceride A lipid containing glycerol and only one fatty acid.

Monosaccharide A single sugar molecule, the simplest form of carbohydrate; examples are glucose, fructose, and galactose.

Monosodium glutamate (MSG) An amino acid used in flavoring foods, which causes allergic reactions in some people.

Monounsaturated fatty acid A fatty acid containing one double bond.

Mutagen A mutation-causing agent.

Negative nitrogen balance Nitrogen output exceeds nitrogen intake.

Niacin (nicotinic acid) One of the B vitamins.

Nitrogen equilibrium (zero nitrogen balance) Nitrogen output equals nitrogen intake.

Nonessential amino acid Any of the 13 amino acids that the body can manufacture in adequate amounts, but which are nonetheless required in the diet in an amount relative to the amount of essential amino acids.

Nutrients Nourishing substances in food that can be digested, absorbed, and metabolized by the body; needed for growth, maintenance, and reproduction.

Nutrition (1) The sum of the processes by which an organism obtains, assimilates, and utilizes food. (2) The scientific study of these processes.

Obesity Condition of being 30 percent above one's ideal body weight.

Oleic acid A monounsaturated fatty acid.

Organic foods Those foods, especially fruits and vegetables, grown without the use of pesticides, synthetic fertilizers, etc.

Osmosis Passage of a solvent through a semipermeable membrane from an area of higher concentration to an area of lower concentration until the concentration is equal on both sides of the membrane.

Osteomalacia Condition in which a loss of bone mineral leads to a softening of the bones; adult counterpart of rickets.

Osteoporosis Disorder in which the bones degenerate due to a loss of bone mineral, producing porosity and fragility; normally found in older women.

Overweight Body weight exceeding an accepted norm by 10 or 15 percent.

Ovo-vegetarian A person who does not eat meat, poultry, fish, milk, or milk products but does eat eggs.
Oxidation The process by which a substrate takes up oxygen or loses hydrogen; the loss of electrons.

Palmitic acid A saturated fatty acid.
Pantothenic acid One of the B vitamins.
Pellagra Niacin deficiency syndrome, characterized by dementia, diarrhea, and dermatitis.
Pepsin A protein-digesting enzyme produced by the stomach.
Peptic ulcer An open sore or erosion in the lining of the digestive tract, especially in the stomach and duodenum.
Peptide A compound composed of amino acids that are joined together.
Peristalsis Motions of the digestive tract that propel food through the tract.
Pernicious anemia One form of anemia caused by an inability to absorb vitamin B_{12}, owing to the absence of intrinsic factor.
pH A measure of the acidity of a solution, based on a scale from 0 to 14: a pH of 7 is neutral; greater than 7 is alkaline; less than 7 is acidic.
Phenylketonuria (PKU) A genetic disease in which phenylalanine, an essential amino acid, is not properly metabolized, thus accumulating in the blood and causing early brain damage.
Phospholipid A fat containing phosphorus, glycerol, two fatty acids, and any of several other chemical substances.
Polypeptide A molecular chain of amino acids.
Polysaccharide A carbohydrate containing many monosaccharide subunits.
Polyunsaturated fatty acids A fatty acid in which two or more carbon atoms have formed double bonds, with each holding only one hydrogen atom.
Positive nitrogen balance Condition in which nitrogen intake exceeds nitrogen output in the body.
Protein Any of the organic compounds composed of amino acids and containing nitrogen; found in the cells of all living organisms.
Provitamins Precursors of vitamins that can be converted to vitamins in the body (e.g., beta-carotene, from which the body can make vitamin A).
Pyridoxine One of the B vitamins (B_6).
Pull date Date after which food should no longer be sold but still may be edible for several days.

Recommended Daily Allowances (RDAs) Standards for daily intake of specific nutrients established by the Food and Nutrition Board of the National Academy of Sciences; they are the levels thought to be adequate to maintain the good health of most people.
Rhodopsin The visual pigment in the retinal rods of the eyes which allows one to see at night; its formation requires vitamin A.
Riboflavin One of the B vitamins (B_2).
Ribosome The cellular structure in which protein synthesis occurs.
Rickets The vitamin D deficiency disease in children characterized by bone softening and deformities.

Saliva Fluid produced in the mouth that helps food digestion.

Salmonella A bacterium that can cause food poisoning.
Saturated fatty acid A fatty acid in which carbon is joined with four other atoms; i.e., all carbon atoms are bound to the maximum possible number of hydrogen atoms.
Scurvy A disease characterized by bleeding gums, pain in joints, lethargy, and other problems; caused by a deficiency of vitamin C (ascorbic acid).
Standard of identity A list of specifications for the manufacture of certain foods that stipulates their required contents.
Starch A polysaccharide composed of glucose molecules; the major form in which energy is stored in plants.
Stearic acid A saturated fatty acid.
Sucrose A disaccharide composed of glucose and fructose, often called "table sugar."
Sulfites Agents used as preservatives in foods to eliminate bacteria, preserve freshness, prevent browning, and increase storage life; can cause acute asthma attacks, and even death, in people who are sensitive to them.

Teratogen An agent with the potential of causing birth defects.
Thiamin One of the B vitamins (B_1).
Thyroxine Hormone containing iodine that is secreted by the thyroid gland.
Toxemia A complication of pregnancy characterized by high blood pressure, edema, vomiting, presence of protein in the urine, and other symptoms.
Transferrin A protein compound, the form in which iron is transported in the blood.
Triglyceride A lipid containing glycerol and three fatty acids.
Trypsin A digestive enzyme, produced in the pancreas, that breaks down protein.

Underweight Body weight below an accepted norm by more than 10 percent.
United States Recommended Daily Allowance (USRDA) The highest level of recommended intakes for population groups (except pregnant and lactating women); derived from the RDAs and used in food labeling.
Urea The main nitrogenous component of urine, resulting from the breakdown of amino acids.
Uremia A disease in which urea accumulates in the blood.

Vegan A person who eats nothing derived from an animal; the strictest type of vegetarian.
Vitamin Organic substance required by the body in small amounts to perform numerous functions.
Vitamin B complex All known water-soluble vitamins except C; includes thiamin (B_1), riboflavin (B_2), pyridoxine (B_6), niacin, folic acid, cobalamin (B_{12}), pantothenic acid, and biotin.

Xerophthalmia A disease of the eye resulting from vitamin A deficiency.

Index

Index

Test Your Knowledge Form

We encourage you to photocopy and use this page as a tool to assess how the articles in *Annual Editions* expand on the information in your textbook. By reflecting on the articles you will gain enhanced text information. You can also access this useful form on a product's book support Web site at *http://www.dushkin.com/online/*.

NAME: _____   DATE: _____

TITLE AND NUMBER OF ARTICLE: _____

BRIEFLY STATE THE MAIN IDEA OF THIS ARTICLE:

_____

LIST THREE IMPORTANT FACTS THAT THE AUTHOR USES TO SUPPORT THE MAIN IDEA:

_____

WHAT INFORMATION OR IDEAS DISCUSSED IN THIS ARTICLE ARE ALSO DISCUSSED IN YOUR TEXTBOOK OR OTHER READINGS THAT YOU HAVE DONE? LIST THE TEXTBOOK CHAPTERS AND PAGE NUMBERS:

_____

LIST ANY EXAMPLES OF BIAS OR FAULTY REASONING THAT YOU FOUND IN THE ARTICLE:

_____

LIST ANY NEW TERMS/CONCEPTS THAT WERE DISCUSSED IN THE ARTICLE, AND WRITE A SHORT DEFINITION:

We Want Your Advice

ANNUAL EDITIONS revisions depend on two major opinion sources: one is our Advisory Board, listed in the front of this volume, which works with us in scanning the thousands of articles published in the public press each year; the other is you—the person actually using the book. Please help us and the users of the next edition by completing the prepaid article rating form on this page and returning it to us. Thank you for your help!

ANNUAL EDITIONS: Nutrition 04/05

ARTICLE RATING FORM

Here is an opportunity for you to have direct input into the next revision of this volume.
We would like you to rate each of the articles listed below, using the following scale:

1. **Excellent: should definitely be retained**
2. **Above average: should probably be retained**
3. **Below average: should probably be deleted**
4. **Poor: should definitely be deleted**

Your ratings will play a vital part in the next revision.
Please mail this prepaid form to us as soon as possible.
Thanks for your help!

RATING	ARTICLE	RATING	ARTICLE
	1. The Changing American Diet: A Report Card		30. A Guide to Rating the Weight-Loss Websites
	2. The 2000 Dietary Guidelines for Americans: What Are the Changes and Why Were They Made?		31. Claims Crazy: Which Can You Believe?
			32. Antioxidants: No Magic Bullet
	3. Rebuilding the Food Pyramid		33. Q & A on Functional Foods
	4. Our Ready-Prepared Ready-to-Eat Nation		34. The Latest Scoop on Soy
	5. We've Got To Stop Eating Like This		35. Food-Friendly Bugs Do The Body Good
	6. Unhappy Meals		36. Herbal Lottery
	7. The Hidden Health Costs of Meal Deals		37. Are Your Supplements Safe?
	8. Moving Towards Healthful Sustainable Diets		38. America's Dietary Guideline on Food Safety: A Plus, or a Minus?
	9. Face the Fats		
	10. Revealing Trans Fats		39. Safe Food From a Consumer Perspective
	11. Building Healthy Bones		40. What You Need to Know Before Your Next Trip to the Supermarket
	12. What You Need to Know About Calcium		
	13. Soaking up the D's		41. Unforgettable Foods: What's Most Likely to Make You Sick
	14. Feast For Your Eyes: Nutrients That May Help Save Your Sight		
			42. Certified Organic
	15. The Vitamin That Does Almost Everything		43. Hooked on Fish? There Might Be Some Catches
	16. Ten Foods That Pack a Wallop		44. Hunger and Mortality
	17. Nutrigenomics		45. Undernourishment, Poverty and Development
	18. Curtains for Heart Disease?		46. Confronting the Causes of Malnutrition: The Hidden Challenge of Micronutrient Deficiencies
	19. Eat Less Live Longer? Does Calorie Restriction Work?		
			47. Agricultural Policies and Programs Can Improve Food Security
	20. The Contribution Of Vegetarian Diets To Health And Disease: A Paradigm Shift?		
			48. Too Much Food for the Hungry
	21. Healthy Eating in Later Years		49. The Promise of Biotechnology in Addressing Current Nutritional Problems in Developing Countries
	22. The Female Athlete Triad: Nutrition, Menstrual Disturbances, and Low Bone Mass		
			50. Assessment of Allergenic Potential of Genetically Modified Foods: An Agenda for Furture Research
	23. Healthy People 2010: Overweight and Obesity		
	24. The Supersizing Of America: Portion Size And The Obesity Epidemic		51. Seeds of Domination
			52. Some Africans Prefer Hunger to a Diet of Gene-Altered Corn
	25. Big Fat Fake: The Atkins Diet Controversy and the Sorry State of Science Journalism		
			53. The Argument for Local Food
	26. Fat Chance: Extra Pounds Can Increase Your Cancer Risk		
	27. Losing Weight: More Than Counting Calories		
	28. Metabolic Effects Of High-Protein, Low-Carbohydrate Diets		
	29. Dietary Dilemmas: Is the Pendulum Swinging Away From Low Fat?		

(Continued on next page)

NO POSTAGE
NECESSARY
IF MAILED
IN THE
UNITED STATES

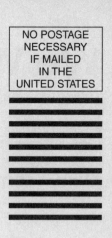

BUSINESS REPLY MAIL
FIRST CLASS MAIL PERMIT NO. 551 DUBUQUE IA

POSTAGE WILL BE PAID BY ADDRESEE

McGraw-Hill/Dushkin
2460 KERPER BLVD
DUBUQUE, IA 52001-9902

IᵢdᵢₗₗₗdᵢllₗₗₗllₗₗₗₗₗₗIlllᵢdₗdᵢdᵢllₗₗₗdᵢdᵢdᵢdII

ABOUT YOU

Name

Date

Are you a teacher? ❐   A student? ❐
Your school's name

Department

Address   City   State   Zip

School telephone #

YOUR COMMENTS ARE IMPORTANT TO US!

Please fill in the following information:
For which course did you use this book?

Did you use a text with this ANNUAL EDITION?   ❐ yes ❐ no
What was the title of the text?

What are your general reactions to the *Annual Editions* concept?

Have you read any pertinent articles recently that you think should be included in the next edition? Explain.

Are there any articles that you feel should be replaced in the next edition? Why?

Are there any World Wide Web sites that you feel should be included in the next edition? Please annotate.

May we contact you for editorial input?   ❐ yes ❐ no
May we quote your comments?   ❐ yes ❐ no